Anemia in the Young and Old

Robert T. Means Jr.
Editor

Anemia in the Young and Old

Diagnosis and Management

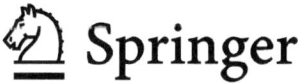 Springer

Editor
Robert T. Means Jr.
James H. Quillen College of Medicine
East Tennessee State University
James H. Quillen College of Medicine
Johnson City, TN
USA

ISBN 978-3-319-96486-7   ISBN 978-3-319-96487-4   (eBook)
https://doi.org/10.1007/978-3-319-96487-4

Library of Congress Control Number: 2018959025

This Springer imprint is published by the registered company Springer Nature Switzerland AG
The registered company address is: Gewerbestrasse 11, 6330 Cham, Switzerland

To my wife,
Stacey W. McKenzie, MD:
my colleague in the most important things.

Preface

The genesis of this book derives from a session presented as part of the educational program at the American Society of Hematology meeting in 2016. Entitled "Anemia in the Young and Old," the session was organized by Dr. David Steensma and consisted of a talk by Dr. Steensma on clonal hematopoiesis of indeterminate potential (CHIP), a talk by Dr. Michael Auerbach on the use of intravenous iron therapy, and a talk by me on pure red cell aplasia (PRCA). It was a very well received session. However, the focus of the session was certainly on adult medicine with a slant toward older patients. CHIP is a syndrome primarily observed in the elderly; while iron deficiency certainly occurs in children, the focus of the talk on that topic was largely on adults; and for my part, I mentioned Diamond Blackfan Anemia and transient erythroblastopenia of childhood solely to say that I was not going to talk about them any further in my presentation. However, sometime after that I was contacted by the publishers of this book and asked if I would consider editing a book with the title "Anemia in the Young and Old." While the topics of CHIP and iron deficiency in adults as well as PRCA are certainly covered, the primary resemblance to the education program session is the title. In preparing this book, the aim was to include authors whose expertise either was in anemic disorders of adults or of children, and the goal of the chapters was to help the readers appreciate the nuances of anemia diagnosis and management in these different populations. For example, iron deficiency is a major contributor to anemia in both children and in the elderly. However, iron deficiency in children has a tendency to be more nutritional in its basis, and iron deficiency in the elderly tends to result primarily from blood loss, usually from some acquired anatomic defect. While it has been proposed that the normal hemoglobin range for the elderly be set lower than the usual World Health Organization (WHO) adult range of >13.0 g/dL for men and 12.0 g/dL for women (as discussed in the chapter on approaches to anemia in the elderly), the WHO normal range for children actually is lower than that (as discussed in the chapter on approaches to anemia in childhood).

I wish to thank Andy Kwan and Dhanapal Palanisamy at Springer for their support of this project, and, of course, the contributors. As always, my primary thanks goes to my wife Stacey and our three children, Casey, Robert, and Patrick, for their support and forbearance in this as in all of my other activities.

Johnson City, TN, USA   Robert T. Means Jr.
June 2018

Contents

Contributors

Amber Afzal Division of Oncology, Department of Internal Medicine, Washington University School of Medicine, St. Louis, MO, USA

Emmanuel Andrès Department of Internal Medicine, Diabetes and Metabolic Disorders, University Hospital of Strasbourg, Strasbourg, France

Alvin N. Eden, MD Department of Pediatrics, New York Medical College, Valhalla, NY, USA

Daniel Guy Division of Oncology, Department of Internal Medicine, Washington University School of Medicine, St. Louis, MO, USA

Jennifer D. Hamm, MD Department of Pediatrics, Division of Pediatric Hematology/Oncology, East Tennessee Children's Hospital, Knoxville, TN, USA

Meagan A. Jacoby Division of Oncology, Department of Internal Medicine, Washington University School of Medicine, St. Louis, MO, USA

Jenny K. McDaniel, MD Department of Pediatrics, Division of Pediatric Hematology/Oncology, St. Jude Affiliate Clinic at Novant Health Hemby Children's Hospital, Charlotte, NC, USA

Robert T. Means Jr., MD James H. Quillen College of Medicine, East Tennessee State University, Johnson City, TN, USA

Suzie A. Noronha, MD Division of Pediatric Hematology/Oncology, Golisano Children's Hospital, University of Rochester Medical Center, Rochester, NY, USA

Yara Perez, MD Department of Pediatrics, New York Medical College, Valhalla, NY, USA

Kendall Presti, BS Department of Pediatrics, New York Medical College, Valhalla, NY, USA

Ariel L. Reinish, MD Division of Pediatric Hematology/Oncology, Golisano Children's Hospital, University of Rochester Medical Center, Rochester, NY, USA

Claudio Sandoval, MD Department of Pediatrics, New York Medical College, Valhalla, NY, USA

Caryn E. Sorge, MD Department of Pediatrics, Division of Pediatric Hematology/ Oncology, University of Kentucky, Lexington, KY, USA

Thomas Vogel, MD Department of Internal Medicine and Geriatrics, University Hospital of Strasbourg, Strasbourg, France

Ilene Weitz, MD Jane Anne Nohl Division of Hematology, USC Keck School of Medicine, Los Angeles, CA, USA

Abrar Zulfiqar, MD Department of Geriatrics, University Hospital of Rouen, Rouen, France

Part I
Approaches

Chapter 1
Introduction: Anemia at the Extremes of Life

Robert T. Means Jr.

Basics of Red Blood Cell Development

The purpose of this section of the chapter is to provide some basic information on the process of erythropoiesis by which red cells come into being and how the critical value of hemoglobin concentration is maintained in a relatively narrow range. If one considers published normal values for the different elements that make up the complete blood count, it is interesting to note that the ratio of the upper limit of normal for hemoglobin concentration to the lower limit for that parameter is approximately 1.3, while the comparable ratios for the white blood count or the platelet count are each roughly 2.4 [1]. This suggests that the physiologic demand for hemoglobin to carry out its physiologic function of delivering oxygen to tissue is much more tightly regulated than the white blood count or the platelet count, important though they are in the defense against infection/inflammation or bleeding/thrombosis.

A detailed discussion of the molecular regulation of erythropoiesis is outside the scope of this work aimed at clinicians. Those who are interested can find detailed discussions elsewhere [2, 3]. The traditional understanding of erythropoiesis has been that a pluripotent hematopoietic stem cell (HSC) capable of self-renewal differentiated into a more restricted but still multipotent progenitor cell with a lower capacity for self-renewal. This progenitor, the colony-forming unit (CFU) – granulocyte/erythroid/monocyte/megakaryocyte (GEMM) – could only give rise to more restricted progenitors of those lineages [4]. A regulated process of proliferation and progressive differentiation led to progenitors restricted to specific lineages with progressively decreased capacity for self-renewal [5]. In the case of erythropoiesis, the restricted progenitors are the erythroid burst-forming unit (BFU-E) and the erythroid colony-forming unit (CFU-E). These progenitors (and indeed, the HSC itself)

R. T. Means Jr., MD
James H. Quillen College of Medicine, East Tennessee State University,
Johnson City, TN, USA
e-mail: MEANSR@mail.etsu.edu

© Springer Nature Switzerland AG 2019   3
R. T. Means Jr. (ed.), *Anemia in the Young and Old*,
https://doi.org/10.1007/978-3-319-96487-4_1

were identified by the number and nature of hematopoietic precursors to which they gave rise in semisolid medium such as methylcellulose [6]. CFU-GEMM, for example, gave rise to large clusters containing a mix of hemoglobinized cells and cells with myeloid, monocytic, or megakaryocytic cytochemical features. BFU-E give rise to large colonies (bursts) of hemoglobinized cells only; CFU-E, having less division potential, give rise to small colonies of erythroid precursors. However, a more recent understanding permitted by the identification of cell surface antigen patterns characteristic of hematopoietic progenitors has demonstrated that the process is not quite as hierarchical as described above [7]. Progenitors limited to one lineage occasionally bud off the erythropoietic tree at earlier stages than the traditional model allowed [7].

The process of erythropoiesis is under regulation of a complex network of hematopoietic growth factors. This includes stem cell factor (SCF), interleukin (IL)-3, transforming forming growth factor (TGF)-α, and insulin-like growth factor (IGF)-1 [7, 8]. However, for the clinician, the most important erythroid growth factor is erythropoietin (Epo) [8]. Epo is the dominant regulator of red cell production from the late BFU-E stage forward and is controlled by a classic feedback loop; anemia is perceived as hypoxia by the Epo-producing cell in the renal cortex, leading to activation of hypoxia-inducible factor (HIF). HIF then activates the Epo enhancer, leading to increased Epo production and consequently to increased red blood cell (RBC) production. As anemia resolves, the Epo-producing cell is adequately oxygenated, HIF is hydroxylated, and Epo production is turned off [9].

Erythroid progenitors are present in the bone marrow at very low concentrations and for the most part are not morphologically distinguishable on Wright-Giemsa stained marrow preparations. In contrast, erythroid precursors, which are terminally differentiated and lack capacity to divide, are abundant and easily identified. The stages of erythroid precursor (or erythroblast) maturation are distinct and morphologically identifiable. A progressive increase in cytoplasmic hemoglobin concentration changes the color of the Wright-Giemsa stained cytoplasm from a deep blue to red/pink, with the cytoplasmic color giving each stage its name (basophilic erythroblast, polychromatophilic erythroblast, orthochromatic erythroblast, nucleated RBC). Fortunately for the color-blind, these cytoplasmic changes are accompanied by nuclear maturation, with the large nucleus with loose chromatin of the basophilic erythroblast progressing to the small dense pyknotic nucleus of the nucleated RBC. These cells then extrude their nuclei through an active process [10]. The RBC after enucleation still contains precipitated RNA that can be identified by supravital staining or flow cytometric techniques. During the period when this RNA is present, the RBC is referred to as a reticulocyte. The proportion of the circulating red cell population represented by reticulocytes can be expressed by a number of different parameters, any of which can serve as a measure of erythropoietic activity [11]. When RBC demand increases (e.g., when anemia is present), the normal response is for the reticulocyte count to increase. A number of factors contribute the late stages of erythroid differentiation/development. B12 is required for nuclear maturation, and iron is a key component of hemoglobin. Testosterone increases erythropoietin production [12], and its deficiency can lead to anemia [13].

The mature anucleate RBC is a biconcave disk, approximately 7 micrometers in diameter with an outer membrane that consists of a lipid bilayer linked to a cytoskeleton by various transmembrane proteins [14, 15]. The content within the RBC membrane consists primarily of hemoglobin but also includes enzymes of intermediary energy metabolism such as glucose-6-phosphate dehydrogenase or pyruvate kinase [16, 17]. The physiologic function of the RBC is to deliver oxygen to tissues, and all aspects of RBC structure, content, and chemistry optimize that function. The biconcave shape of the RBC optimizes passage of the cell through the circulation and facilitates gas exchange across the capillary endothelium. The generation of 2,3-diphosphoglycerate (2,3-DPG) in the course of RBC metabolism regulates hemoglobin oxygen affinity [18], while other metabolic mechanisms support hemoglobin and red cell structural integrity by maintaining optimal intracellular redox conditions and osmotic stability [19, 20].

Mature RBCs circulate in the peripheral blood for 100 to 120 days, and approximately 1% of the body's red cells are lost and replaced each day under normal conditions. When more RBCs are required (bleeding, hypoxia), the marrow has substantial capacity to upregulate erythropoiesis. Senescent RBCs are removed from the circulation by macrophages in the spleen, liver, and bone marrow [21, 22].

Definition and Basic Processes of Anemia

If one were to define anemia in a pure functional or physiologic sense, anemia would be defined as an insufficient RBC mass to deliver appropriate oxygen to peripheral tissues. WHO has tried to apply such a physiologic definition by providing modifiers that, for example, increase the lower limit of the normal hemoglobin range in people dwelling at high altitudes [23].

Since methods to assess effective peripheral oxygen delivery at a tissue level are not available at a clinically practical level, anemia is defined for practical purposes by a surrogate measure estimating red cell mass to be lower than the population norm. Any of three surrogate measures on whole blood are used. All are concentrations and so can be altered by factors that expand or contract plasma volume. All are routinely reported by electronic hematology analyzers.

The oldest but least used although perhaps most reproducible measure is the RBC concentration in cells per liter (10^{12}/L) ("red cell count"). The most commonly used measure, particularly in more developed countries, is hemoglobin concentration, typically expressed as grams of hemoglobin per deciliter (g/dL) in the United States and as grams per liter (g/L) in countries using Systeme Internationale (SI) units. The WHO hemoglobin cutoffs for anemia are expressed as hemoglobin concentration [23]. The last measure is the hematocrit, also called the *packed cell volume (PCV)*, which as originally conceived represents the proportion of blood volume occupied by RBCs, expressed as a percent or as a decimal. Originally, it was determined by centrifuging a standard volume specimen of venous or capillary blood in a graduated tube and reading off the percentage of the blood column comprised of (packed) red blood cells. The graduated tube was called a "hematocrit," hence the name [24]. That approach is still used routinely in resource-poor environments [25]. In electronic counters, hematocrit is calculated by multiplying the measured RBC concentration by the measured mean RBC volume (MCV) and then applying a correction factor to normalize to a standard volume.

Underproduction (or *hyporegenerative*) anemia refers to anemia associated with an inappropriately low reticulocyte response. Anything that interferes with erythroid development prior to the egress of the reticulocyte from the bone marrow will typically result in underproduction anemia. A few examples (which will be discussed in specific chapters) would be clonal disorders of erythropoiesis, interfering with the orderly progression of the HSC to the erythroid precursors; congenital marrow failure disorders, typically impacting the molecular regulation of erythropoiesis; Epo deficiency, as is seen in the anemia of chronic kidney disease; or B12 or iron deficiency, interfering with erythroid precursor nuclear maturation or hemoglobin synthesis, respectively.

Anemia with an appropriate (or increased) reticulocyte response results from RBC loss after leaving the marrow results from blood loss or from hemolysis and reflects a problem with red cell structure or contents. Hemolysis, whether acquired or congenital, results from defects in hemoglobin (as in the hemoglobinopathies), in red cell metabolic integrity (as when glucose-6-phosphate deficiency impedes the appropriate response to oxidative stress), or red cell structure (whether intrinsic from structural protein defects or extrinsic from a membrane-directed autoantibody).

References

1. Kratz A, Ferraro M, Sluss PM, Lewandrowski KB. Case records of the Massachusetts General Hospital. Weekly clinicopathological exercises. Laboratory reference values. N Engl J Med. 2004;351(15):1548–63.
2. Tumburu L, Thein SL. Genetic control of erythropoiesis. Curr Opin Hematol. 2017;24(3):173–82.
3. Gnanapragasam MN, Bieker JJ. Orchestration of late events in erythropoiesis by KLF1/EKLF. Curr Opin Hematol. 2017;24(3):183–90.
4. Nakahata T, Ogawa M. Identification in culture of a class of hematopoietic colony-forming units with extensive capability to self-renew and generate multipotential hemopoietic colonies. Proc Natl Acad Sci U S A. 1982;79:3843–7.
5. Leary AG, Ogawa M, Strauss LC, Civin CI. Single cell origin of multilineage colonies in culture. Evidence that differentiation of multipotent progenitors and restriction of proliferative potential of monopotent progenitors are stochastic processes. J Clin Invest. 1984;74(6):2193–7.
6. Eaves AC, Eaves CJ. Erythropoiesis in culture. Clin Haematol. 1984;13:371–91.
7. Dulmovits BM, Hom J, Narla A, Mohandas N, Blanc L. Characterization, regulation, and targeting of erythroid progenitors in normal and disordered human erythropoiesis. Curr Opin Hematol. 2017;24(3):159–66.
8. Muta K, Krantz SB, Bondurant MC, Wickrema A. Distinct roles of erythropoietin, insulin-like growth factor, and stem cell factor in the development of erythroid progenitor cells. J Clin Investig. 1994;94:34–43.

9. Jelkmann W. Regulation of erythropoietin production. J Physiol. 2011;589.(Pt 6:1251–8.
10. Koury ST, Koury MJ, Bondurant MC. Cytoskeletal distribution and function during the maturation and enucleation of mammalian erythroblasts. J Cell Biol. 1989;109(6 Pt 1):3005–13.
11. Piva E, Brugnara C, Spolaore F, Plebani M. Clinical utility of reticulocyte parameters. Clin Lab Med. 2015;35(1):133–63.
12. Bachman E, Travison TG, Basaria S, et al. Testosterone induces erythrocytosis via increased erythropoietin and suppressed hepcidin: evidence for a new erythropoietin/hemoglobin set point. J Gerontol A Biol Sci Med Sci. 2014;69(6):725–35.
13. Ferrucci L, Maggio M, Bandinelli S, et al. Low testosterone levels and the risk of anemia in older men and women. Arch Intern Med. 2006;166(13):1380–8.
14. Narla M, Gallagher PG. Red cell membrane: past, present, and future. Blood. 2008;112(10):3939–48.
15. Daniels G. Functions of red cell surface proteins. Vox Sang. 2007;93(4):331–40.
16. Prchal JT, Gregg XT. Red cell enzymes. Hematology Am Soc Hematol Educ Program. 2005:19–23.
17. van Wijk R, van Solinge WW. The energy-less red blood cell is lost: erythrocyte enzyme abnormalities of glycolysis. Blood. 2005;106(13):4034–42.
18. Yonetani T, Park SI, Tsuneshige A, Imai K, Kanaori K. Global allostery model of hemoglobin. Modulation of O(2) affinity, cooperativity, and Bohr effect by heterotropic allosteric effectors. J Biol Chem. 2002;277(37):34508–20.
19. Siems WG, Sommerburg O, Grune T. Erythrocyte free radical and energy metabolism. Clin Nephrol. 2000;53(1 Suppl):S9–17.
20. Joiner CH, Lauf PK. Ouabain binding and potassium transport in young and old populations of human red cells. Membr Biochem. 1978;1(3–4):187–202.
21. Bratosin D, Mazurier J, Tissier JP, et al. Cellular and molecular mechanisms of senescent erythrocyte phagocytosis by macrophages. A review. Biochimie. 1998;80(2):173–95.
22. Landaw SA. Factors that accelerate or retard red blood cell senescence. Blood Cells. 1988;14(1):47–67.
23. WHO. Haemoglobin standards for the diagnosis of anaemia and assessment of severity. 2011; www.who.int/vmnis/indicators/haemoglobin.pdf.
24. Means RTJ. It all started in New Orleans: Wintrobe, the hematocrit and the definition of normal. Am J Med Sci. 2011;341(1):64–5.
25. Isah AY, Amanabo MA, Ekele BA. Prevalence of malaria parasitemia amongst asymptomatic pregnant women attending a Nigerian teaching hospital. Ann Afr Med. 2011;10(2):171–4.

Chapter 2
Diagnostic Approach to Anemia in Childhood and Adolescents

Jenny K. McDaniel and Caryn E. Sorge

Anemia is the most common reason for pediatric hematology consultation [25]. Based on World Health Organization estimates in 2011, approximately 43% of children have anemia during childhood (WHO 2011). Outside of the neonatal period, anemia in childhood is seen most frequently in toddlers and then again in adolescence, both periods of rapid growth accompanied by potential challenges with nutritional intake. The primary focus of this chapter is to give an overview of the potential etiologies of anemia in the pediatric population and focus on the clinical and laboratory features that may accompany them.

Identifying patients with anemia is important due to the potential effects long-standing, untreated anemia can have on children. General consequences of anemia commonly include fatigue, decreased exercise tolerance, and headache. Anemia and its underlying cause can also affect growth and have many other potential impacts on overall health. The identification and treatment of patients with iron deficiency is of utmost importance given the associated risk of adverse neurodevelopment effects, although investigation regarding the impact of iron repletion on these effects is ongoing [3, 4, 10, 20, 22, 28, 29, 32, 39, 48].

The definition of anemia varies significantly with age and gender, and there are also variations in the normal ranges based on ethnicity. When evaluating a patient for anemia, it is important to ensure the proper normative reference ranges are being used. The definition of anemia in the pediatric population is a reduction in

J. K. McDaniel, MD
Department of Pediatrics, Division of Pediatric Hematology/Oncology,
St. Jude Affiliate Clinic at Novant Health Hemby Children's Hospital, Charlotte, NC, USA
e-mail: jkmcdaniel@novanthealth.org

C. E. Sorge, MD (✉)
Department of Pediatrics, Division of Pediatric Hematology/Oncology,
University of Kentucky, Lexington, KY, USA
e-mail: caryn.sorge@uky.edu

© Springer Nature Switzerland AG 2019
R. T. Means Jr. (ed.), *Anemia in the Young and Old*,
https://doi.org/10.1007/978-3-319-96487-4_2

hemoglobin or hematocrit more than two standard deviations below the mean for patient's age, gender, and ethnicity.

The World Health Organization and American Academy of Pediatrics recommend universal screening for anemia in patients at 1 year of age. Additionally, The AAP recommends additional screening in children with risk factors for anemia including abnormal growth, poor feeding, or dietary concerns [3].

History

When approaching a patient with anemia, there are several historical considerations that can be helpful in quickly narrowing the differential diagnosis including a thorough dietary history to evaluate for potential nutritional deficiencies, history of blood loss, and the presence of pica. Coexisting diseases such as autoimmune diseases or inflammatory disorders predispose patients to anemia of chronic disease. Recent infections can also significantly impact the bone marrow's ability to produce normal blood cells. A history of jaundice or dark urine may indicate a red cell destructive process. The presence of fever, weight loss, or night sweats may accompany anemia related to underlying malignancy. In many cases of chronic anemia, clinical findings may not be apparent until hemoglobin falls below 8 g/dL. History of fatigue, dizziness, irritability, and decreased energy may be obtained from the history.

In cases of heritable causes of anemia, the family history can also be informative. The diagnosis may be clear based on a family history of anemia if the underlying cause is known. There could also be a history of vague symptoms in family members that become congruent when a diagnosis is determined in the presenting patient. Additional questions to address include whether family members have required red blood cell transfusions or if they have had complications such as splenomegaly or splenectomy, gallstones or cholecystectomy, or either neonatal or episodic jaundice.

Key Exam Components

A thorough physical exam should be performed in patients undergoing evaluation for anemia. In cases of severe anemia, vital sign abnormalities such as tachycardia and tachypnea may be present; in severe cases, especially in the setting of acute blood loss, hypotension may be present. Generalized pallor may be appreciated. In hemolytic anemias, patients may appear jaundiced and have scleral icterus. Significant lymphadenopathy could indicate infectious etiology but also could be present in malignant disorders. Hepatosplenomegaly can be found in oncologic processes, hemolytic anemias, or long-standing anemias resulting in extramedullary hematopoiesis.

Laboratory Data

Anemia can be the consequence of many underlying pathologic processes. To help narrow the differential diagnosis, several different classification methods can be used. The initial laboratory evaluation should include a complete blood count with red cell indices and differential. A reticulocyte count and peripheral smear should also be performed.

In patients with anemia, the red cell indices often will narrow the differential diagnosis and help guide the additional evaluation indicated. The mean corpuscular volume (MCV) denotes the average size of the red blood cells. The mean corpuscular hemoglobin (MCH) and mean corpuscular hemoglobin concentration (MCHC) indicate the hemoglobin content of the red blood cells. The red blood cell distribution width (RDW) is a measure of the heterogeneity of red blood cell sizes.

Classifying anemia by red cell size is also helpful in narrowing the differential. The definitions of microcytic, normocytic, and macrocytic vary with age in the pediatric population, so it is important to ensure the appropriate reference ranges are being used (Table 2.1).

In addition to red cell size, another helpful indication to help delineate the underlying cause is by evaluating the marrow response to anemia. In cases of nutritional deficiencies or bone marrow pathology, the marrow cannot appropriately increase red cell production to compensate for the anemia. However, in cases of red cell destruction or blood loss, the bone marrow should be able to respond to anemia with an increased reticulocytosis.

The reticulocyte count is helpful to understand the underlying pathogenic process. Reticulocytes are young anuclear red blood cells that indicate an active marrow undergoing erythropoiesis. Anemia with reticulocytosis can be seen with blood loss or peripheral destruction of the red blood cells. Anemia without reticulocytosis indicates poor marrow response which could be related to infections, inadequate nutrition, or other red cell production inadequacies including infiltrative marrow processes. There are caveats to these generalities, for example, in acute blood loss,

Table 2.1 Normative hematologic values based on age and sex

Age	Hemoglobin (g/dL)	Hematocrit (%)	MCV (fL)
6–23 m	12.0	36	78
24 m–4y	12.5	38	79
5–7y	13.0	39	81
8–11y	13.5	40	83
12–18y			
Male	14.5	43	88
Female	14.0	41	90
>/=18y			
Male	15.5	47	90
Female	14.0	41	90

Data compiled from two sources. Brugnara et al. [9] and Gajjar and Jalazo [18]

reticulocytosis may take several days to develop. Additionally, in some conditions of peripheral red cell destruction, the reticulocytes may also be a target of destruction.

Interpreting the reticulocyte response can be challenging in some cases. The percentage of reticulocytes must be taken in context for the degree of anemia present in the patient. To correct for this, either the absolute reticulocyte count can be used or the reticulocyte percentage observed can be corrected for the degree of anemia. The reticulocyte percentage can be corrected as follows: patient hematocrit/normal hematocrit x reticulocyte percentage multiplied by a correction factor for the degree of patient's anemia. A corrected reticulocyte percentage <2% indicates inadequate compensatory reticulocytosis. A corrected reticulocyte percentage >3% indicates compensatory production of reticulocytes to replace the lost or destroyed red blood cells.

There are many helpful clues that can be gained through examination of the peripheral smear that may reveal potential causes for the patient's anemia. Relative red cell size and hemoglobin content can be observed visually to compare to the red cell indices. The presence of spherocytes, schistocytes, blister cells, sickle cells, targets, basophilic stippling, Heinz bodies, polychromasia, anisocytosis, poikilocytosis, Howell-Jolly bodies, acanthocytes, and many other red cell forms can be seen which may aid in understanding the etiology of the anemia.

Spherocytes are red blood cells with absent central pallor. When they are numerous, they can be detected on the red blood cell indices as increased mean corpuscular hemoglobin concentration. Spherocytes are found in hereditary spherocytosis but also can be seen in other types of hemolytic anemias such as G6PD. In hemolytic anemias, spherocytes are seen due to the progressive loss of membrane during the removal of antibodies by macrophages. Schistocytes are fragmented red blood cells that result from intravascular hemolysis as seen in microangiopathic hemolytic anemias, autoimmune hemolytic anemias, and other types of hemolytic anemias. They result from the mechanical destruction or shearing of red blood cells within the circulation. Blister cells are red blood cells with a peripheral area of clearing that gives the red blood cell a blistered appearance. These cells are precursors to bite cells and are seen in G6PD and other oxidative hemolytic anemias. Sickle cells are crescent or C-shaped red blood cells associated with hemoglobin S mutation. This mutation causes the hemoglobin to crystalize and the red blood cells lose their deformability making them more prone to hemolysis and limiting their ability to flow freely through the circulation.

Aside from laboratory testing on the patient, obtaining labs including a complete blood cell count and peripheral smear on family members can be useful in making the diagnosis of certain hereditary conditions such as thalassemia and hereditary spherocytosis.

Imaging Considerations

In most cases, imaging is not necessary in patients with anemia. However, in certain situations, particularly when concerned for underlying malignant process, it may be helpful to consider.

A chest X-ray may be obtained to evaluate for mediastinal adenopathy or mass. Pulmonary hemosiderosis also can result in abnormal findings on chest X-ray.

Abdominal ultrasonography may be useful to evaluate for hepatosplenomegaly or masses. In hemolytic anemias, splenomegaly or gallstones may be detected.

The use of computed tomography (CT) can also detect adenopathy, masses, and hepatosplenomegaly and may also be useful to evaluate for occult bleeding. Radiation exposure should be taken into account when using CT; the use of MRI can decrease radiation exposure and allow for improved diagnostic quality.

Specialized testing such as radioactively tagged red blood cell radionuclide scans is occasionally useful in patients with occult gastrointestinal bleeding not detected by other means, such as stool guaiac testing or direct visualization on during procedures such as colonoscopy.

Procedures

Bone marrow aspirate and biopsy rarely are needed if anemia is isolated. They are, however, warranted when there are additional abnormalities in additional cell lines such as thrombocytopenia and/or neutropenia.

Microcytosis

The most common cause of anemia in childhood worldwide is iron deficiency anemia. Iron is recycled after the breakdown of red blood cells and the absorption of iron is limited to 1–2 mg daily. Hepcidin which is found in the wall of the intestines helps maintain iron stores and prevents deficiency as well as toxicity from excess iron [11].

Iron deficiency is the reduction in iron stores prior to the development of anemia. There are three phases of iron deficiency, each with varying laboratory values associated with them. Initially you may only see a decrease in ferritin that indicates decreased tissue iron stores. During this initial phase, you may not see any change in hemoglobin/hematocrit or even serum iron levels. As the deficiency becomes more severe, the reticuloendothelial macrophage iron stores are depleted, and this is when you will see a drop in serum iron levels and total iron-binding capacity increases. During this phase the hemoglobin/hematocrit remains normal. Finally true iron deficiency anemia develops at which time microcytosis and hypochromia develop. These features are the result of erythropoiesis occurring after iron stores were limited [2]. Other findings of iron deficiency anemia include decreased RBC count and increased RDW, and on peripheral smear you may see anisocytosis. Reticulocyte count in iron deficiency is typically low to normal depending on the stage at which it is being evaluated.

So as you can see, the clinical and laboratory findings occur on a spectrum, and only in the late phases of iron deficiency do you see the typical laboratory findings of microcytosis and true anemia. This demonstrates the importance of using a screening dietary history so that deficiency can be picked up prior to the development of anemia.

When taking a dietary history, both quality and quantity are important when discussing dietary sources of iron. Heme which comes from animal tissues is the most easily absorbed form of iron. Plant-derived iron is poorly absorbed [36]. Though breastmilk has a low concentration of iron, the bioavailability of the iron within breastmilk is greater than that of cow's milk [21]; the high content of calcium in cow's milk contributes to the decreased absorption of iron [14]. Iron content however is not the only reason cow's milk contributes to the development of iron deficiency. Drinking large volumes of cow's milk contributes to decreased consumption of iron-rich foods. Along with this, increased consumption can also cause irritation in the gastrointestinal tract that leads to chronic micro-hemorrhage which again contributes to the development of iron deficiency [35]. With all of this in mind, childhood is a peak time for the development of iron deficiency because not only are there behavioral aspects to the dietary contributors but this is also a time of rapid growth during which demands for iron are much higher.

In children and adolescents, blood loss must be considered as a cause of their iron deficiency. Epistaxis, GI blood loss, menstrual bleeding, and hematuria can be sources and must be reviewed in taking a history. In adolescent females, you must obtain a thorough menstrual history and can consider suppressing menstrual bleeding if not corrected with oral supplementation. Occult gastrointestinal (GI) blood loss is often overlooked but simple to rule out with stool studies. If by history there is concern for more significant GI blood loss, then GI consultation with colonoscopy should be used to evaluate the underlying cause of iron deficiency anemia. In younger patients with concerns for occult blood loss, stool parasite testing should be performed. History of hematuria can also indicate blood loss contributing to iron deficiency; urinalysis with microscopy can confirm this.

If, after treating a patient with appropriate dosed oral iron, there is no improvement in your red cell indices, you must confirm that your diagnosis of iron deficiency is correct. Other considerations can be lead poisoning, some forms of sideroblastic anemia, chronic inflammation, thalassemia, ongoing blood loss, poor compliance with medication, or very rarely defects in iron absorption.

Oral iron challenge can determine if compliance is the underlying issue. If a witnessed oral challenge indicates that oral iron is not being absorbed, then further evaluation is necessary. GI causes should be ruled out. Iron-refractory iron deficiency anemia (IRIDA) is a rare disorder. These patients do not respond to oral iron replacement and only partially respond to IV iron. Germline mutations in TMPRSS6 have been identified in these populations, which leads to inappropriately high levels of hepcidin. TMPRSS6 testing can be performed if your suspicion is high for IRIDA [17].

Though lead poisoning is rare in today's day and age given the removal of lead-based paints from the market, lead levels should be obtained and confirmed normal in patients with persistent microcytic anemia.

Anemia of chronic disease (also called "anemia of inflammation") often initially masquerades as iron deficiency as a microcytic hypochromic anemia. Inflammation caused by chronic diseases affects the utilization of iron stores through upregulation of hepcidin. A thorough history should help to rule out significant chronic inflammation. Symptoms such as unexplained rashes, joint pain, or swelling or GI symptoms such as abdominal pain, hematochezia, or melena potentially indicting Crohn's or ulcerative colitis should warrant the appropriate referral. Elevated inflammatory markers such as C-reactive protein, sedimentation rate (which may be falsely elevated in severe anemia), and ferritin can indicate an underlying inflammatory condition.

Thalassemia

Thalassemia is another common cause of microcytic hypochromic anemia in childhood. It is caused by the impaired production of globin chains, alpha or beta, resulting in alpha thalassemia and beta thalassemia. The scope of the disease will be discussed in subsequent chapters, and the focus now will be on the diagnosis thalassemia. Within the spectrum of each type of thalassemia, there is also a spectrum of laboratory and clinical findings that are found.

For any microcytosis consult, thalassemia should be included in the differential. The minor phenotypes of both thalassemia subtypes can present with microcytosis, but the degree of anemia is variable. In homozygous forms anemia is severe and these patients are transfusion dependent.

Family history including ethnic origin is important in aiding in the differential. Beta thalassemia occurs primarily in patients of Mediterranean and Southeast Asian descent. Alpha thalassemia is also seen predominantly in Southeast Asians but also those of African descent. Family history including history of stillborn births is important and may indicate a severe form of alpha thalassemia as a result of 4 gene deletion and subsequent hydrops fetalis. Depending on the age of the patient, there may be clinical indications of extramedullary hematopoiesis in patients with thalassemia including splenomegaly or bony changes.

Thalassemia is a process that includes both ineffective erythropoiesis and destruction of red cells. In beta thalassemia trait, red cell indices will show a mild microcytic, hypochromic anemia with a normal RDW, elevated RBC count, and normal MCHC. In contrast to iron deficiency, these patients will likely have normal iron studies.

Peripheral smear findings include target cells, basophilic stippling, and elliptocytes [15]. Due to the potential for hemolysis, there may be hyperbilirubinemia, low haptoglobin, and an elevated LDH. On hemoglobin electrophoresis, an elevated A2 greater than 3.5% will be seen due to the impaired beta production [1]. In the setting of severe iron deficiency there are mixed reports on the interpretation of HgbA2. Historically, it has been reported that iron deficiency does falsely lower the HgbA2 in patients with beta thalassemia minor [24]; however, other reports stated that there was not a significant decrease in HgbA2 in patients with concomitant iron deficiency and beta thalassemia minor [1]. To delineate these iron studies including ferritin, TIBC and transferrin saturation can be obtained at the time of other testing for thalassemia in select populations where the potential for thalassemia is high. Confirmation would be obtained through globin gene analysis.

In severe forms of beta thalassemia, persistent fetal hemoglobin can delay the diagnosis. Severe anemia in these patients is expected, and these patients are transfusion dependent. Hemoglobin electrophoresis in these patients depicts elevated fetal hemoglobin with an elevated HgbA2 and varying degrees of decreased HgbA. Bone marrow evaluation can show erythroid hyperplasia. Iron studies in these patients including serum iron levels and ferritin and transferrin saturation are elevated. TIBC is only slightly elevated. Parents of these patients will be found to have a microcytic hypochromic anemia.

It is important to monitor for iron overload in these patients and the complications that accompany iron overload. Ferritin levels can be monitored on regular intervals and T2* MRI is currently widely accepted as a measure for both liver and cardiac iron monitoring. Iron overload and the chelation therapy necessary to treat it can cause multiple complications in these patients, and therefore it is important that they are monitored by an ophthalmologist and audiologist. Oftentimes, endocrinology consultation is necessary to manage the endocrinopathies (hypogonadism, hypoparathyroidism, diabetes, and hypothyroidism) that are associated with iron overload [13].

The use of hemoglobin electrophoresis can differentiate between alpha thalassemia trait and beta thalassemia trait. In the neonate, a small amount of Hgb Barts may be present. Unlike in beta thalassemia, there is no elevation of fetal hemoglobin in alpha thalassemia. Therefore if your patient has hypochromia, microcytosis, and erythrocytosis in the setting of normal iron studies and normal HgbA2, then alpha thalassemia is likely the diagnosis. Alpha-globin gene analysis can be performed to confirm and educate your patient and their families.

Hgb H seen on hemoglobin electrophoresis outside of the neonatal period is an indication of three gene deletion alpha thalassemia. When Hgb Barts reaches levels of 80–90%, then the patient has four gene deletions. These patients are high risk of intrauterine death or hydrops fetalis.

Normocytic

Much like with microcytosis, the approach to normocytic anemia follows a stepwise fashion. In normocytic anemia, the MCV falls within two standard deviations of the mean based on age. This category can be divided by the reticulocyte response to the normocytic anemia. An elevated reticulocyte panel is a clear indication that the marrow is functioning normally in response to the anemia. Reticulocytosis is a sign of a destructive process that is affecting the red blood cells. The differential for a normocytic anemia with normal or low reticulocyte count is vast and includes infection, anemia of chronic disease, or underlying marrow pathology such as transient erythroblastopenia of childhood or Diamond-Blackfan anemia or malignancy.

A detailed history will allow you to determine whether your destructive process is either acute blood loss/hemorrhage or hemolysis. Acute blood loss will typically cause a normocytic anemia; however, if the blood loss becomes chronic, it can become microcytic.

In regard to hemolysis, a detailed history of the events leading up to the discovery of anemia is important. History recent infections, jaundice, and dark urine are all indications of a hemolytic process. Certain types of hemolysis can be triggered by medications or environmental exposures. One should obtain a family history of hematologic disorders such as hemoglobinopathies (sickle cell disease), membrane defects (hereditary spherocytosis, hereditary elliptocytosis), and enzyme defects (pyruvate kinase deficiency, G6PD deficiency).

Physical examination is the next step in evaluating your patient with normocytic anemia secondary to hemolysis. Scleral icterus is an indication of hyperbilirubinemia. Splenomegaly can be seen in autoimmune hemolytic anemia. Right upper quadrant pain can be a clinical finding of gallstones which are caused by hemolysis.

There are two main types of hemolysis, extravascular vs intravascular hemolysis. Where the hemolysis occurs is determined by the underlying cause of red blood cell destruction and affects the results of laboratory testing. Intravascular hemolysis occurs within the vessels. During the destruction of the red blood cells, hemoglobin is released into the circulation. With destruction of the cells, lactate dehydrogenase will be elevated. The released hemoglobin is then bound by haptoglobin to allow for clearance through the liver and eventually circulating haptoglobin becomes depleted. Free hemoglobin in the circulation results in hemoglobinuria or methemoglobinuria and can also cause injury to the kidney.

Extravascular hemolysis occurs when red blood cells are engulfed by macrophages in the reticuloendothelial system and destroyed. The by-products released from red blood cell destruction are released into the reticuloendothelial system and the hemoglobin is converted into bilirubin. Intravascular hemolysis is classically complement-mediated or related to mechanical trauma, whereas extravascular hemolysis involves antibody-mediated opsonization and phagocytosis of red blood cells. Often in hemolytic anemias, there may be components of both types of hemolysis.

A direct antiglobulin test (DAT) will categorize your patient into one of these two processes. A DAT is a direct way of visualizing agglutination that develops after a reagent is added to the patient's blood. In this test, the patient's red blood cells are washed and antibodies against IgG, IgM, and complement are added under varying conditions. If antibodies are present, the reaction should cause agglutination. The occurrence of agglutination with the various reagents can help differentiate the type of autoimmune hemolytic anemia.

Hereditary hemolytic anemias include disorders of red cell membranes and red cell enzyme defects. Family history can be helpful in detecting these hereditary disorders in most cases; however, some will not have any pertinent history to aid in the diagnosis.

Red cell membrane disorders include hereditary spherocytosis (HS) which is often suspected when a peripheral smear shows spherocytosis, DAT is negative, and there is a strong family history. These patients may not have anemia or may be mildly anemic with an elevated reticulocyte count. During an acute phase of hemolysis, splenomegaly may be present on exam. Other laboratory findings include an elevated MCHC and typically a normal MCV. By history these patients often have jaundice during the neonatal period. If there is a strong family history with the findings consistent with HS, then no further testing is necessary [7]. The gold standard for diagnosing HS is the incubated osmotic fragility testing. In atypical cases where osmotic fragility testing is normal, measurement of affected protein levels, spectrin, ankyrin-1, band 3 protein, or protein 4.2, can be obtained commercially [37]. Hereditary elliptocytosis has similar laboratory and clinical findings as hereditary spherocytosis except on peripheral smear the major finding is elliptocytes. The proteins involved include alpha-spectrin, beta-spectrin, protein 4.1, and glycophorin C [19, 45].

The hereditary hemolytic anemias associated with enzyme defects also present with findings consistent with hemolysis (elevated reticulocyte count, hyperbilirubinemia) and like HS are DAT negative. Unlike HS these patients do not have spherocytes on peripheral smear and have normal osmotic fragility testing. During the work-up of these patients, membranopathies and hemoglobinopathies must be ruled out as the cause of the hemolysis. In that case then assays can be performed to quantify the activity of enzymes that you suspect are involved with the most common being pyruvate kinase deficiency [50].

Glucose 6 phosphate dehydrogenase (G6PD) deficiency is a unique hemolytic anemia in that patients typically are clinically well without anemia and hemolysis except for when they are challenged with an oxidative agent or stressor; the most common being medication, fava beans or an infection [5]. Hemolysis is present after exposure to these and laboratory findings are consistent with what has been described with hemolysis prior. On peripheral smear, spherocytes and bite cells may be present. Outside of exposure to the known agents that cause hemolysis, patients are clinically well and typically do not have anemia. Diagnosis is often made by measuring enzyme activity or testing for known mutations in the gene encoding G6PD. It is important that enzyme activity is measured during steady state [31].

Sickle cell disease (SCD) is a hemoglobinopathy that results in decreased deformability of the red blood cells thus impairing their ability to freely flow through circulation. When these cells become sickled, they cause vascular occlusion which can cause a myriad of symptoms depending on the site involved. Sickle cells have a shorter life-span than normal red blood cells, and their less deformable structure and propensity toward vascular occlusion all can cause increased hemolysis. These patients have a normal alpha-chain globin and an abnormal beta chain that is caused by an amino acid substitution of a valine for a glutamic acid in the sixth position on the beta chain [16]. There are two genes encoding beta globin chain synthesis, and when both have this mutation, that is known as hemoglobin S disease. Hemoglobin S is more commonly seen in patients of African descent. In the USA, patients with sickle cell are usually diagnosed by state newborn screens that detect the abnormal hemoglobin. Abnormal hemoglobin findings are confirmed and quantified on hemoglobin electrophoresis. Early detection with newborn screens improved morbidity and mortality in these patients [33]. Patients who have only sickle cell trait, meaning only one beta globin gene contains the S mutation, do not have anemia, and their hemoglobin electrophoresis shows 40% or less hemoglobin S. Those with sickle cell disease, or both beta globin genes containing the S mutation, have a higher percentage of hemoglobin S and have varying degrees of the associated symptoms including hemolytic anemia, pain crises, risk for life-threatening infection, risk for splenic sequestration, and risk for neurologic events, to name a few [30, 38]. These patients require management by pediatric hematologists who are familiar with necessary interventions and best therapies. Hemoglobin S can also combine with other abnormal hemoglobins such as hemoglobin C, beta thalassemia, and hemoglobin O, among others. These multiple chain hemoglobinopathies can present with varying degrees of severity and are detected on hemoglobin electrophoresis.

In patients with normocytic anemia and normal to low reticulocyte count, starting with a history can be beneficial. Viral and bacterial infections can cause anemia in this setting. Viral testing including parvovirus, Epstein-Barr virus (EBV), and cytomegalovirus (CMV) can present in this fashion. These patients will recover their hemoglobin on their own oftentimes without treatment. If the anemia is severe and there is no indication of an appropriate reticulocyte response, then transfusion is necessary.

Past medical history of chronic illnesses dictates further evaluation. Anemia of renal disease can be detected by screening renal function. If this is normal, then iron, TIBC, and ferritin should be drawn. In anemia of chronic disease, you will see low serum iron and TIBC with elevated ferritin indicating increased or normal iron stores [49].

If there is no history to indicate recent infection or anemia of chronic disease and the hemoglobin, in the setting of low reticulocyte count, one should consider a bone marrow evaluation. Erythroid hypoplasia on bone marrow would indicate the possibility of Diamond-Blackfan anemia (DBA) vs transient erythroblastopenia of childhood (TEC). TEC as the name indicates is a transient red cell aplasia. The cause of TEC is unknown. Bone marrow evaluation shows a normocellular marrow with decreased erythroid precursors. This is similar to what is seen in the marrow of patients with DBA. To differentiate between DBA and TEC, one can measure fetal hemoglobin. Elevated fetal hemoglobin is typically seen in DBA and is normal in TEC. If your suspicion is high for DBA, then you should also measure erythrocyte adenosine deaminase activity [27, 46].

Malignancy including leukemia and metastatic solid tumors can present with a normocytic anemia with normal or low reticulocyte count. History of fever, weight loss, night sweats, and bone pain are all indications of a malignant process. In the setting of leukemia, oftentimes other cell lines are affected. If thrombocytopenia is present, often patients will have a history of easy bruising or bleeding. On exam lymphadenopathy and/or hepatosplenomegaly may be present. In the case of metastatic disease from a solid tumor, evaluation for palpable masses is important. Performing a peripheral smear may show blasts. Bone marrow evaluation, including aspirate and biopsy, should be sent for morphologic evaluation, flow cytometry, and cytogenetics. If negative for leukemia, biopsy can evaluate for presence of solid tumor. If there is concern for metastatic involvement, then further evaluation is needed to determine the location and type of primary tumor.

Neonatal Anemia

Anemia is common in the neonatal period and there is increased risk of anemia in premature infants. This is often multifactorial, but potential causes include decreased iron stores, immune-mediated destruction, blood loss related to phlebotomy or other causes, marrow suppression related to medication or infections, and less commonly due to underlying defects in red blood cell synthesis or stability.

Hemolytic Disease of the Newborn

Immune-mediated destruction of red blood cells in the neonate is unique as it is caused by maternal antibodies against fetal red blood cell antigens. Maternal sensitization to the antigen can occur during pregnancy or potentially from a previous blood transfusion. The maternal antibodies of the IgG subtype can be transported across the placenta and enter fetal circulation during pregnancy. Once in the fetal circulation, these antibodies attack fetal red blood cells that express these antigens and cause hemolysis. Infants often present with jaundice shortly after birth.

The major cause of immune-mediated hemolytic disease in neonates is due to Rh blood group incompatibility between mother and fetus. Classically this is due to antibodies to the D antigen; however other Rh antigens including C, c, E, and e are also potential triggers. At-risk pregnancies are those in which the mother is Rh D negative, and the fetus inherits the D antigen from the father and thus is Rh D positive.

There can also be incompatibilities related to the ABO blood group when the mother and father have different blood types. This can be seen in women with blood type O, A, or B if the fetus has a different blood type. The hemolytic disease related to ABO incompatibility is usually not as severe as that related to Rh incompatibility because there is less expression of the ABO blood group antigens in fetal red blood cells. Additionally, unlike Rh antigens, the ABO blood group antigens are also expressed by other fetal tissue types thus decreasing the chances of the maternal antibody binding the target antigens on red blood cells. There can be maternal antibodies directed against other antigens of Kell, Duffy, Kidd, MNS, or s blood group antibodies, though these are less common.

Pregnant women are screened for blood type, Rh status, and presence of antibodies with an indirect antibody screen during pregnancy. Obtaining a history of previous pregnancies allows for you to predict whether mom has been sensitized if she is Rh negative. The use of anti-D IgG in women at risk has dramatically reduced the incidence and severity of Rh sensitization and hemolytic disease related to Rh incompatibility. This is typically given around 28 and 34 weeks of gestation and at delivery and may also be given during other events in pregnancy with risk of sensitization [8]. Knowing whether mom has received anti-D IgG in all previous pregnancies can help you predict risk and severity for this child. In patients who are at high risk, then monitoring during pregnancy should be undertaken by an experienced obstetrician. If treatment is necessary during pregnancy, the use of intrauterine transfusion can be performed and in some cases hydrops can be reversed [43].

In the neonate, assessment should include a complete blood count and blood group typing including the presence of antibodies. These patients should also have their bilirubin monitored closely given the risk of hyperbilirubinemia and the adverse effects associated. In patients where hyperbilirubinemia is detected, the use of phototherapy has been useful and oftentimes exchange transfusion can be avoided [23].

Macrocytic

Macrocytosis is defined as a larger than normal red blood cell. Macrocytic anemias in children are unusual. Examination of the peripheral smear is helpful to evaluate for megaloblastic anemia detected by the presence of hypersegmented neutrophils.

The nutrient deficiencies that can cause macrocytic anemia with hypersegmented neutrophils are specifically B12 or folate. Like all forms of anemia, a detailed history including a dietary history including restrictions may indicate the underlying cause as patients who are strict vegans can be B12 deficient. This is also true of exclusively breastfed infants of mothers who are strict vegans or have a B12 deficiency themselves [6, 42]. Animal products are the only natural source for B12. Besides dietary restrictions, malabsorption of B12 can also occur. Though pernicious anemia is not common in the pediatric patient population, it can occur. Past medical history of short gut secondary to surgical management of necrotizing enterocolitis as a neonate can lead to B12 deficiency if the ileum was involved in the resection. In teens with inflammatory bowel disease (IBD), B12 deficiency can be seen if there has been prolonged, untreated inflammation with resulting malabsorption [42].

In infants with B12 deficiency, exam findings can be extensive including poor growth and development, hypotonia, irritability, lethargy, tremors, and coma. Beyond these neurologic symptoms, they can also develop abnormal skin pigmentation, sparse hair, hepatosplenomegaly, and failure to thrive [6]. This is because B12 plays a vital role in the development and initial myelination of the central nervous system [42]. In older adolescents neurologic symptoms if present include neuropathy or gait disturbances.

Clearly the next logical step in evaluating these patients is a serum B12 and folate level. There is controversy regarding the measurement of B12 and the incidence of false positives. A B12 level less than 150 pg/L [26] can be an indication of

B12 deficiency. To confirm B12 results, methylmalonic acid (MMA) levels and homocysteine levels are used. In B12 deficiency, MMA and homocysteine are elevated [12]. If these are not elevated, then likely the low B12 level is not clinically significant [40].

If B12 deficiency is identified, then the cause of the deficiency must be determined. Again the differential includes poor dietary intake and malabsorption from either anatomical issues (ileal resection or IBD) or from antibodies to intrinsic factor (pernicious anemia). These antibody levels can be drawn and measured. If malabsorption is thought to be the cause of deficiency, then parental therapy is traditionally the preferred method of treatment [12]; however there are reports that high-dose oral replacement therapy is an option [42]. Response to therapy should be monitored. You should expect increased reticulocyte count within 3–4 days of starting replacement therapy. Serum levels should normalize and anemia should normalize within 4–8 weeks [12]. Concomitant treatment with folic acid is sometimes necessary. If you are not seeing the typical response to therapy and there is reported compliance, then you must consider other causes of anemia. Improvement in neurologic findings can take much longer to occur, however some of these symptoms can be irreversible [44]. If the cause of deficiency is irreversible, then lifelong treatment is necessary; otherwise if reversible, then treatment can be stopped once deficiency is corrected [12].

Folate, unlike B12, is available in fruits, vegetables, and meats; however poor dietary intake is still the main cause of deficiency. However, like iron deficiency, periods of rapid growth are times when requirements are increased. Unlike B12, folate deficiency can occur quickly. Malabsorption is also a cause of folate deficiency, and this can be seen in IBD. Drugs that have antifolate effect are also a risk factor for developing folate deficiency [34]. The presence of these risk factors should be reviewed in your history.

As with B12 deficiency, symptoms of folate deficiency are similar except for the finding of neurologic symptoms. Should your patient develop neurologic symptoms with the treatment of folate deficiency, B12 level should be checked and B12 deficiency should be treated.

Similar to B12 deficiency, thrombocytopenia and neutropenia can be present in folate deficiency. Both serum and erythrocyte folate levels can be checked. Serum folate levels can decrease significantly in a short time frame, however erythrocyte levels decrease slowly. In folate deficiency, homocysteine is elevated and MMA is normal.

Treatment for folate deficiency should be initiated once confirmed and continued until correction of deficiency. Diet modifications should be made if intake is deemed the cause of the deficiency. Response to therapy should be expected as with B12.

Other potential causes of macrocytic anemia include bone marrow disorders, liver disease, hypothyroidism, and hemolysis or hemorrhage with compensatory reticulocytosis.

If the reticulocyte count is normal or low and there is no presence of hypersegmented neutrophils, then one should seriously consider bone marrow evaluation to rule out bone marrow pathology such as a bone marrow failure (inherited or acquired). The measurement of fetal hemoglobin is often an indication of a stressed marrow. Physical exam is important to evaluate for the presence of congenital anomalies that would indicate an inherited bone marrow failure syndrome such as Fanconi anemia. Fanconi anemia would show a hypocellular marrow for age. Dyskeratosis congenita is associated with the classic triad of skin pigmentation, nail dystrophy, and oral leukoplakia [47]. If on bone marrow evaluation there is solely a red cell aplasia, then one can consider Diamond-Blackfan anemia or congenital dyserythropoietic anemia (CDA); however this can also present with normocytic anemia. For most inherited bone marrow failure syndromes, specific testing can be performed. This includes telomere length for dyskeratosis congenita and chromosome breakage for Fanconi anemia. Specific gene testing can also be sent for further evaluation, and once confirmed family members should also be screened and, if positive, undergo gene testing.

Bone marrow evaluation for severe aplastic anemia shows a hypocellular marrow and varying degrees of involvement of other cell lines. Causes of aplastic anemia include hepatitis, infection, or drug. Work-up for this includes evaluation of liver function, hepatitis panel, and viral studies (EBV, CMV, HIV, and parvovirus) [41].

Hypothyroidism and liver disease typically present with mild anemia that is less profound than those with underlying marrow pathology. History of hypothyroidism symptoms such as fatigue, cold intolerance, weight gain, dry skin, and hair loss may be present. Screening thyroid-stimulating hormone and measurement of free T4 can be done. Liver disease can also be seen as the underlying cause. Screening liver function tests that showed elevated liver function without other cause warrants a referral to a gastroenterologist.

In general, macrocytic anemias warrant earlier referral to a pediatric hematologist for evaluation.

References

1. Amid A, Haghi-Ashtiani B, Kiby-Allen M, Hagh-Ashtiani MT. Screening for thalassemia carriers in populations with a high rate of iron deficiency: revisiting the applicability of the mentzer index and the effect of iron deficiency on hb A2 levels. Hemoglobin. 2015;39(2):141. https://doi.org/10.3109/03630269.2015.1024321.
2. Andrews NC, Ullrich CK, Fleming MD. Disorders of iron metabolism and sideroblastic anemia. In: Orkin S, Nathan D, Ginsburg D, Look AT, Fisher D, Lux S, editors. Nathan and Oski's hematology of infancy and childhood. Philadelphia: Saunders; 2009. p. 521–70.
3. Baker RD, Greer FR. Committee on Nutrition American Academy of PediatricsDiagnosis and prevention of iron deficiency and iron-deficiency anemia in infants and young children (0–3 years of age). Pediatrics. 2010;126(5):1040–50.
4. Beard JL. Why iron deficiency is important in infant development. J Nutr. 2008;138(12):2534–6.
5. Belfield KD, Tichy EM. Review and drug therapy implications of glucose 6 phosphate dehydrogenase deficiency. Am J Health-Syst Pharm. 2018;75:97–104.
6. Black MM. Effects of vitamin B12 and folate deficiency on brain development in children. Food Nutr Bull. 2008;29(2 Suppl):S126–31.

7. Bolton-Maggs PHB, Langer JC, Iolascon A, Tittensor P, King MJ. Guidelines for the diagnosis and management of hereditary spherocytosis- 2011 update. Br J Haematol. 2011;156:37–49.
8. Bowman JK. RhD hemolytic disease of the newborn. N Engl J Med. 1998;339:1775–7.
9. Brugnara C, Oski FA, Nathan DG. Diagnostic approach to the anemic patient. In: Orkin S, Nathan D, Ginsburg D, Look AT, Fisher D, Lux S, editors. Nathan and Oski's hematology of infancy and childhood. Philadelphia: Saunders; 2009. p. 455–66.
10. Bruner AB, Joffe A, Duggan AK, Casella JF, Brandt J. Randomized study of cognitive effects of iron supplementation in non-anemic iron-deficient adolescent girls. Lancet. 1996;348(9033):992–6.
11. Camaschella C. Iron-deficiency anemia. N Engl J Med. 2013;372:1832–43.
12. Carmel R. How I treat cobalamin (vitamin B12) deficiency. Blood. 2008;112:2214–21.
13. Chahkandi T, Norouziasl S, Farzad M, Ghanad F. Endocrine disorders in beta thalassemia major patients. Int J Pediatr. 2017;5(8):5531–8. https://doi.org/10.22038/ijp.2017.21937.1834.
14. Conrad ME, Barton JC. Factors affecting iron balance. Am J Hematol. 1981;10:199–225.
15. Cunningham MJ, Sankaran VG, Nathan DG, Orkin SH. The thalassemias. In: Orkin S, Nathan D, Ginsburg D, Look AT, Fisher D, Lux S, editors. Nathan and Oski's hematology of infancy and childhood. Philadelphia: Saunders; 2009. p. 1015–106.
16. Fernandes Q. Therapeutic strategies in sickle cell anemia: the past present and future. Life Sci. 2017;178:100–8.
17. Finberg KE, Heeney MM, Campagna DR, Aydinok Y, Pearson HA, Hartman KR, Mayo MM, Samuel SM, Strouse JJ, Markianos K, Andrews NC, Fleming MD. Mutations in TMPRSS6 cause iron-refractory iron deficiency anemia (IRIDA). Nat Genet. 2008;40(5):569–71. https://doi.org/10.1038/ng.130.
18. Gajjar R, Jalazo E. Hematology. In: Engorn B, Flerlage J, editors. The harriet lane handbook: a manual for pediatric house officers. Philadelphia: Elsevier; 2015. p. 305–33.
19. Gallagher PG. Hereditary elliptocytosis: spectrin and protein 4.1R. Semin Hematol. 2004;41(2):142–64.
20. Grantham-McGregor S, Ani C. A review of studies on the effect of iron deficiency on cognitive development in children. J Nutr. 2001;131(2S-2):649S–66S.
21. Hallberg L, Rossander-Hulten L, Brune M, Gleerup A. Bioavailabilty in man of iron in human milk and cow's milk in relation to their calcium content. Pediatr Res. 1992;31(5):524–7.
22. Halterman JS, Kaczorowski JM, Aligne CA, Auinger P, Szilagyi PG. Iron deficiency and cognitive achievement among school-aged children and adolescents in the United States. Pediatrics. 2001;107(6):1381–6.
23. Hansen TW. Acute management of extreme neonatal jaundice-the potential benefits of intensified phototherapy and interruption of enterohepatic bilirubin circulation. Acta Pediatr. 1997;86:843–6.
24. Jameel T, Baig M, Ahmed I, Hussain MB, Alkhamaly MD. Differentiation of beta thalassemia trait from iron deficiency anemia by hematological indices. Pak J Med Sci. 2017;33(3):665–9. https://doi.org/10.12669/pjms.333.12098.
25. Johnston DL, Murto K, Kurzawa J, Liddy C, Keely E, Lai L. Use of electronic consultation to improve access to care in pediatric hematology/oncology. J Pediatr Hematol Oncol. 2017;39(7):e367–9.
26. Langan RC, Goodbred AJ. Vitamin B12 deficiency:recognition and management. Am Fam Physician. 2017;96(6):384–9.
27. Leguit RJ, van den Tweel JG. The pathology of bone marrow failure. Histopathology. 2010;57:655–70.
28. Logan S, Martins S, Gilbert R. Iron therapy for improving psychomotor development and cognitive function in children under the age of three with iron deficiency anaemia. Cochrane Database Syst Rev. 2001;(2):CD001444.
29. Lozoff B, Jimenez E, Hagen J, Mollen E, Wolf AW. Poorer behavioral and developmental outcome more than 10 years after treatment for iron deficiency in infancy. Pediatrics. 2000;105(4):e51.

30. Madden NA, Jones GL, Kalpatthi R, Woods G. Practice patterns of stroke screening and hydroxyurea use in children with sickle cell disease: a survey of health care providers. J Pediatr Hematol Oncol. 2014;36:e382–6.
31. Mason PJ, Bautista JM, Gilsanz F. G6PD deficiency: the genotype-phenotype association. Blood Rev. 2007;21(5):267–83.
32. McCann JC, Ames BN. An overview of evidence for a causal relation between iron deficiency during development and deficits in cognitive or behavioral function. Am J Clin Nutr. 2007;85(4):931–45.
33. Minkovitz CS, Grason H, Ruderman M, Casella JF. Newborn screening progams and sickle cell disease. A public health services and systems approach. Am J Prev Med. 2016;51(1S1):S39–47.
34. Moll R, Davis B. Iron, vitamin B12, and folate. Medicine. 2017;45(4):198–203.
35. Oski F. Whole cow milk feeding between 6 and 12 months of age? Go back to 1976. Pediatr Rev. 1990;12(6):187–9.
36. Oski F. Iron deficiency in infancy and childhood. N Engl J Med. 1993;329(3):190–3.
37. Perrotta S, Gallagher PG, Mohandas N. Hereditary spherocytosis. Lancet. 2008;372:1411–26.
38. Reeves SL, Tribble AC, Madden B, Freed GL, Dombkowski KJ. Antibiotic prophylaxis for children with sickle cell anemia. Pediatrics. 2018;141(3):1–9.
39. Sachdev H, Gera T, Nestel P. Effect of iron supplementation on mental and motor development in children: systematic review of randomised controlled trials. Public Health Nutr. 2005;8(2):117–32.
40. Savage DG, Lindenbaum J, Stabler SP, Allen RH. Sensitivity of serum methylmalonic acid and total homocysteine determinations for diagnosing cobalamin and folate deficiencies. Am J Med. 1994;96(3):239–46.
41. Scheinberg P, Young NS. How I treat acquired aplastic anemia. Blood. 2012;120:1185–96. https://doi.org/10.1182/blood-2011-12-274019.
42. Stabler SP. Vitamin B12 deficiency. N Engl J Med. 2013;368(2):149–60. https://doi.org/10.1056/NEJMcp1113996.
43. van Kamp IL, Klumper F, Bakkum R, Oepkes D, Meerman RH, Scherjon SA, Kanhai H. The severity of immune fetal hydrops is predictive of fetal outcome after intrauterine treatment. Am J Obstet Gynecol. 2001;185:668–73.
44. Vasconcelos OM, Poehm EH, McCarter RJ, Campbell WW, Quezado ZMN. Potential outcome factors in subacute combined degeneration review of observational studies. J Gen Intern Med. 2006;21:1063–8. https://doi.org/10.1111/j.1525-1497.2006.00525.x.
45. Vaya A, Suescun M, Pardo A, Fuster O. Erythrocyte deformability and hereditary elliptocytosis. Clin Hemorheol Microcirc. 2014;58:471–3.
46. Vlachos A, Ball S, Dahl N, Alter BP, Sheth S, Ramenghi U, Meerpohl J, Karlsson S, Liu JM, Leblanc T, Paley C, Kang EM, Leder EJ, Atsidaftos E, Shimamura A, Bessler M, Glader B, Lipton JM, Participants of Sixth Annual Daniella Maria Arturi International Consensus Conference. Diagnosing and treating Diamond Blackfan anaemia:results of an international clinical consensus conference. Br J Haematol. 2008;142(6):859–76. https://doi.org/10.1111/j.1365-2141.2008.07269.x.
47. Vulliamy TJ, Dokal I. Dyskeratosis congenita: the diverse clinical presentation of mutations in telomerase complex. Biochimie. 2008;90:122–30. https://doi.org/10.1016/j.biochi.2007.07.017.
48. Walter T, De Andraca I, Chadud P, Perales CG. Iron deficiency anemia: adverse effects on infant psychomotor development. Pediatrics. 1989;84(1):7–17.
49. Weiss G, Goodnough LT. Anemia of chronic disease. N Engl J Med. 2005;352:1011–23.
50. Zaninoni A, Fermo E, Vercellati C, Consonni D, Marcello AP, Zanella A, Cortelezzi A, Barcellini W, Bianchi P. Use of laser assisted optical rotational cell analyzer (LoRRca MaxSis) in the diagnosis of RBC membrane disorders, enzyme defects, and congenital dyserythropoietic anemias: a monocentric study of 202 patients. Front Physiol. 2018;9(451):1–12. https://doi.org/10.3389/fphys.2018.00451.

Chapter 3
Approach to Anemia in the Elderly

Robert T. Means Jr.

General Principles

Is Anemia "Normal" in the Elderly?

The incidence of anemia (defined by the World Health Organization (WHO) as a hemoglobin <13.0 g/dL in adult men and <12.0 g/dL in adult women [1]) increases after the age of 50. For individuals over the age of 65 in the United States, approximately 10% of both men and women are anemic, although the vast majority of cases are mild with hemoglobin concentrations >11.0 g/dL [2]. In a report of 19,758 elderly adults followed at a hospital in Austria, 21.7% of patients between 64 and 69 years were anemic, rising to a 37.0% prevalence over age 90 [3].

This high frequency of anemia has led many to wonder if anemia of mild degree should be considered a non-pathologic process in the elderly [4, 5], possibly due to the characteristic age-associated decline in renal function [6] or in testosterone concentration [7]. Figure 3.1 shows overall hemoglobin concentration data (median with 5th and 95th percentiles) for men and women above age 50 from the National Health and Nutrition Examination Survey (NHANES) III [8]. While there is a statistically significant trend toward decline with age for both men and women from age 50 (author's analysis), median values generally remain in the WHO-defined normal range. In the Austrian population cited above, the mean hemoglobin for each 5-year age range stayed above 13.0 g/dL until after age 85 [3]. The presence of comorbidities increases the prevalence of anemia [9].

The question, "What do you consider anemia in an older person?" is common in discussions on anemia evaluation. The answer is "The same as anemia in other adults" [10, 11]. Increasing prevalence of anemia in the elderly is strongly associated

R. T. Means Jr., MD
James H. Quillen College of Medicine, East Tennessee State University,
Johnson City, TN, USA
e-mail: MEANSR@mail.etsu.edu

© Springer Nature Switzerland AG 2019
R. T. Means Jr. (ed.), *Anemia in the Young and Old*,
https://doi.org/10.1007/978-3-319-96487-4_3

Fig. 3.1 Hemoglobin ranges by age decile over age 50 (median and 5th, 95th percentiles shown). (Data from National Health and Nutrition Examination Survey (NHANES) III [8]). (**a**) Women; (**b**) men

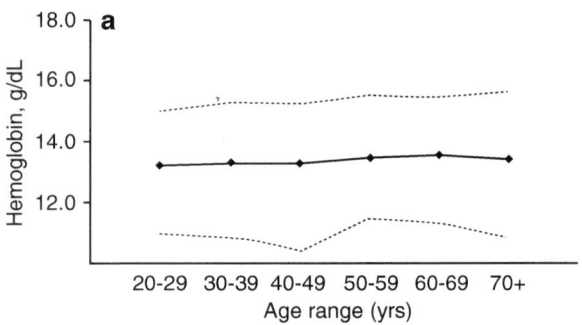

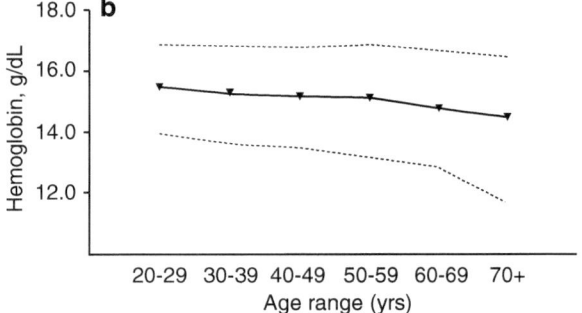

with increasing prevalence of various comorbidities [9]. The actual question that should be asked is "When should anemia be evaluated in the elderly?" Approaches to that issue will be addressed below.

Significance of Anemia in the Elderly

Table 3.1 lists various adverse conditions that are seen more commonly in elderly patients with anemia than in elderly patients without anemia. In a series of unselected geriatric patients discharged from a hospital in 2008, the absence of anemia was associated with a lower risk of death during 5.5 years of post-discharge follow-up [10]. It is unclear whether anemia is the cause of the complication or morbidity per se or a sign of an underlying condition that caused the anemia. It is likely that each circumstance holds true in specific situations. For example, one study of 632 nursing home residents showed no improvement in fall risk with anemia therapy, suggesting anemia was not the cause of increased risk [24], while an almost identically sized study of community-living elderly women showed an improvement in mobility scores with anemia treatment [4]. The etiology of anemia may also make a difference in morbidity and mortality risk [25].

Table 3.1 Adverse outcomes or indicators associated with anemia in the elderly	Mortality [12–15]
	Hospitalization [13]
	Frailty [16]
	Recurrent falls [17]
	Stroke (in women) [18]
	Osteoporotic fractures (in men) [19]
	Increased WHO disability score [20]
	Decreased ADL score [21, 22]
	Decreased mobility score [4]
	Decreased muscle strength [23]
	Decreased HRQoL score [21]

WHO World Health Organization, *ADL* activities of daily living, *HRQoL* health-related quality of life

Etiologies of Anemia in the Elderly

Table 3.2 lists etiologies of anemia in elderly patients reported in four different series from four different centers in three Western countries. To some extent, the differences in the series reflect the study methodology underlying each report. The results based on data taken from the NHANES III study [2] are based on laboratory survey data and therefore only include diagnoses that can be made with clinical laboratory results and not those that may require a tissue diagnosis. The other three series are derived from practice sites and will reflect the nature of the referral base of that practice and to some extent the population demographics. The studies from Chicago [26] and from Italy [27] have a significant number of hemoglobinopathy/thalassemia patients included in the category "Other." The study from Poland [9] includes a significant number of patients with chemotherapy- or radiation therapy-induced anemia in "Other." The variation in the proportion of individuals reported with anemia due to renal insufficiency among the studies may also reflect referral and management patterns for chronic kidney disease patients. A study from Brazil reported that nearly all of the anemic participants in the São Paulo Aging and Health Study had anemia attributable to either renal disease (62%) or the anemia of inflammation/chronic disease (AICD; 35%) [28].

Despite specific differences between the studies cited in Table 3.2 and other reports in the literature, the general trend is that the vast majority of cases of anemia in the elderly fall into three categories. These are nutritional deficiency anemias, primarily iron, vitamin B12, or folate; anemias resulting from chronic systemic syndromes such as the anemia of renal insufficiency/chronic kidney disease or AICD; and the entity referred to as "unexplained anemia of the elderly (UAE)." Clonal disorders of hematopoiesis, whether rising to the level of a myelodysplastic syndrome or detectable by molecular markers of clonality only [29], represent a small but significant portion of these etiologies.

Nutritional anemias, particularly iron, B12, and to a lesser extent folate, are more common in older patients. These may reflect changes in the gastrointestinal tract

Table 3.2 Distribution of anemia etiologies in elderly patients. Data from four studies

Etiologies	Frequency (%)			
Country of report origin	USA-1 [2]	USA-2 [26]	Italy [27]	Poland [9]
Iron deficiency	16.6	25.3	16.0	13.0
B12 and/or folate-deficiency anemia	14.3	<1	9.5	7.1
Iron and B12 and/or folate-deficiency anemia	3.4	–	–	2.4
Anemia of inflammation/chronic disease (AICD)	19.7	9.8	17.4	33.1
Anemia of renal insufficiency	8.2	3.4	15.0	1.2
Anemia of renal insufficiency and AICD	4.3	–	–	–
Unexplained anemia of elderly (UAE)	33.6	43.7	26.4	28.4
Clonal hematopoietic disorder	–	7.5	1.8	–
Other	–	10.3	14.4	14.8

Disorders represented by "Other" vary widely between centers, reflecting population demographics, study design, and referral patterns for each center. In two reports, it includes a significant proportion of thalassemia/hemoglobinopathy patients; in one of the other reports, it includes anemia due to blood loss and to cancer treatment

with aging, including achlorhydria [30], changing dietary patterns [31], or other factors [32, 33]. When anemia attributed to renal insufficiency is removed, most of the remaining cases of mild anemia can be attributed to either AICD or UAE.

AICD is characterized by low serum or plasma iron despite adequate or increased iron stores and is typically seen in association with inflammatory, infectious, or neoplastic diseases [34]. UAE is mild anemia not attributable to blood loss, renal disease, nutritional deficiency, or AICD. The precise laboratory definition varies depending on specific cut points chosen as normal values [35]. Both are attributable to effects of the cytokine mediators of inflammation [36, 37] and are discussed in Part II, Chap. 7.

Diagnostic Approach to Anemia in the Elderly

Who Needs an Evaluation, and How Much of an Evaluation?

Anemia is typically a marker of disease rather than a disease itself, and so it is a general rule that anemia should be evaluated when it is detected. Severe anemia (defined as requiring transfusion or significantly limiting activities) should be evaluated in a thorough and comprehensive manner under nearly all circumstances. In elderly patients with mild anemia, there may be circumstances when diagnostic evaluation might be limited, if performed at all. For example, it may be reasonable to limit anemia evaluation in a bedbound patient with mild anemia and a limited life span. In an elderly patient, again with a limited life span diagnosed with iron deficiency, it may be reasonable not to perform a colonoscopy seeking a source of blood loss if the patient would not consider treatment of an identified malignancy. If a frail patient has anemia under circumstances suggesting a low-grade myelodysplastic syndrome for which the appropriate management is observation, it may be reasonable to forgo bone marrow aspiration and biopsy. However, such decisions should not be made by the provider unilaterally but rather after an informed discussion with the patient (and in most cases the patient's family as well). Engaging the family in such decisions is particularly important in patients who are near the end of life.

Laboratory Approach to Diagnosis

This chapter focuses on the approach to diagnosis in individuals in whom the primary hematologic issue is anemia. The guidance provided is less applicable to patients in whom anemia is only one element of a spectrum of hematologic findings, as in aplastic anemia or acute leukemia. In circumstances where those diagnoses are major considerations, examination of the peripheral blood film followed by bone marrow examination is likely the best first step.

Table 3.3 lists the initial diagnostic studies with anemia, particularly elderly individuals. The purpose of this testing panel is to identify the major causes of anemia in the elderly, namely, nutritional anemias (essentially vitamin B12 deficiency, folate deficiency, and iron deficiency), anemia of renal insufficiency, and AICD. The table also lists second-line tests that may be indicated, including how to address equivocal results. The panel will also identify of hemolysis, although this is typically

Table 3.3 Laboratory approach to anemia in the elderly

Initial testing	
Hematology: complete blood count	
Routine serum chemistry: creatinine, blood urea nitrogen, estimated glomerular filtration rate, lactate dehydrogenase, total bilirubin	
Serum iron parameters: iron, total iron-binding capacity or transferrin, ferritin	
Nutritional anemia parameters: serum B12, red blood cell folate	
Secondary testing	
Indication	**Test**
Equivocal B12 results	Serum methylmalonic acid
Equivocal iron results	Serum soluble transferrin receptor
Suspicion of hemolysis (elevated bilirubin, lactate dehydrogenase	Reticulocyte count, direct antiglobulin test, peripheral blood film; other tests as indicated by clinical circumstances
Abnormal position sense, neutropenia, other tests negative	Serum or plasma copper, ceruloplasmin
Other tests negative in a man	Serum testosterone
Other tests negative with macrocytosis and/or other cytopenias	Bone marrow examination or molecular profiling for clonal hematopoiesis
Isolated normocytic anemia with reticulocyte count 10,000/μL or less	Bone marrow examination for pure red cell aplasia

uncommon in the elderly. Laboratory criteria for the diagnosis of iron deficiency, B12/folate deficiency, and AICD are outlined in the chapters devoted to those topics. Anemia due to renal insufficiency/chronic kidney disease is effectively ruled out by an estimated glomerular filtration rate greater than 45 mL/min/1.73 sq. m [38]. Epidemiologic studies have suggested that a more definitive criterion for this diagnosis in the elderly would be a measured creatinine clearance less than 30 mL/min [6].

Since the vast majority of etiologies of mild anemia seen in the elderly are underproduction anemias associated with decreased reticulocyte production, it is not this author's practice to include a reticulocyte count routinely in the initial evaluation of anemia in the elderly. In patients with severe isolated normocytic anemia at levels where transfusion is a consideration, I do obtain a reticulocyte count to address the possibility of pure red cell aplasia. In individuals in whom hemolysis is suspected, direct antiglobulin testing (Coombs test), a reticulocyte count and a peripheral blood film should be obtained. The peripheral blood film may provide indicators of disorders such as thrombotic thrombocytopenic purpura or evidence of morphology-based hemolytic disorders such as spur cell anemia. While hereditary disorders of red cell metabolism or membrane structure typically present in childhood, occasionally a diagnosis is not made until the patient is an adult. Erythrocyte glucose-6-phosphate dehydrogenase levels decline with patient age, making the red cells of older adults more susceptible to hemolysis under conditions of oxidative stress [39].

Individuals not categorized by these initial tests would typically fall into the category referred to as UAE or represent clonal disorders of hematopoiesis. When the anemia observed is normocytic, it is reasonable to assign it to that category. UAE is associated with fewer comorbidities and better survival than anemias attributed to more definable ideologies in the elderly [25]. When the anemia is macrocytic, or if it is associated with cytopenias in the white cell or platelet lineage (and B12 deficiency has been ruled out), a clonal marrow disorder should be considered. Traditionally, these patients would have been considered for bone marrow examination with cytogenetics and flow cytometry. This is still a reasonable approach in the appropriate patient setting. The recent description of the entity referred to as clonal hematopoiesis of indeterminate potential (CHIP) provides an opportunity to make a diagnosis from peripheral blood rather than from bone marrow [29]. CHIP panels are available through both research laboratories and commercial reference laboratories, with analysis for various clonal mutations carried out by next-generation sequencing. However, costs for these assays can be considerable, and in many areas of the United States, third-party payers do not cover them. CHIP is discussed in a separate chapter later in the book.

In male patients with presumed UAE, the diagnosis of testosterone deficiency should be considered. In one multicenter study of men with low testosterone, 54% of men with presumed UAE had an increase in hemoglobin >1 g/dL after testosterone treatment for 12 months compared to 15% of such men treated with placebo [40]. It may therefore be reasonable to consider measuring testosterone in UAE patients and considering a trial of testosterone if low: however nearly half of UAE patients with low testosterone had minimal response. In patients with anemia, leukopenia, and problems with gait or position sense, copper deficiency should be considered, particularly if the patient has had bariatric surgery or has dentures and uses a zinc-containing adhesive [41–46].

Management

As in patients of all ages, the management of anemia is determined by the specific diagnosis. Management of specific syndromes is discussed in the chapters devoted to those syndromes. As has been discussed earlier, aggressiveness of management and therapeutic modalities employed may need to be adjusted to reflect the elderly patient's overall condition. However, such decisions should only be made in consultation with the patient and the patient's family.

References

1. WHO. Haemoglobin standards for the diagnosis of anaemia and assessment of severity. 2011; www.who.int/vmnis/indicators/haemoglobin.pdf.
2. Guralnik JM, Eisenstaedt RS, Ferrucci L, Klein HG, Woodman RC. Prevalence of anemia in persons 65 years and older in the United States: evidence for a high rate of unexplained anemia. Blood. 2004;104(8):2263–8.
3. Bach V, Schruckmayer G, Sam I, Kemmler G, Stauder R. Prevalence and possible causes of anemia in the elderly: a cross-sectional analysis of a large European university hospital cohort. Clin Interv Aging. 2014;9:1187–96.
4. Chaves PH, Xue QL, Guralnik JM, Ferrucci L, Volpato S, Fried LP. What constitutes normal hemoglobin concentration in community-dwelling disabled older women? J Am Geriatr Soc. 2004;52(11):1811–6.
5. Cappellini MD, Motta I. Anemia in clinical practice-definition and classification: does hemoglobin change with aging? Semin Hematol. 2015;52(4):261–9.
6. Ble A, Fink JC, Woodman RC, et al. Renal function, erythropoietin, and anemia of older persons: the InCHIANTI study. Arch Intern Med. 2005;165(19):2222–7.
7. Yeap BB, Beilin J, Shi Z, et al. Serum testosterone levels correlate with haemoglobin in middle-aged and older men. Intern Med J. 2009;39(8):532–8.
8. Hollowell JG, van Assendelft OW, Gunter EW, Lewis BG, Najjar M, Pfeiffer C. Hematological and iron-related analytes – reference data for persons aged 1 year and over: United States, 1988–94. Vital and health statistics Series 11, Data from the national health survey. 2005;(247):1–156.
9. Michalak SS, Rupa-Matysek J, Gil L. Comorbidities, repeated hospitalizations, and age >/= 80 years as indicators of anemia development in the older population. Ann Hematol. 2018;97:1337.
10. Bien B, Bien-Barkowska K, Wojskowicz A, Kasiukiewicz A, Wojszel ZB. Prognostic factors of long-term survival in geriatric inpatients. Should we change the recommendations for the oldest people? J Nutr Health Aging. 2015;19(4):481–8.
11. Mindell J, Moody A, Ali A, Hirani V. Using longitudinal data from the health survey for England to resolve discrepancies in thresholds for haemoglobin in older adults. Br J Haematol. 2012;160(3):368–76.
12. Patel KV, Guralnik JM. Prognostic implications of anemia in older adults. Haematologica. 2009;94(1):1–2.

13. Riva E, Tettamanti M, Mosconi P, et al. Association of mild anemia with hospitalization and mortality in the elderly: the health and anemia population-based study. Haematologica. 2009;94(1):22–8.
14. Chalmers KA, Knuiman MW, Divitini ML, Bruce DG, Olynyk JK, Milward EA. Long-term mortality risks associated with mild anaemia in older persons: the Busselton health study. Age Ageing. 2012;41:759.
15. Wu CY, Hu HY, Chou YJ, Huang N, Chou YC, Li CP. What constitutes normal hemoglobin concentrations in community-dwelling older adults? J Am Geriatr Soc. 2016;64(6):1233–41.
16. Juarez-Cedillo T, Basurto-Acevedo L, Vega-Garcia S, et al. Prevalence of anemia and its impact on the state of frailty in elderly people living in the community: SADEM study. Ann Hematol. 2014;93(12):2057–62.
17. Bowling CB, Muntner P, Bradbury BD, et al. Low hemoglobin levels and recurrent falls in U.S. men and women: prospective findings from the REasons for geographic and racial differences in stroke (REGARDS) cohort. Am J Med Sci. 2013;345(6):446–54.
18. Panwar B, Judd SE, Warnock DG, et al. Hemoglobin concentration and risk of incident stroke in community-living adults. Stroke. 2016;47(8):2017–24.
19. Valderrabano RJ, Lee J, Lui LY, et al. Older men with anemia have increased fracture risk independent of bone mineral density. J Clin Endocrinol Metab. 2017;102(7):2199–206.
20. Bryce RM, Salas A, Acosta D, et al. The prevalence, correlates and impact of anaemia among older people in Cuba, Dominican Republic, Mexico, Puerto Rico and Venezuela. Br J Haematol. 2012;160(3):387–98.
21. Bailey RA, Reardon G, Wasserman MR, McKenzie RS, Hord RS. Association of anemia with worsened activities of daily living and health-related quality of life scores derived from the minimum data set in long-term care residents. Health Qual Life Outcomes. 2012;10:129.
22. Bang SM, Lee JO, Kim YJ, et al. Anemia and activities of daily living in the Korean urban elderly population: results from the Korean Longitudinal Study on Health and Aging (KLoSHA). Ann Hematol. 2012;92(1):59–65.
23. Penninx BW, Pahor M, Cesari M, et al. Anemia is associated with disability and decreased physical performance and muscle strength in the elderly. J Am Geriatr Soc. 2004;52(5):719–24.
24. Reardon G, Pandya N, Bailey RA. Falls in nursing home residents receiving pharmacotherapy for anemia. Clin Interv Aging. 2012;7:397–407.
25. Shavelle RM, MacKenzie R, Paculdo DR. Anemia and mortality in older persons: does the type of anemia affect survival? Int J Hematol. 2012;95(3):248–56.
26. Artz AS, Thirman MJ. Unexplained anemia predominates despite an intensive evaluation in a racially diverse cohort of older adults from a referral anemia clinic. J Gerontol A Biol Sci Med Sci. 2011;66(8):925–32.
27. Tettamanti M, Lucca U, Gandini F, et al. Prevalence, incidence and types of mild anemia in the elderly: the "Health and Anemia" population-based study. Haematologica. 2010:haematol.
28. Santos IS, Scazufca M, Lotufo PA, Menezes PR, Benseñor IM. Causes of recurrent or persistent anemia in older people from the results of the São Paulo Ageing & Health Study. Geriatr Gerontol Int. 2012.
29. Steensma DP, Bejar R, Jaiswal S, et al. Clonal hematopoiesis of indeterminate potential and its distinction from myelodysplastic syndromes. Blood. 2015;126(1):9–16.
30. Bhutto A, Morley JE. The clinical significance of gastrointestinal changes with aging. Curr Opin Clin Nutr Metab Care. 2008;11(5):651–60.
31. Drewnowski A, Shultz JM. Impact of aging on eating behaviors, food choices, nutrition, and health status. J Nutr Health Aging. 2001;5(2):75–9.
32. Metz J. Haematological implications of folate food fortification. S Afr Med J [Suid-Afrikaanse tydskrif vir geneeskunde]. 2013;103(12 Suppl 1):978–81.
33. Wee AK. Serum folate predicts muscle strength: a pilot cross-sectional study of the association between serum vitamin levels and muscle strength and gait measures in patients >65 years old with diabetes mellitus in a primary care setting. Nutr J. 2016;15(1):89.
34. Weiss G, Goodnough L. Anemia of chronic disease. N Engl J Med. 2005;352(10):1011–23.

35. Eisenga MF, Stam SP, Bakker SJL. Redefining unexplained anemia in elderly. JAMA Intern Med. 2017;177(9):1394–5.
36. Ferrucci L, Semba RD, Guralnik JM, et al. Proinflammatory state, hepcidin and anemia in older persons. Blood. 2010:blood-2009.
37. Means RT. Pathogenesis of the anemia of chronic disease: a cytokine-mediated anemia. Stem Cells. 1995;13:32–7.
38. Astor BC, Muntner P, Levin A, Eustace JA, Coresh J. Association of kidney function with anemia: the Third National Health and Nutrition Examination Survey (1988–1994). Arch Intern Med. 2002;162(12):1401–8.
39. Rodgers GP, Lichtman HC, Sheff MF. Red blood cell glucose-6-phosphate dehydrogenase activity in aged humans. J Am Geriatr Soc. 1983;31(1):8–11.
40. Roy CN, Snyder PJ, Stephens-Shields AJ, et al. Association of testosterone levels with anemia in older men: a controlled clinical trial. JAMA Intern Med. 2017;177(4):480–90.
41. Abdel-Mageed AB, Oehme FW. A review of the biochemical roles, toxicity and interactions of zinc, copper and iron: I. Zinc. Vet Hum Toxicol. 1990;32(1):34–9.
42. Afrin LB. Fatal copper deficiency from excessive use of zinc-based denture adhesive. Am J Med Sci. 2010;340(2):164–8.
43. Freeland-Graves JH, Lee JJ, Mousa TY, Elizondo JJ. Patients at risk for trace element deficiencies: bariatric surgery. J Trace Elem Med Biol. 2014;28(4):495–503.
44. Gabreyes AA, Abbasi HN, Forbes KP, McQuaker G, Duncan A, Morrison I. Hypocupremia associated cytopenia and myelopathy: a national retrospective review. Eur J Haematol. 2013;90(1):1–9.
45. Gregg XT, Reddy V, Prchal JT. Copper deficiency masquerading as myelodysplastic syndrome. Blood. 2002;100(4):1493–5.
46. Petrosyan I, Blaison G, Andres E, Federici L. Anaemia in the elderly: an aetiologic profile of a prospective cohort of 95 hospitalised patients. Eur J Intern Med. 2012;23(6):524–8.

Part II
Specific Disorders

Chapter 4
Inherited Bone Marrow Failure Syndromes

Jennifer D. Hamm and Caryn E. Sorge

Introduction

A variety of underlying pathologies can present with anemia, i.e., nutritional deficiencies, hemoglobin defects, membrane defects, enzyme disorders, hemolysis, renal failure, infection, anemia of chronic disease, and metabolic conditions [23, 31]. One potential cause with vast implications is anemia as the presenting symptoms of an inherited bone marrow failure syndrome (IBMFS) [7]. The Canadian Inherited Marrow Failure Registry found that of their 124 registered patients with a bone marrow failure diagnosis, 45 presented with anemia and of those, 34 were single-cell cytopenia at presentation [137]. Bone marrow failure encompasses conditions that can be either inherited or acquired. IBMFS include a variety of genetic mutations that lead to hematopoietic failure and an increased risk of malignancies. Many are associated with congenital malformations; however, the penetrance of these is variable and cytopenias may be the only presenting symptom [7, 9].

This chapter will focus on inherited bone marrow failure syndromes that have a propensity to present with anemia during childhood. The anemia can be either isolated or in combination with other cytopenias. Of the inherited bone marrow failure syndromes, Diamond-Blackfan anemia (DBA), Pearson syndrome (PS), and the congenital dyserythropoietic anemias (CDA) tend to present with isolated anemia, while Fanconi anemia and dyskeratosis congenita can present with

J. D. Hamm, MD
Department of Pediatrics, Division of Pediatric Hematology/Oncology,
East Tennessee Children's Hospital, Knoxville, TN, USA
e-mail: JDHamm@etch.com

C. E. Sorge, MD (✉)
Department of Pediatrics, Division of Pediatric Hematology/Oncology,
University of Kentucky, Lexington, KY, USA
e-mail: caryn.sorge@uky.edu

© Springer Nature Switzerland AG 2019
R. T. Means Jr. (ed.), *Anemia in the Young and Old*,
https://doi.org/10.1007/978-3-319-96487-4_4

pancytopenia [137]. In contrast, Shwachman-Diamond syndrome (SDS), GATA2 deficiency, and severe congenital neutropenia (SCN) tend to present with iso-lated neutropenia, while congenital amegakaryocytic thrombocytopenia (CAMT) and thrombocytopenia absent radii (TAR) present with isolated thrombocytope-nia [137]. Figure 4.1 demonstrates an easy-to-use algorithm for inherited bone marrow failure syndromes and how they may present.

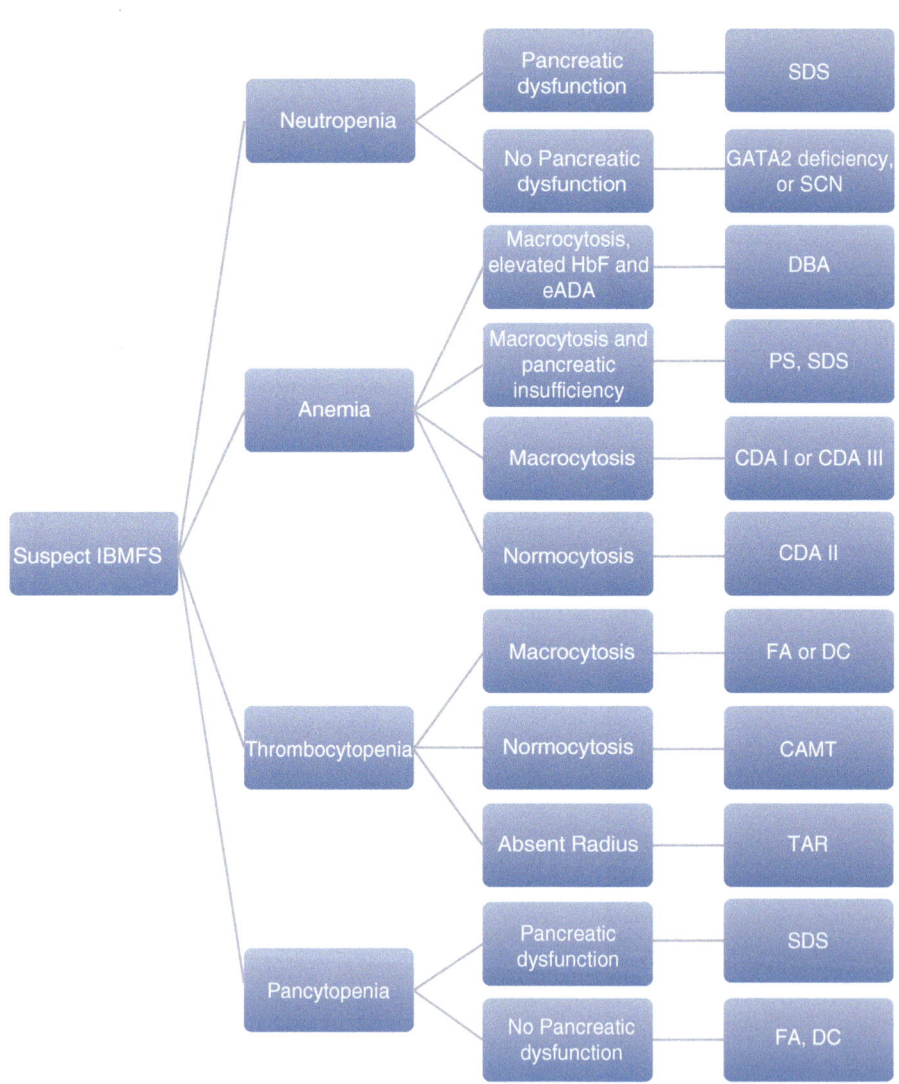

Fig. 4.1 A suggested flowchart to help clinicians think through IBMFS. Many patients will have clinical heterogeneity and may not follow these exact patterns, but these generalities can help guide initial considerations

Thrombocytopenia

There are two inherited bone marrow failure syndromes that tend to present with isolated thrombocytopenia, and these include congenital amegakaryocytic thrombocytopenia (CAMT) and thrombocytopenia with absent radii (TAR). At times, Fanconi anemia (FA) can initially present with thrombocytopenia, but unlike CAMT and TAR, FA will evolve to affect the other hematopoietic cell lines and is therefore discussed in the section that includes pancytopenia. This section will focus on a better understanding of both CAMT and TAR.

In both CAMT and TAR, patients typically present as neonates with varying degrees of thrombocytopenia which can lead to an increased risk of bleeding, including intracranial or mucous membrane bleeding. Statistically, thrombocytopenia will be detected at birth in 70% of patients with CAMT [19] and in the neonatal period for 60% of patients with TAR [84].

Given the percentage of patients that will present either at birth of within the neonatal period, these disorders should be included in the differential diagnosis for any neonate with thrombocytopenia, with or without bleeding manifestations. Other considerations should include neonatal infections, sepsis, neonatal alloimmune thrombocytopenia, neonatal autoimmune thrombocytopenia, or even development of a thrombus. One helpful difference when considering the possible etiologies is that CAMT is not associated with characteristic dysmorphology; whereas, TAR does have dysmorphic features.

Congenital Amegakaryocytic Thrombocytopenia

Despite the classic description of CAMT presenting with an isolated thrombocytopenia, it can also progress over time to a severe aplastic anemia with resultant pancytopenia. Inherited in an autosomal recessive fashion, CAMT results from mutations of the c- MPL gene that encodes for the thrombopoietin (TPO) receptor. With this mutation, cells cannot respond to TPO, a step crucial for the development of normal megakaryocytes [59]. The majority of patients are described to have either homozygous or compound heterozygous mutations of the c-MPL gene [19]; however, some patients do not exhibit a mutation here but are thought to have other mutations that affect the TPO pathway [59]. Commonly seen with autosomal recessive conditions, consanguinity has been reported among patients with CAMT [19, 85].

CAMT is divided into two categories based upon their exact type of c-MPL genetic mutation and their corresponding phenotypes. CAMT I is seen with homozygous nonsense, deletions, or frameshift mutations and is associated with a more severe thrombocytopenia that can rapidly progress to pancytopenia and marrow exhaustion. These types of mutations lead to a total loss of TPO receptor function. On the other hand, CAMT II is a result of homozygous or compound heterozygous missense mutations, and these patients tend to have a milder clinical course and can even have a steady rise in the platelet count, above 50×10^9/L, during the first year of life. However, despite this perceived improvement, these patients will ultimately develop pancytopenia like those with CAMT I. This difference is thought to be due to some allowance of residual function of the TPO receptor [61]. It is possible for these patients to remain undiagnosed until they present with pancytopenia, typically after the first year of life, making this diagnosis a consideration in the setting of an older child with pancytopenia [24].

CAMT should be considered in any pediatric patient presenting with petechiae and bleeding and can be screened for with a complete blood count. Most patients with CAMT will have severe thrombocytopenia; however, a platelet count greater than 100×10^9/L should not exclude this possibility. Once CAMT is suspected, a bone marrow evaluation is warranted. This should show normal cellularity with reduced or absent megakaryocytes in patients with CAMT [19, 59]. Early in the disease process, megakaryocyte pathology may be subtle and serial marrows maybe necessary to definitively diagnose CAMT [60]. With progression of CAMT, subsequent bone marrow evaluations can show hypocellular marrows due to the failure of hematopoiesis in a majority of patients [19].

Supportive care with platelet transfusions is necessary to prevent bleeding in patients with CAMT. As stated above, patients with CAMT are at increased risk of complete bone marrow failure, but they are also at increased risk of developing a myelodysplasia or myeloid leukemia [59]. These two consequences are the driving force behind an attempt at a cure. Currently, the only curative treatment is hematopoietic stem cell transplantation. Ideally, a transplant in this setting should occur prior to the onset of pancytopenia to minimize prior antigen exposure through blood products. HLA matched, unaffected sibling donors are ideal [3, 92]; however, successful transplants have been reported using sibling donors who are heterozygous carriers of a c-MPL mutation [104]. Due to the lack of other modalities for treatment, matched unrelated donors have been used with success when sibling donors are not available [91]; however, outcomes when compared to matched sibling donors is much poorer secondary to more toxic preparative regimens and increased percentages of engraftment failure [98].

Thrombocytopenia with Absent Radii

As the name implies, patients with TAR present with thrombocytopenia in the setting of absence of radii. Platelet counts are usually below 50×10^9/L. The severity of thrombocytopenia is greatest at birth with tendencies to improve over the course of the first year. There is a risk of bleeding due to thrombocytopenia, and therefore platelet transfusions are necessary but should become less frequent as the disease course improves [144]. TAR differs from Fanconi anemia in that the thumbs are typically present, although they may be hypoplastic [4]. In 98% of TAR cases, both radii are affected [84]. The radii malformations are pathognomonic for TAR; however, it is important to remember that other dysmorphic features can occur and include both skeletal and non-skeletal abnormalities. For example, humeral and ulnar involvement is described in several patients [144] and lower extremities defects are reported in about 46% of patients [69]. Short stature, facial dysmorphisms, cardiac abnormalities, gastrointestinal (gastroenteritis and cow's milk allergy) pathology, genitourinary abnormalities, and capillary hemangiomas are also described [144].

TAR affects approximately 1 in 240,000 live births and is inherited in an autosomal recessive fashion [4]. Studies have shown that the c-MPL gene is normally expressed in patients with TAR, but there is still no response to thrombopoietin, leading to the thought that TAR is a result of a signaling defect in this pathway [20]. So far, no known genetic mutation exists to help diagnose patients with TAR; however, the HOX family of genes, including c-MPL, HOXA10, HOXA11, and HOXD11, have all been determined to not play a role in patients with TAR [54, 144].

Thrombocytopenia and the absent radii are all that is necessary to make a diagnosis of TAR. However, if a bone marrow evaluation is undertaken, it will likely show decreased megakaryocytes. As above, treatment includes supportive care with platelet transfusions to minimize risk of serious bleeding during infancy along with orthopedic care. Unlike CAMT, patients with TAR do not progress to bone marrow failure. However, there are reports of leukemias, both lymphoid and myeloid, in patients with history of TAR, warranting continued monitoring after resolution of thrombocytopenia [32, 64, 81].

Pure Red Cell Aplasia

Pure red cell aplasias (PRCA) are a group of disorders that present with anemia, reticulocytopenia, and reduced or absent erythroid progenitor cells within the bone marrow [100]. There are many potential etiologies of PRCA, some inherited and some acquired. The most common inherited form is Diamond-Blackfan anemia (DBA); however, Pearson marrow-pancreas syndrome (PS) can also present similarly and is at times difficult to differentiate from DBA [58]. In contrast, there are several acquired forms of PRCA, and these can be thought of in terms of a primary red cell disorder versus anemia secondary to other underlying pathology. For example, a primary acquired PRCA includes transient erythroblastopenia of childhood (TEC), whereas an acquired secondary PRCA could be associated with underlying autoimmune disorders, malignancies, infections, or medications, for example [100]. This chapter will focus on inherited forms of PRCA.

Diamond-Blackfan anemia is the prototype of inherited PRCA. However, other considerations are Pearson marrow-pancreas syndrome (PS) as well as congenital dyserythropoietic anemia (CDA). The underlying cause of these disorders is very distinct and oftentimes they will have dissimilar clinical presentations; however, the severity of each lies within a clinical spectrum which can make distinguishing them from one another challenging at times.

Diamond-Blackfan Anemia

DBA is an inherited bone marrow failure syndrome (IBMFS) characterized by red blood cell failure and oftentimes is associated with congenital anomalies and a predilection toward development of malignancies [148]. While the first published clinical case describing DBA is thought to have occurred in 1936 by pediatrician, Hugh Josephs, the specific characterization of DBA is attributed to Louis Diamond and Kenneth Blackfan, two pediatricians who published a paper on DBA in 1938 [46, 82]. With time, the description of DBA has evolved to include a spectrum of diseases that have much heterogeneity, not only in their clinical presentation but also in their underlying genetic mutations [36]. This evolving description of DBA has now led to the idea of a "classical" form of DBA and a "nonclassical" form, and some cases are starting to be identified later in childhood or even adulthood [97, 147].

Because of the evolving description of DBA, defining the true incidence is currently a moving target; however, classical DBA is thought to affect about 7/1,000,000 live births, and when nonclassical DBA is considered, the overall incidence of DBA is thought to be between 1/100,000 and 1/200,000, evenly distributed between ethnicities and genders [147]. Of the IBMFS, DBA is considered one of the four most frequently identified, in addition to Fanconi anemia, dyskeratosis congenita, and Shwachman-Diamond syndrome [7].

Another evolving aspect of DBA involves the numbers and types of underlying mutations now being identified as having a causative role in the disease. Genetic mutations are now found in about 70% of patients diagnosed with DBA, and of these, almost all are found in ribosomal proteins that result in pre-ribosomal RNA maturational defects [36]. This has led to classifying DBA as a "ribosomopathy" [101]. Interestingly, two other well-known IBMFS are now known to involve ribosomal mutations: Shwachman-Diamond syndrome and dyskeratosis congenita [154].

The first genetic mutation thought to cause the DBA phenotype was linked to chromosome 19q13, which codes for ribosomal protein S19 (RPS19) [67]. It is now known that ribosomes have 80 functional proteins, and at least 21 of these have been implicated as the causative mutation of DBA: RPS19, RPS24, RPS17, RPL5, RPL11, RPS10, RPS26, RPS7, RPS15A, RPS26, RPS27, RPS28, RPS29, RPL9, RPL15, RPL18, RPL26, RPL27, RPL31, RPL35, and RPL35A [36]. Ninety percent of cases can be attributed to six of these proteins, RPS19, RPL5, RPS26, RPL11, RPL35A, and RPS24, with RPS19 accounting for 25% of cases [36, 55].

Essential to protein synthesis, ribosomes are cellular organelles composed of ribosomal RNA and proteins that form two subunits, a larger 60S and a smaller 40S subunit [154]. The connection between ribosomal mutations and the phenotypes seen with DBA remains to be completely elucidated; however, there are several interesting connections that have been demonstrated thus far. Several studies have shown that erythroid cells in patients with Diamond-Blackfan anemia lack the ability to have an erythroid expansion and terminal differentiation in response to erythropoietin, and it seems this is a result of a defect downstream from the erythropoietin receptor itself that traps erythroid progenitor cells in the proerythroblast form [105, 107]. The normal erythropoiesis process requires the rate of RNA synthesis to exceed the rate of cellular proliferation, a step that is blocked by the RPS19 deletion [55, 133]. Furthermore, cells that lack RPS19 have been shown to have stabilization of p53, cell cycle delay in the G1 phase, and reduced levels of key transcriptional proteins, leading to speculation that the decreased ribosomal biogenesis ultimately leads to nucleolar stress and p53-mediated apoptosis [133]. This thought was supported in a study that blocked RNA polymerase I at the proerythroblast stage, resulting in p53 activation and terminal differentiation [28].

In recent years, two mutations have been identified as causative for DBA that are not involved in genes for ribosomal proteins: GATA-1 and TSR2 [65, 110, 124]. The GATA-1 protein is part of a family of transcription factors, of which three (GATA-1, GATA-2, and GATA-3) are known to impact hematopoiesis [53]. More specifically, GATA-1 has been shown to have a role as a transcriptional regulator in ribosome biosynthesis, linking mutations in GATA-1 to impaired ribosomal biogenesis [10]. The TSR2 mutation was identified through a study of patients with Treacher Collins syndrome (TCS), a disorder that presents with craniofacial dysmorphogenesis and is also known to involve ribosome biogenesis [38, 65]. Through the use of Sanger sequencing in six families with both TCS and another mandibulofacial dysostosis along with DBA, two families were found to have RPS26 gene mutations, two were found to have RPS28 mutations, and one family had a TSR2 gene mutation that was thought to be causative [65]. Importantly, the gene product of TSR2 binds directly to RPS26, linking this mutation to ribosomal function [65].

About 55% of mutations seen in DBA are thought to be de novo while 45% are found to be familial [36]. Of the familial cases, all of the ribosomal protein mutations found thus far inherited in a heterozygous pattern leading to speculation that the homozygous inheritance pattern is lethal [36]. There may be some X-linked inheritance patterns as the only non-ribosomal protein mutations, TSR2 and GATA-1, are both located on the X chromosome [65].

Establishing the diagnosis of DBA takes into account the potential for genetic mutations, the patient's clinical course, as well as the family history. With regard to a patient's clinical presentation, age at presentation can be very helpful. The Diamond-Blackfan Anemia Registry of North America reported that as many as 50% of patients present within 3 months of life, 75% by 6 months of life, and 92% by 1 year of life [148]. A report from the United Kingdom found that 72.5% of patients presented prior to 3 months of age [17]. Another key element is the potential for congenital anomalies to be present.

Early reports associated DBA with hypertelorism, broad and flat nasal bridges, triphalangeal thumbs, or heart defects [1, 33, 76]. Since these reports, large registries have now shown that up to 47% of patients will have at least one congenital anomaly and about 25% will have more than one anomaly [147]. Of these, craniofacial anomalies are most common, representing about 50% of the anomalies seen, and include hypertelorism, a broad, flat nasal bridge, cleft palate, high-arched palate, microcephaly, micrognathia, microtia, low-set ears, low hairline, ptosis, and epicanthal folds [147]. Thumb anomalies and genitourinary anomalies are each reported to occur in up to 19% of patients, while cardiac anomalies are seen in up to 15% [147]. Other reported anomalies include congenital glaucoma, cataracts, strabismus, short or webbed necks, Sprengel deformity, Klippel-Feil anomaly, and syndactyly [147]. Approximately 25% of patients will have low birth weight, and about 30% are thought to have short statures with heights below the third percentile for age [147]. Some described anomalies seem to have a higher correspondence to particular gene mutations. For example, RPL5 mutations are thought to be associated with abnormal thumbs, cleft palate, and cardiac defects, RPL11 mutations are also associated with thumb anomalies, whereas RPS26 mutations are associated with skeletal defects [36]. Despite these correlations, patients with DBA within the same family and therefore having the same mutations often have different levels of clinical severity, leading to an incompletely understood genotype-phenotype correlation.

When DBA is suspected, further laboratory data should be obtained. A complete blood count (CBC), reticulocyte count, fetal hemoglobin (HbF), and an erythrocyte adenosine deaminase activity (eADA) level should be obtained. Patients that have DBA will mostly commonly have a macrocytic anemia with an inappropriately low reticulocyte count [147]. The eADA is elevated in 80–85% of cases, and importantly, it is not affected by prior transfusion [147]. Given the variability in presentation, criteria exist to help in the diagnostic approach. These criteria are broken down into diagnostic criteria and supporting criteria, and different combinations can lead to a diagnosis of classical, nonclassical, or probable DBA (Table 4.1) [147].

Another consideration when establishing the diagnosis of DBA includes consideration of other entities that can present similarly. In particular TEC, PS, and infectious causes, such as parvovirus B19, should be considered and ruled out [100, 148]. There are some very helpful differences between these entities. For example, TEC will spontaneously resolve within 1–2 months, and it should present with normal fetal hemoglobin levels and normal erythrocyte adenosine deaminase activity and typically has normal MCV levels [94, 147]. A bone marrow evaluation can be quite helpful in differentiating these entities. Both DBA and TEC can show a bone marrow with normal cellularity but decreased erythroid precursors; however, when TEC begins to recover, the bone marrow could show increased erythropoietic activity [94, 147]. If the patient has parvovirus B19 causing anemia, the bone marrow might show enlarged proerythroblasts with intranuclear inclusions and some dyserythropoiesis [94]. The bone marrow in patients with PS will often show vacuolization, hypocellularity, and ringed sideroblasts [141]. Table 4.2 demonstrates some of these differences based upon the most common clinical findings.

Once a patient meets criteria to establish a diagnosis of DBA, an echocardiogram and renal ultrasound should be obtained given the risk of congenital malformations involving these organ systems [147]. Additionally, immediate family members should be evaluated with a thorough history, complete blood count, eADA, and HbF level [147]. Given the potential inheritance pattern of DBA, referral to a geneticist or genetic counselor may be of some value as well.

Table 4.1 Diagnostic criteria for Diamond-Blackfan anemia

Diagnostic criteria
Anemia presenting at less than 1 year of age
Macrocytic anemia without significant other cytopenias
Reticulocytopenia
Normal marrow cellularity with a paucity of erythroid precursors
Supporting criteria
Major
Gene mutation known to be associated with DBA
Positive family history
Minor
Elevated erythrocyte adenosine deaminase activity
Congenital anomalies known to be associated with DBA
Elevated HbF
No evidence of other inherited bone marrow failure syndromes
Making the diagnosis
Classical DBA: all four diagnostic criteria are met
Nonclassical DBA: some diagnostic criteria are met plus a DBA gene mutation
Probable DBA if:
3 diagnostic criteria plus a family history
2 diagnostic criteria plus 3 minor supporting criteria
Family history plus 3 minor supporting criteria

Several treatment options exist for patients with DBA; however, corticosteroids, red blood cell transfusions, and hematopoietic stem cell transplant provide the primary options. While stem cell transplant is the only curative option, others are often utilized in hopes of improving the patient's anemia and perhaps leading to a remission, as defined by maintenance of an adequate hemoglobin level without treatment for at least 6 months [148]. When choosing which treatment option to utilize, age of the patient, severity of the anemia, and clinical acuity must be considered.

Corticosteroid therapy will provide an initial response in about 80% of patients, and of those that do initially respond, some will eventually stop responding and go on to need transfusions, some will require long-term steroid exposure, and about 20% of patients will be able to stop therapy while maintaining transfusion independence [147]. The mechanism by which steroids improve anemia in patients with DBA is not completely understood; however, cellular studies have demonstrated that sensitivity for the erythropoietin-stimulated erythroid burst is greatly improved by steroid exposure [105]. Because significant long-term morbidity is associated with chronic steroid use at young ages, it is recommended to delay use of steroids until at least 1 year of age [136, 148, 156]. As such, most patients will need initial therapy with RBC transfusions and some will ultimately need chronic RBC transfusions. Given this, iron overload must be considered, particularly because patients

Table 4.2 Characteristics of DBA, TEC, parvovirus B19 infections, and PS

	DBA	TEC	Parvovirus B19	PS
Anemia	PRCA, macrocytic	PRCA, normocytic	PRCA, normocytic	PRCA, but often with other cytopenias, sideroblastic
Age at presentation	<1 year	3 months–4 years	Any age	<1 year
Genetic mutations	Sporadic, heterozygous, rare X-linked	Not inherited	Not inherited	Sporadic or mitochondrial DNA inheritance
Bone marrow	Normal cellularity Decreased erythroid precursors	Normal cellularity, decreased or increased erythroid precursors	Enlarged proerythroblasts with vacuoles	Hypocellular, sideroblasts, vacuolization
Supportive laboratory studies	Increased HbF, elevated erythrocyte ADA activity, reticulocytopenia	Normal HbF, normal erythrocyte ADA activity, reticulocytopenia	Normal HbF, normal erythrocyte ADA activity, parvovirus DNA present	Metabolic acidosis Increased lactate
Supportive Clinical information	Congenital anomalies present	No congenital anomalies	Infectious symptoms present. Known to have decreased RBC survival	Diarrhea

with DBA are not utilizing iron stores for erythropoiesis [147]. Other treatments that have been attempted with varying degrees of success include androgens, erythropoietin, interleukin-3 therapy, cyclosporine, metoclopramide, valproic acid, leucine, 6-mercaptopurine, cyclophosphamide, vincristine, and intravenous immunoglobulin therapy [147].

The role of hematopoietic stem cell transplant is somewhat controversial because of the risks involved in the procedure itself along with the potential long-term complications of transplant. With experience, outcomes are improving, and currently, patients less than 9 years of age, receiving a transplant from a matched sibling, tend to do best. Data from the DBA registry gives an overall survival of about 90% when these criteria are met; however, overall survival when alternative donors are used is about 32% therapy [147]. As the best outcomes have been with use of sibling donors, donors must be thoroughly screened when being considered for transplant, and this should include checking eADA, HbF, and MCV [147].

Other than the congenital malformations and the anemia associated with DBA, patients are at an increased risk of myelodysplastic syndrome, leukemia, aplastic anemic, and development of solid tumors, such as osteogenic sarcoma, soft tissue sarcomas, lymphomas, breast cancer, hepatocellular carcinoma, gastric cancer, and colon cancer [147]. Because of this and the potential for treatment-related side effects, routine clinical and laboratory monitoring is appropriate and needs to be followed through with bone marrow evaluations if CBCs demonstrate significant concerns. Taking all things into consideration, patients with DBA currently have a decreased life expectancy. Statistics from the DBA registry indicate that only about 75% of patients survive to the age of 40 [96].

Pearson Marrow-Pancreas Syndrome

Pearson marrow-pancreas syndrome, or Pearson syndrome (PS), was first described in 1979 when a case series of four unrelated children with severe, refractory macrocytic anemia, varying degrees of neutropenia and thrombocytopenia, exocrine pancreatic dysfunction, and bone marrow evaluations demonstrating vacuolizations and ringed sideroblasts was first published [112]. Since that first case series, it has become apparent that PS is truly a multisystem disease with clinical heterogeneity and an estimated incidence of approximately 1/1,000,000 live births [86].

Another important characteristic of PS is that patients tend to have a metabolic acidosis with high lactate to pyruvate ratios. This finding led a group to perform molecular analysis of the mitochondrial DNA of five patients with PS, demonstrating that all five had abnormalities in their mitochondrial DNA [122]. Furthermore, all tissues sampled seemed to have a proportion of mitochondrial DNA with defects and another proportion without defects, leading to the interpretation that PS is a multisystem disorder resulting from mitochondrial heteroplasmy [122]. Importantly, this same study demonstrated that patients with Shwachman-Diamond syndrome, another bone marrow failure syndrome with exocrine pancreatic dysfunction, did not have defects in mitochondrial DNA [122]. Given the severity of PS and the presence of the underlying defect being a mitochondrial DNA deletion, most cases are de novo in nature and not directly inherited from an affected family member.

Similar to DBA, clinical findings outside of the severe anemia can vary greatly. Children with PS have progressive and often fatal multisystem disease with liver, kidney, pancreatic, and central nervous system involvement [50]. Many associated symptoms are described and include proximal myopathy, seizures, ataxia, other movement disorders, skin disorders, proximal renal tubular acidosis, hepatomegaly, splenomegaly, diabetes mellitus, adrenal insufficiency, growth impairment, ventricular wall thickness, cardiac depolarization disorders, prolonged QT, and ophthalmic complications [14, 50, 121]. A cohort of 11 patients from Italy found that increased serum lactate and alanine and increased urine lactate, fumarate, and malic acid, along with an increased fetal Hb and erythropoietin level, are common [50]. This same study demonstrated normal triglycerides, normal cholesterol, and normal transaminases; however, two of the children had elevated gamma-glutamyl transferase levels [50]. Additionally, some patients that seem to survive the early hematologic manifestations progress and clinically transform into other syndromes, particularly Kearns-Sayre syndrome and Leigh syndrome [93, 99, 125]. Interestingly, no correlation has been identified between the type or size of mitochondrial DNA mutations and the range of phenotypes observed [103].

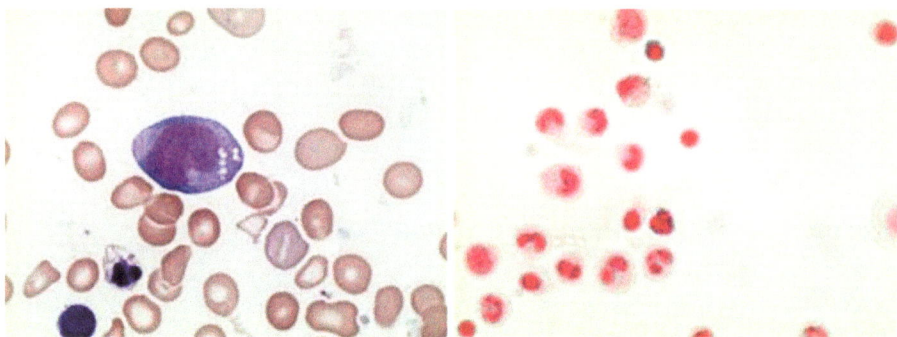

Fig. 4.2 Demonstration of vacuolization of red blood cell precursors as well as ringed sideroblasts [115]. Used with permission

Bone marrow evaluations can be very helpful when working through the potential causes of congenital anemia. Findings of PS include vacuolization of both myeloid and erythroid precursors, hypocellularity, and ringed sideroblasts [141]. A recent review of the literature found that patients with PS tend to have progression of bone marrow abnormalities when comparing evaluations done prior to 30 days of life and those done between 31 and 90 days old, followed by some degree of stabilization [141]. Vacuoles were seen in 58.3% of cases done prior to 30 days of life, 84.6% of those done between 31 and 90 days of life, and 80% of those done after 91 days of life. Altered cellularity was observed in 25% of cases less than 30 days old, 46.2% done between 31 and 90 days of life, and 40% of cases evaluated after 90 days of life [141]. The classic ringed sideroblast was only seen in 25% of cases evaluated prior to 30 days, in 38.4% of those done between 31 and 90 days, and in 50% of those done after 91 days of life [141]. (Fig. 4.2).

When considering the differential diagnosis of congenital anemia, both DBA and PS must be considered and given the clinical overlap between patient's signs and symptoms in both disease processes, distinguishing the diagnosis can be difficult at times. When DBA is diagnosed based on clinical signs and symptoms and because of the apparent lack of pancreatic insufficiency, sideroblasts, or metabolic acidosis, it has been demonstrated that as many as 2% of these patients will actually have PS when testing for mitochondrial DNA deletions is undertaken [58]. This finding should warrant consideration of PS in patients clinically thought to have DBA, but without the supporting family history or an underlying genetic mutation for DBA.

Pearson syndrome invariably leads to a premature death. Earlier reports suggest that most deaths occur by the age of 3 years with very few patients living into young adulthood [50, 103]. The Italian cohort of 11 patients suggests that death may be more common between 5 and 11 years of age and with more recent improvements in supportive care [50]. The ultimate cause of death is somewhat variable; however, sepsis, renal failure, and metabolic derangements are relatively common [50]. Given the rarity and the relatively quick progression to death, treatment strategies are difficult to study and currently no fundamental treatment exists. Corticosteroids and erythropoietin have been shown largely ineffective [50, 58]. Management largely consists of supportive care through transfusional support for anemia, GCSF for neutropenia, pancreatic supplements, and nutritional changes for the metabolic acidosis [86].

Congenital Dyserythropoietic Anemia

The congenital dyserythropoietic anemias are a rare group of hereditary disorders characterized by ineffective erythropoiesis and distinct morphologic findings within the bone marrow [70]. The first use of the term CDA was in 1966 by Crookston et al. who described cases that would later be classified as CDA type II [35]. In 1968, criteria for classifying the CDA family into three types, CDA I, CDA II, and CDA III were proposed and these criteria are still utilized [73]. However, since this initial classification was proposed, several patients have been described who meet the general diagnostic criteria for CDA but who don't necessarily fit into one of the three proposed types, and so there are now CDA variants [27]. There does not seem to be a gender or ethnicity preference; however, most patients described in the literature are of European or Middle Eastern descent, including 712 cases enrolled on the German CDA registry and 206 enrolled on the Italian registry as of the year 2011 [78].

Although there are several differences between each type of CDA, there are also some commonalities. In general, patients with any type of CDA will show signs and symptoms of increased hemoglobin (Hb) turnover with elevated bilirubin and low haptoglobin; however, they should also have an inappropriately low reticulocyte count [78]. Bone marrow evaluation will always show hypercellularity because of increased erythroblasts giving a decreased myeloid to erythroid ratio [78]. Extramedullary hematopoiesis is also seen in each type, particularly presenting as paravertebral masses, most commonly in the thoracic spinal area [71]. Age of onset is also very similar with most patients presenting in the neonatal period or early childhood, although there are many case reports describing hydrops fetalis as part of several types of CDA [90, 134]. All types of CDA are inherited with type I and II having an inheritance pattern of autosomal recessive, types III and IV demonstrating autosomal dominant inheritance, and the variant forms showing either autosomal recessive or an X-linked pattern [78].

Congenital Dyserythropoietic Anemia Type 1

CDA I is characterized by a macrocytic anemia with megaloblastic changes, chromatin bridges between erythroblasts representing ineffective erythropoiesis, and electron-lucent areas within the chromatin giving a characteristic "Swiss cheese" appearance on electron microscopy [41, 119] (Figs. 4.3 and 4.4) [116]. Taken from the available European data, the incidence of CDA I is approximately 0.24/1,000,000 [78].

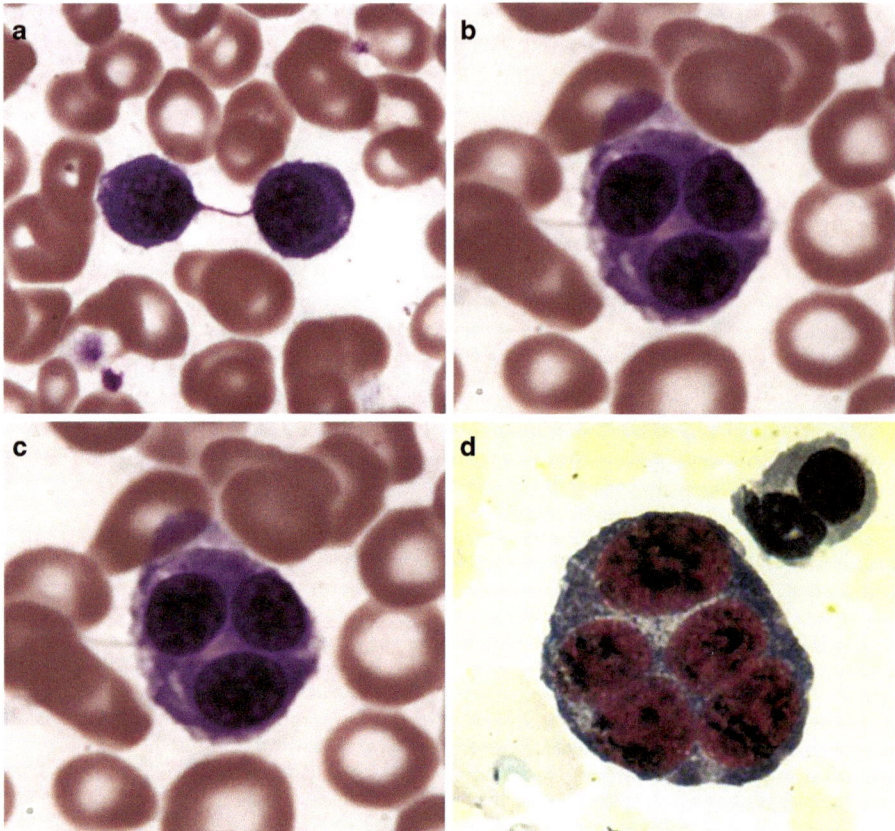

Fig. 4.3 Light microscopy of bone marrow erythroblasts obtained by aspiration, indicating the spectrum of nuclear abnormalities. (**a**) Internuclear chromatin bridging in CDA-1. (**b**) Binuclearity in CDA-2. (**c**) Trinuclearity, as observed in all CDA types. (**d**) Multinuclearity in CDA-3. (Courtesy of H. Heimpel, Ulm, Germany) [116]

Clinically, patients with CDA I have varying degrees of anemia with hemoglobin levels typically ranging between 7 and 11 g/dL throughout life; however, there are also cases reported needing chronic transfusional support [78]. Many cases will present in the neonatal period with one study finding that as many as 64% of patients will show symptoms as a neonate with symptoms including hepatomegaly, jaundice, small for gestational age, pulmonary hypertension, and transient thrombocytopenia [131]. Other symptoms reported in the literature include splenomegaly, gallstones, retinal angioid streaks, and dysmorphic features seen in up to 14% of patients, particularly affecting the patient's digits [56, 78, 116].

Once clinically suspected, CDA type I can be confirmed through genetic testing as up to 90% of patients will have a genetic mutation in gene CDAN1 (chromosome 15q15.1q15.3) which encodes a protein, codanin-1 [42, 123]. The exact function of codanin-1 is yet to be completely understood, but studies would suggest that

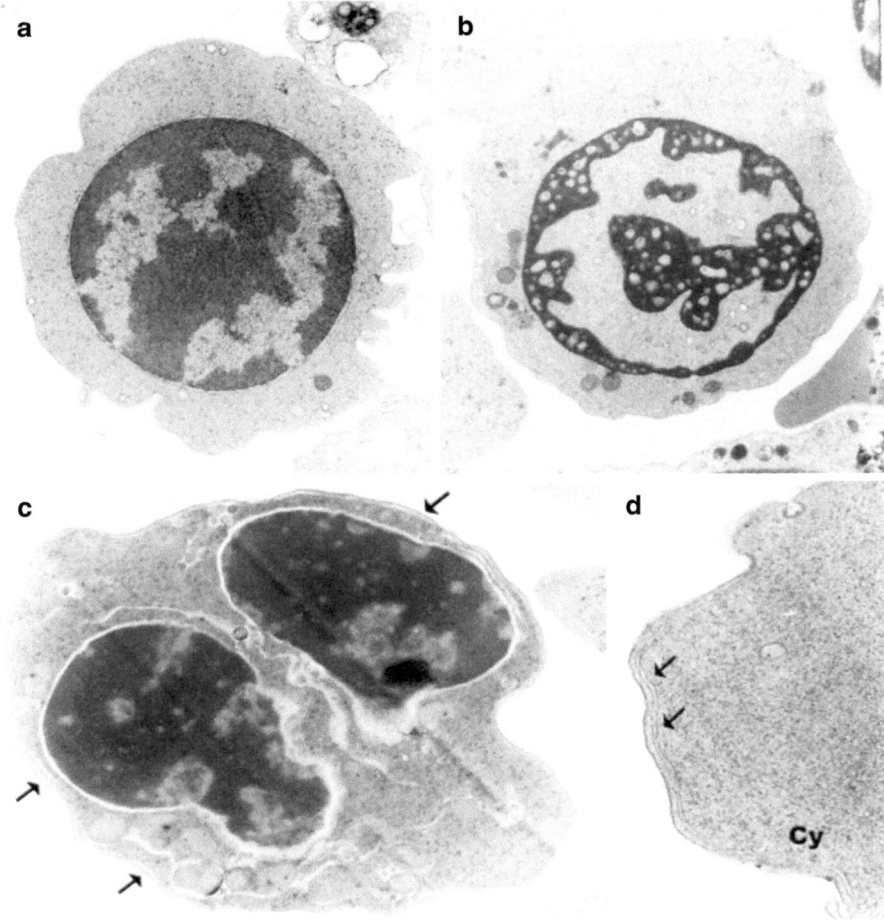

Fig. 4.4 Electron microscopy of bone marrow erythroblasts obtained by aspiration showing the specific abnormalities observed in CDA-1 and CDA-2. (**a**) Normal erythroblast. The nucleus is composed of heterochromatin (high electron density) and euchromatin (low electron density). (**b**) CDA-1 erythroblast with characteristic "Swiss cheese" (spongy) heterochromatin. (**c**) CDA-2 binucleate erythroblast. Arrows show characteristic "double membrane." (**d**) CDA-2 erythroblast cytoplasmic membrane (detail). Arrows show double membrane (possibly peripheral cisternae of smooth endoplasmic reticulum) running parallel (40–60 nm interval) to cytoplasmic membrane of erythroblasts. Cy cytoplasm [116]

codanin-1 is a cell-regulated protein active in the S phase of the cell cycle [106]. Consistent with this, codanin-1 has been shown to interact with anti-silencing function 1 (Asf1), a histone chaperone active during DNA replication [13].

Complications are relatively common and are typically associated with the known anemia and ineffective erythropoiesis. A study looking at 32 Bedouin adult CDA type I patients with a mean age of 34 years demonstrated that 8 out of 9 patients had osteoporosis, 21 out of 30 had cholelithiasis, 5 out of 6 had pulmonary arterial hypertension, and many had signs of iron overload as demonstrated by 9 out of 24 having hypothyroidism, 6 out of 32 having diabetes mellitus, and of the 13 patients that underwent T2* MRI, all had increased liver iron, but none had increased cardiac iron levels [130]. Six of these patients underwent splenectomy, of which five had improvement in their anemia; however, these are the same six patients that developed pulmonary arterial hypertension [130]. In this cohort, 3 patients died between the age of 46 and 56, 2 from sepsis, and 1 from pulmonary hypertension [130]. Another study looked at morbidity and mortality of 21 patients with CDA I enrolled on the German CDA registry [72]. From this data, 20 patients reported feeling that they had less fitness as compared to their classmates or feelings of moderate fatigue [72]. Other associated difficulties included leg ulcers, 2 patients required regular red cell transfusions, 4 developed cholelithiasis, and 20 patients had iron overload [72]. The oldest living patient at the time of this study was 55 years old and 5 patients had died between the ages of 31 and 56 years, 3 from heart and liver disease with 2 of these having confirmed severe iron overload, 1 from squamous cell carcinoma of the ear, and 1 from sepsis [72].

Therapy for patients with CDA I consists mainly of red blood cell transfusions, interferon α-2a or interferon α-2b, and management of complications. Many patients undergo splenectomy and only some will have improvement in their anemia, and many will have increased mortality from pulmonary hypertension or sepsis [72, 130]. Three children with CDA type I have reportedly undergone stem cell transplant. Prior to transplant, all were dependent on red cell transfusions and two had iron overload as defined by ferritin values >1000 µg/L [16]. Matched sibling donors were utilized and all three engrafted well had normal posttransplant bone marrow morphology, and at least at 2 years posttransplant, all three were transfusion independent [16].

Congenital Dyserythropoietic Anemia Type II

CDA II, also known as hereditary erythroblastic multinuclearity with positive acidified serum test (HEMPAS), is the most common type of CDA, being about three times more common than CDA type I [41, 78]. It is characterized by a normocytic anemia with a positive acidified serum test, increased agglutination with anti-I antibodies, and erythroblasts that have two or more nuclei [119] (Figs. 4.3 and 4.4) [116]. With the acidified serum test, also called the Ham test, red blood cells should lyse when placed in an acidic environment [108]. Another common finding in CDA type II is impaired glycosylation on all erythrocyte membranes [41].

Like CDA type I, CDA type II has an autosomal recessive inheritance pattern [78]. Patients typically present a little older as compared to CDA type I, with an average age of presentation of 18–20 years [116]. The anemia is typically mild, 90% of patients will have hyperbilirubinemia, 70% will have splenomegaly, and 45% will have hepatomegaly [116]. As with CDA type 1, patients are at increased risk of an aplastic crisis in association with parvovirus B19 infection [116]. Patients with CDA type II are also at increased risk of iron overload with 50% of patients having ferritin values >1000 µg/L by 50 years of age [116].

To help diagnose patients with CDA type II, analysis of erythrocyte membrane proteins by sodium dodecyl sulfate polyacrylamide gel electrophoresis (SDS-PAGE) should show a narrower band size and faster migration of band 3 and band 4.5 proteins [78]. The increased destruction of erythrocytes in patients with CDA type II has been associated with hypoglycosylation of band 3, causing an increased clusterization of the band 3 protein on the cell surface, leading to increased destruction within the spleen [57, 78] (Fig. 4.5). Molecular testing is also available to look for a mutation in the SEC23B gene, located on the short arm of chromosome 20 [129]. This gene encodes for a cytoplasmic coat protein (COP) II and is involved in the transport of correctly folded products that bud from the endoplasmic reticulum and get transported to the Golgi apparatus, a pathway that is critical for membrane homeostasis, localization of proteins within cells, and secretion of extracellular factors [78].

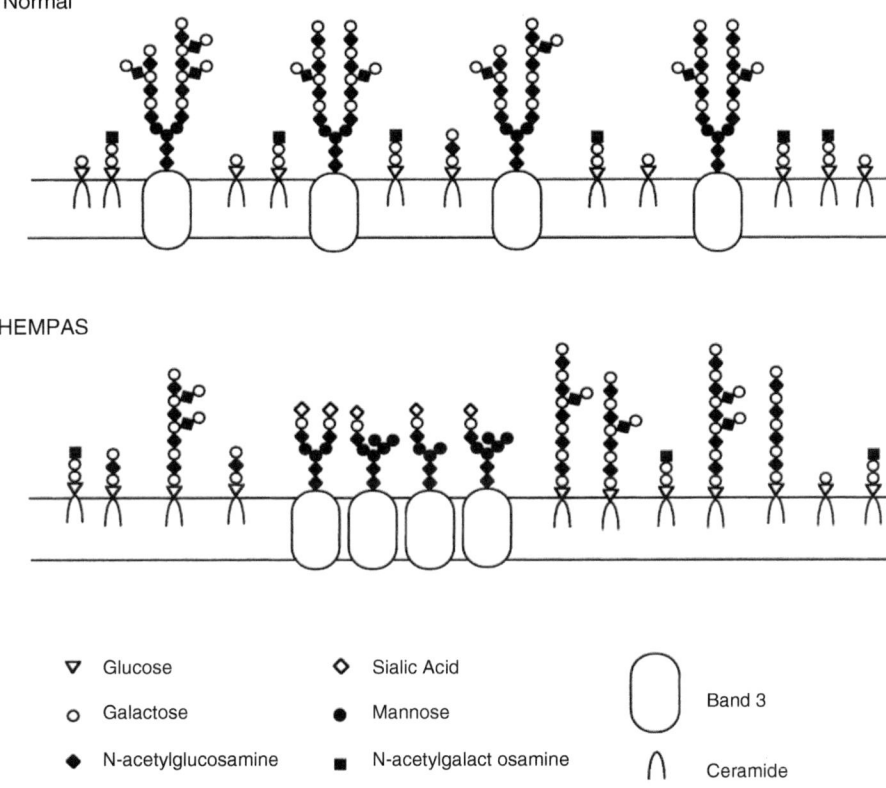

Fig. 4.5 Erythrocyte membrane glycoproteins and glycolipids in normal and HEMPAS. In normal erythrocyte, glycoproteins, such as band 3, are glycosylated by polylactosamines. Although polylactosaminyl ceramides are present in small quantity in normal erythrocytes, the majority of erythrocyte glycolipids belong to the globo-series with short carbohydrate chains. In HEMPAS, glycoproteins lack polylactosamines, whereas lacto-series glycolipids including polylactosaminyl-ceramides are accumulated [57]. Used with permission

The majority of patients will have mild disease; however, 10–20% of patients will have severe anemia requiring intervention [102]. Treatment largely consists of red blood cell transfusions and treatment for iron overload. Unlike CDA type I, splenectomy can be of more utility in CDA type II because the anemia does tend to improve; however, the procedure still has several risks associated with it and should only be considered in cases of severe anemia and transfusion dependence [79]. Some patients have opted to undergo stem cell transplant and several cases are now reporting success for patients with CDA type II [29, 102, 146].

Congenital Dyserythropoietic Anemia Type III

CDA type III is the most rare of the classical types of CDA (I-III) with only about 60 cases described globally with a large proportion of these being from a single Swedish family that has at least 34 members known to have CDA type III [41, 95]. CDA III has an autosomal dominant inheritance pattern and presents with a macrocytic anemia and giant erythroblasts that contain up to 12 nuclei [41, 119] (Figs. 4.3 and 4.4) [116]. Most cases tend to be mild, without the need for transfusions and without signs of iron overload [41]. There is an association with monoclonal gammopathies, multiple myeloma, and retinal angioid streaks [155]. The genetic defect occurs in the KIF23 gene on chromosome 15q23 which encodes mitotic kinesin-like protein 1 (MKLP1) and leads to failure of cytokinesis [95].

Nonclassical Types of Congenital Dyserythropoietic Anemia

Several variants of CDA have been described that don't seem to fit into the classic three groups [78]. CDA type IV is a variant of CDA type II that does not share the serum test results but also has bone marrow morphology similar to CDA type II [78]. The other types include CDA with prominent erythroblastosis after splenectomy, CDA with intraerythrocytic inclusions, CDA with thrombocytopenia, and a much more rare form of CDA without dysplasia [78].

Neutropenia

There are several inherited genetic mutations recognized as causing congenital neutropenia. Some of these mutations present with the classically thought of severe congenital neutropenia (SCN), while others associated with disorders such as Barth disease, WHIM syndrome, or Cohen syndrome and still others are only recently being recognized. The focus of this section will be severe congenital neutropenia (SCN) and Shwachman-Diamond syndrome (SDS); however, the clinician should recognize that broad differential diagnosis is encompassed by isolated neutropenia.

Severe Congenital Neutropenia

SCN encompasses a group of disorders that all present with severe neutropenia in the neonatal period. Within this group, Kostmann syndrome seems to be the prototype. Kostmann syndrome was first described in the 1950s and was defined by the presence of an absolute neutrophil count of <200/μL within the first few weeks of life, maturational arrest of granulopoiesis at the promyelocyte stage, and death due to bacterial infections [88, 89]. Sadly, 11 of the first 14 reported patients died during their first year of life because of these infections [48].

Kostmann syndrome is a specific form of SCN, inherited in an autosomal recessive fashion that has been associated with mutations in the gene encoding the HAX1 mitochondrial protein which is critical in maintaining the mitochondrial membrane potential and protecting cells from apoptosis [87]. Classically, patients with this form of SCN will progress to have neurologic involvement, whereas other forms of SCN do not have this particular progression [48]. Another genetic cause of SCN has been linked to mutations in the neutrophil elastase (ELANE) gene and is inherited in an autosomal dominant pattern [48]. This particular gene is also known to have involved mutations in patients with cyclic neutropenia, suggesting that cyclic neutropenia and SCN may represent disorders on a continuum [40, 48, 74].

The SCN as a result with either HAX1 mutations or ELANE mutations encompass the disorders classically thought of as SCN; however, there are several other disorders which should be considered when thinking through congenital neutropenia. In 2003, mutations involving gene GFI1 which encodes for a transcriptional repressor oncoprotein Gfi1 were found to repress the ELANE protein, leading to SCN that is inherited in an autosomal dominant manner and is associated with lymphopenia as well [48, 113]. Wiskott-Aldrich syndrome is a relatively well-known syndrome of microthrombocytopenia, immune dysfunction, and eczema that is inherited in an X-linked pattern from a mutation in the WAS gene. Since Wiskott-Aldrich syndrome was defined, a different mutation in the same gene has been shown to lead to an X-linked inheritance of SCN that is associated with monocytopenia [48].

A congenital neutropenia disorder that does not show maturational arrest on bone marrow evaluation is that of WHIM syndrome, which refers to warts, hypogammaglobulinemia, infections, and myelokathexis. Given the component of myelokathexis, a patient with this will have trapped white blood cells and increased cellularity [66]. WHIM syndrome is inherited in an autosomal dominant pattern, involves a mutation of the CXCR4 gene that encodes a chemokine receptor, and is also associated with lymphopenia and thrombocytopenia [48]. Genetic defects in the G6PC3 gene are now known to cause SCN and be inherited as an autosomal recessive disorder associated with superficial venous dermatologic findings, atrial cardiac defects, and uropathy [48].

Several other diseases exist that can present with a congenital neutropenia, but with no maturation arrest on bone marrow evaluation. These include Barth disease, an X-linked disorder that can cause congenital neutropenia in the setting of hypertrophic cardiomyopathy, and Hermansky-Pudlak syndrome type 2, which is autosomal recessive inheritance of an AP3B1 gene mutation and is associated with albinism [48]. These also include autosomal recessive mutations in the AP14 gene that are associated with albinism and autosomal recessive mutations in the 16ORF57 gene that is also associated with poikiloderma [48]. Glycogen storage type 1b and Cohen syndrome can have congenital neutropenia associated with them [48]. Some authors would classify Shwachman-Diamond syndrome (SDS) (also known as Shwachman-Bodian-Diamond syndrome) as a congenital neutropenia. For this chapter, SDS will be discussed in the next section.

More recently, GATA2 mutations have been identified in up to 10% of patients with congenital neutropenia and/or aplastic anemia. GATA2 deficiency encompasses a large variation in phenotypes that encompass increased risk of infection, cytopenias, myelodysplasia, myeloid leukemias, pulmonary alveolar proteinosis, and lymphedema with the typical age of presentation occurring in adolescence [77]. In 2011, GATA2 mutations were found to be the underlying cause of several different clinical entities, including MonoMAC syndrome, DCML (dendritic cell, monocyte, B and NK lymphoid deficiency), familial AML, and Emberger syndrome (lymphedema and myelodysplasia or leukemia) [77]. GATA2 is a hematopoietic transcription factor, and when mutated, it predisposes to myelodysplasia or AML at very high rates [77]. In fact, 6 of 14 GATA2 deficiency patients identified on the French Severe Chronic Neutropenia Registry had progression to MDS/AML [77].

No matter the underlying cause of SCN, the consequences of congenital neutropenia are similar with infection being a leading cause of morbidity and mortality. Omphalitis may be the presenting symptom that leads to screening with a complete blood count [39]. The preferential sites of infection seem to be skin, mucosa, and pulmonary regions [48]. Patients with untreated SCN almost always have erosive, hemorrhagic, and painful gingivitis associated with papules of the tongue and cheek mucosa after the age of 2 years [48]. It is important to recognize that signs and symptoms of infection may not be typical in the setting of severe neutropenia.

In 1989, a case series was published showing successful use of recombinant human granulocyte colony-stimulating factor (G-CSF) to stimulate neutrophil maturation resulting in higher absolute neutrophil counts was reported [26]. This treatment also resulted in resolution of preexisting chronic infections and reduced the need for antibiotics [26]. For this case series, side effects from treatment included medullary pain, splenomegaly, and elevation of leukocyte alkaline phosphatase [26]. Since this first report, G-CSF has become a critical tool in helping patients with congenital neutropenia, particularly those forms not associated with other immunodeficiency conditions. An area of concern regarding G-CSF therapy continues to be the possibility of malignant transformation, but it is difficult to differentiate the underlying increased risk of malignancy with SCN disorders versus the risk that G-CSF may add to that. The decision to utilize G-CSF must balance the risk of bacterial sepsis and death with the potential of malignant transformation.

An international registry was created with the goal of better understanding the risks and benefits of using G-CSF [49]. This registry was able to collect prospective data from 231 patients with various forms of SCN starting in 1994 and published data in 2005 [49]. In that time period, eight patients died of sepsis and none of these were receiving G-CSF. There were 13 cases of myelodysplastic syndrome or acute leukemia with an incidence of 2.7% at 10 years of treatment and 8.1% at 20 years of treatment exposure. These occurred only in patients with classic SCN of SDS, and when broken down, the risk of leukemia did increase with the degree of G-CSF exposure for the patients with SCN [49]. This has led some to argue that hematopoietic stem cell transplantation (HSCT) should be considered when high doses of G-CSF are needed to prevent sepsis [39].

Current indications for HSCT in the setting of SCN include G-CSF resistance as defined by use of >20 μg/kg/day for more than 1 month without neutrophil normalization, patients with high dosing needs of G-CSF as defined by at least 10 μg/kg/day of G-CSF for at least 3 months per year, patients with recurrent bacterial infections and have a matched family donor, patients with GATA2 mutations and a matched donor available, or those that have undergone transformation to myelodysplasia or leukemia [43].

Shwachman-Bodian-Diamond Syndrome

SDS is a disease characterized by exocrine pancreatic insufficiency, impaired hematopoiesis, and a predisposition to development of leukemia [30]. Similar to DBA, SDS is classified as a "ribosomopathy," but unlike DBA, SDS is always inherited as an autosomal recessive disorder with the exception of about 10% of cases that seem to be de novo mutations [94, 154]. This condition is named after two pediatricians, Harry Shwachman and Louis Diamond, along with an ophthalmologist, Martin Bodian, who were all involved in publishing some of the earliest descriptions of SDS in 1964 [154]. Bodian helped report two patients with congenital hypoplasia of the exocrine pancreas, while Shwachman and Diamond described three patients that had been managed at a cystic fibrosis clinic because of their underlying pancreatic insufficiency, but unlike the patients with cystic fibrosis, these patients also had bone marrow hypoplasia and did not have respiratory complications [25, 132].

After cystic fibrosis, SDS is now known to be the second leading cause of exocrine pancreatic dysfunction in children and has an estimated incidence reported as high as 1/76,563. In 2001, the underlying genetic defect for patients with SDS was mapped to chromosome 7 [63]. Since then, the specific gene has been identified as the SBDS gene, and 90% of patients with SDS are now known to carry one of three common pathogenic SBDS mutations, 183_184TA > CT, 258 + 2T > C, or a combination of these two [154]. Additionally, many novel sequence variations have been identified in patients who are compound heterozygotes with one of the three common gene mutations [154]. Still, about 5–10% of patients with a clinical diagnosis of SDS will not have a mutation identified in the SDBS gene [154]. To that, biallelic mutations in the DNAJ homolog subfamily C member 21 (DNAJC21) gene as well as mutations in the gene encoding for elongation factor-like GTPase 1 (EFL1) have now been associated with patients that have the phenotype of SDS, but not an underlying mutation in SDBS [45, 139, 145]. The following paragraph describes how all three of these gene products are an integral part in ribosome biogenesis.

Specifically, the SDBS gene encodes a protein that acts as an allosteric regulator of the enzyme EFL1 to then disassociate eukaryotic initiation factor 6 (eIF6) from the cytoplasmic pre-60S ribosomal subunit. When mutations occur in the SDBS gene, eIF6 does not disassociate the pre-60S ribosomal subunit, prohibiting it from binding to the 40S subunit to form the final 80S ribosome [154]. There is also a compelling link between the DNAJC21 mutations and ribosomal synthesis as it the encoded protein from DNAJC21 associates with the rRNA necessary for maturation of the 60S ribosomal subunit [145]. As in DBA, these mutations in ribosomal processing lead to activation of p53, resulting in apoptosis. There are now over 13 disorders known to be a result of ribosomal pathway mutations, but it remains to be seen how mutations that all seem to inhibit ribosomal assembly can end up leading to different diseases with distinct phenotypes.

Most patients with SDS will be diagnosed in early childhood. The most common hematologic abnormality is neutropenia which is seen in 88–100% of patients when defined by an absolute neutrophil count <1500 /μL; however, only a third of these patients will have chronic neutropenia while the others will have intermittent neutropenia [30]. Anemia, which can be normocytic or macrocytic, has been described in 42–82% of patients, while thrombocytopenia is reported in 24–88% of patients [30]. Pancytopenia has also been reported [68]. Elevated HbF levels are seen in approximately 80% of patients [30]. Bone marrow evaluations are less helpful as patients can have normal-appearing marrow or marrow that has very subtle signs of dysplasia. Some bone marrow evaluations might show reduction of trabecular bone volume similar to osteoporosis with decreased osteoid, osteoblasts, and osteoclasts [94].

Similarly to patients with SCN, these patients are at increased risk of infections from neutropenia; however, it has also been shown that the neutrophils of patients with SDS don't have normal neutrophil chemotaxis [138]. As such, the risk of infection is not only in quantity but also in the quality of the neutrophils. Lymphocyte defects have also been described with some patients having decreased B cells, low immunoglobulin G levels, decreased B-cell proliferation, decreased levels of natural killer cells, decreased T lymphocytes, decreased T-cell proliferation, as well as inverse ratios of CD4 to CD8 cells [30].

As with many other IBMFS, SDS can progress to aplastic anemia, myelodysplastic syndrome (MDS), or acute myeloid leukemia (AML). Several registries have reported data, but given the small numbers and other confounding factors, estimating the true rate of malignant transformation is very difficult. One registry reported numbers as high as 36% by age 30 years, and this is similar to another registry that estimated rate of transformation to MDS or AML as 1% per year [75].

Exocrine pancreatic dysfunction caused from the absence of pancreatic acinar cells is a key feature of SDS and commonly presents as early as infancy with malabsorption, steatorrhea, failure to thrive, and low levels of fat soluble vitamins [30]. Patients with SDS should have a normal sweat chloride test but may have low fecal elastase levels, low pancreatic trypsinogen, and low pancreatic isoamylase levels [30]. Caution should be used when interpreting these test results as fecal elastase can be normal, pancreatic trypsinogen tends to normalize after the age of 3 years even if the patient has SDS, and isoamylase levels can be low in children less than 3 years of age even if they do not have SDS [30]. Pancreatic imaging can be helpful as it most often shows a small, structurally abnormal pancreas that has largely been replaced by fat [30]. One report suggested that the frequency of this finding by MRI was high enough that SBDS gene mutations were unlikely when this was not found [143]. It is important to note though that this study was a small cohort of 14 patients with SDS [143]. Fortunately, about 50% of patients will show spontaneous improvement in pancreatic exocrine function, while pancreatic endocrine function most commonly remains intact [30]. Hepatomegaly, elevation of serum transaminases, periportal and portal inflammatory infiltration with or without fibrosis, and steatosis can all occur early in childhood but seem to resolve after about the age of 3 years; however, older patients can have cholestasis and hepatic microcysts [30].

Another common finding in patients with SDS is that of skeletal abnormalities. About half of patients with SDS will have metaphyseal dysostosis, most commonly involving the femoral head, but other sites are reported [2, 30, 62] (Fig. 4.6). Rib cage abnormalities are also relatively common with a few case reports of severe rib cage dysmorphology leading to neonatal respiratory distress [37]. Consistent with the bone marrow pathology that can be seen, low turnover osteopenia and osteoporosis have also been reported [30, 75].

Cardiac manifestations are also reported in patients with SDS. Specifically, myocardial fibrosis has been found at autopsy and ventricular dysfunction has been described, particularly during exercise studies [30, 142, 143]. With vast variations, neurocognitive impairment is becoming more recognized in patients with SDS [75]. There are also reports of insulin-dependent diabetes, growth hormone deficiency, hypogonadotropic hypogonadism, hypothyroidism, urinary tract anomalies, renal tubular acidosis, eczema, ichthyosis, cleft palate, and renal calculi in patients with SDS [30, 68].

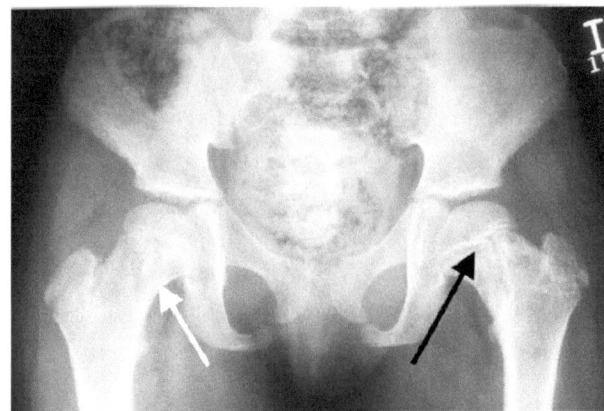

Fig. 4.6 Pelvis radiograph of patient with SDS. There is prominent sclerosis and lucency of both proximal metaphysis (black arrow) and femoral necks (white arrow). These changes extend into the subtrochanteric regions. The acetabular roofs are horizontal [83]. Used with permission

Establishing a diagnosis can be difficult at times due to the clinical heterogeneity of SDS. When considering this diagnosis, it is important to consider and try to exclude other syndromes that could present similarly, such as cystic fibrosis, Pearson's syndrome, FA, DC, and SCN. Several diagnostic studies could be helpful, and the following tests should be considered: a complete blood count, reticulocyte count, bone marrow aspirate, and biopsy to include cytogenetic studies and iron staining, trypsinogen if the patient is less than 3 years old, pancreatic isoamylase if greater than 3 years old, fecal elastase, a 72 h fecal fat test, fat soluble vitamin levels, and genetic analysis [30]. It is important to remember that the genetic mutation is not necessary to establish a diagnosis of SDS. Other testing that could be helpful include hepatic transaminase levels, gamma-glutamyl transferase, albumin level, prealbumin level, prothrombin time (PT), partial thromboplastin time (PTT), immunoglobulin levels (IgA, IgG, and IgM), T and B lymphocyte subset analysis, pancreatic imaging, X-ray evaluation for skeletal involvement, and an echocardiogram [30, 120].

In 2002, an international conference developed guidelines to help in management decisions for patients with SDS [120]. These guidelines recommend that initial follow-up occurs every 1 to 3 months to help the patient and family adjust to the diagnosis and provide educational review [120]. Every 6–12 months, complete physical exams, assessment of pubertal development, developmental progress, and evaluation of nutritional status should be completed [120]. These visits should include a minimum laboratory evaluation of a complete blood count, serum concentrations of vitamin A, vitamin E, 25-OH-vitamin D, and PT/PTT to help assess the potential for vitamin K deficiency since serum levels of vitamin K are not as reliable [120]. Comprehensive care should include pediatric gastroenterologist, pediatric hematologist, and may need to include a registered nutritionist, orthopedic physician, developmental specialist, or other subspecialist as indicated by symptoms. Most patients will develop normal pancreatic function by the age of 4 years; therefore, ongoing need for pancreatic enzyme supplementation should also be assessed periodically [120]. Bone marrow evaluation with aspirate and biopsy to include cytogenetic testing is recommended yearly given the increased risk of MDS, acute leukemia, and other clonal disease [30].

Treatment for patients with SDS should include G-CSF for those patients that are neutropenic and have recurrent or severe infections [30]. As discussed in the section on SCN, malignant transformation is a concern; however, data is inconclusive as to the effect G-CSF may have in development of leukemia, so it should not be held based upon this concern, particularly with the risks associated with infections and immune dysfunction [30]. About half of the patients with SDS will need pancreatic enzyme supplementation for some period of time [30].

Hematopoietic stem cell transplantation (HSCT) should be considered in the context of disease severity. The primary causes of death during infancy are malabsorption, infections, and thoracic dystrophy, whereas older patients succumb to hemorrhage, infection, and hematologic complications [30]. Limited data is available regarding use of HSCT in patients with SDS, but several cases have described complications, such as congestive heart failure, cardiac hypokinesia, pancarditis, severe graft versus host disease, and severe hepatic toxicity [30]. Transplant-related mortality is high at 30–40% thought due to intensive conditioning regimens and increased toxicity seen in patients with SDS [43]. Because of these considerations and the relatively high mortality rate, no clear guidelines have been established as to when to consider HSCT, but certainly, HSCT should be considered with worsening cytopenias, increased need for transfusions, or transformation to MDS or leukemia [43].

Pancytopenia

Pancytopenia is defined as an abnormal decrease in in all three hematopoietic cell lines, but varying degrees in each cell line may be present at presentation. While the differential is broad and includes multiple causes of impaired production, destruction, or a combination of both, this chapter will focus on pancytopenia secondary to inherited bone marrow failure syndromes (IBMFS). Of the IBMFS, Fanconi anemia (FA) and dyskeratosis congenita are the two most likely to present with some degree of pancytopenia.

Fanconi Anemia

Fanconi anemia is an IBMFS that is associated with congenital abnormalities as well as a predisposition to cancer. The congenital abnormalities associated with FA include café au lait spots, short stature, hypoplastic or absent thumbs, male hypogonadism, microcephaly, microphthalmia, renal anomalies, low birth weight, developmental disabilities, and hearing loss (Table 4.3). Patients with FA may also have a common syndrome known as VACTERL that includes vertebral anomalies, anal atresia, cardiac abnormalities, tracheaesophageal fistula, and renal and radial limb anomalies [15]. A fraction of patients with FA will not have any associated abnormalities [5, 51]. Like many of the other IBMFS, this spectrum of clinical presentation necessitates consideration of FA with or without the presence of dysmorphology, particularly in the setting of pancytopenia.

In the United States, the incidence is reported as 1 in 300 live births with an increased incidence in Ashkenazi Jews and Afrikaners [5, 15, 51]. In the vast majority of cases, FA is inherited in an autosomal recessive pattern; however, one of the genes known to rarely cause FA is inherited in an X-linked fashion [5, 24].

There are 16 distinct genes associated with FA (FANCA, FANCB, FANCC, FANCD1/BRCA2, FANCD2, FANCE, FANCF, FANCG, FANCI, FANCJ/BRIP1, FANCL, FANCM, FANCN/PALB2, FANCO/RAD51C, FANCP/SLX4, FANCQ) [153]. These genes play a role in DNA repair by correcting DNA interstrand cross-links. The most common gene mutation involved is FANCA. FANCB is the only gene known to be associated with FA that is found on the X chromosome [135].

Table 4.3 Congenital malformations in patients in the International Fanconi Anemia Registry (IFAR) [15]

Skin	Café-au-lait spots hyper- and hypopigmentation
Growth	Intrauterine growth retardation, short stature, endocrine abnormalities
Eyes	Microphthalmia, short or almond-shaped palpebral fissures, ptosis, epicanthal folds, hyper-and hypotelorism, strabismus, cataracts
Thumb and radius	Thenar hypoplasia, absence or hypoplasia of radius and/or thumb, floating thumb, bifid thumb, digitalized thumb/abnormal thumb placement
Other skeletal	Dysplastic or absent ulna, micrognathia, frontal bossing, spina bifida, Klippel-Feil, vertebral anomalies, absent clavicles, Sprengel's deformity, Perthes disease, congenital hip dysplasia/dislocation, scoliosis, rib abnormalities, clubfoot, sacral agenesis (hypoplasia), leg length discrepancy, kyphosis, brachydactyly, arachnodactyly, humeral abnormality, craniosynostosis
Kidney and urinary tract	Ectopic, horseshoe, rotated, hypoplastic or absent, dysplastic, hydronephrosis, hydroureter, urethral stenosis, reflux
Ears	Deafness (usually conductive), abnormal or absent pinna, prominent ears, abnormally positioned ears (low set or posteriorly rotated), small or absent ear canals, absent tympanic membrane, microtia, fused ossicles
Genital	Males: micropenis, penile/scrotal fusion, undescended or atrophic or absent testes, hypospadias, chordee, phimosis, azospermia Females: bicornuate uterus, aplasia or hypoplasia of vagina and uterus, atresia of vagina, hypoplastic uterus, hypoplastic/absent ovary, hypoplastic/fused labia
Cardio-pulmonary	Patent ductus arteriosus, ventricular septal defect, pulmonic or aortic stenosis, coarctation of the aorta, double aortic arch, cardiomyopathy, tetralogy of Fallot, pulmonary atresia
Gastrointestinal	Esophageal atresia, duodenal atresia, anal atresia, tracheoesophageal fistula, annular pancreas, intestinal malrotation, intestinal obstruction, duodenal web, biliary atresia, foregut duplication cyst
Central nervous system (CNS)	Microcephaly, hydrocephalus. Bell's palsy, CNS arterial malformations, abnormal pituitary, absent septum pellucidum/corpus callosum, hyperreflexia, neural tube defection, Arnold-Chiari malformation, moyamoya, single ventricle

The Fanconi anemia pathway is shown in Fig. 4.7. When interstrand cross-links develop in DNA due to stress, replication and transcription are unable to occur. FANCM's role is to recognize these interstrand cross-links and to form an anchor complex with FAAP24, MHF1, and MHF2. FANCA, FANCB, FANCC, FANCE, FANCF, FANCG, and FANCL along with FAAP20 and FAAP100 make up the core complex. The core complex adds a single ubiquitin to FANCD2 and FANCI which allows for formation of a heterodimer, ID2, which is a critical component of DNA repair [80, 153]. Downstream repair factors, FANCD1/BRCA2, FANCJ, FANCN, and FANCO, are activated by the monoubiquitination step and also play an important role in repair. Mutations within these latter genes are associated with increased risk of breast cancer and ovarian cancer [153].

The hematologic manifestations of FA occur at a median age of 7 years with BMF occurring in 90% of patients by age 40 years [6, 15]. Laboratory findings concerning for FA include varying degrees of cytopenias, with thrombocytopenia

Fig. 4.7 Schematic of the complexes in the Fanconi anemia pathway. The FANCI/FANCD2 (ID2) complex is depicted in blue/green. The core complex is shown in gold, and the anchor complex shown in pink/purple. Downstream repair factors are in gray. Each complex is thought to exist separately but converge at sites of DNA interstrand cross-links (*red lines*). Abbreviation: Ub ubiquitin [153]. Used with permission

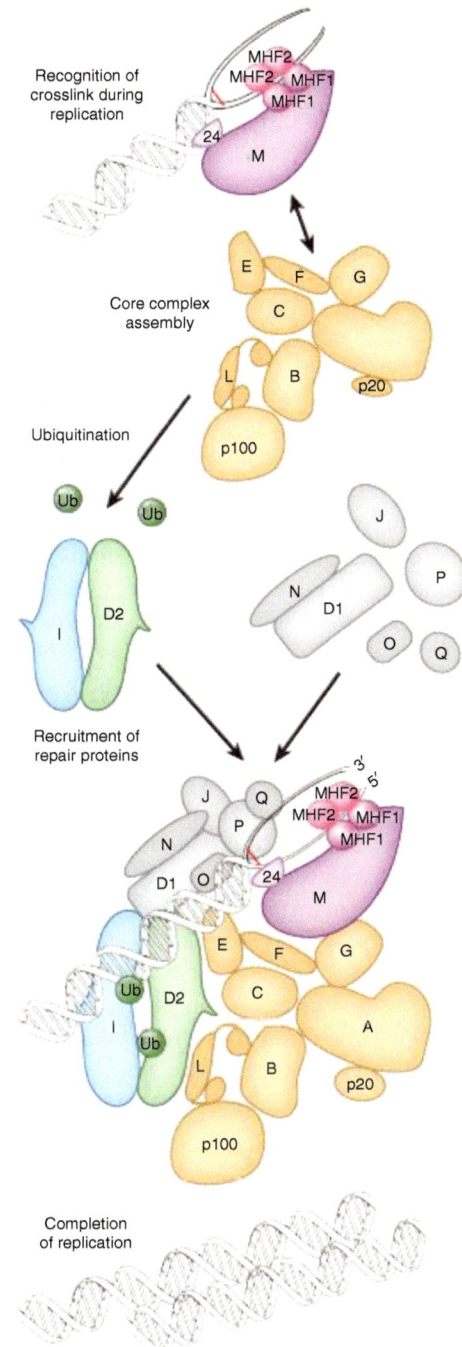

typically occurring first. In addition to the cytopenias, macrocytosis, elevated fetal hemoglobin, and elevated red blood cell membrane "i" antigens can also be present. These latter findings are nonspecific to FA as they can be seen as part of many bone marrow failure syndromes. Sometimes, FA is not diagnosed until development of myelodysplasia (MDS) or acute myeloid leukemia (AML) [15].

Patients with FA are 800 to 1000 times more likely to develop cancer in their lifetime when compared to the general population [24]. More specifically, in patients with FA, the incidence of leukemia or MDS by 25 years of age is 10% and 5%, respectively [6]. By 40 years of age, the risk of developing MDS or AML is reported as high as 52% [15]. Compared to the general population, patients with FA have a 500- to 700-fold increased risk of head and neck cancer, particularly squamous cell carcinoma [15]. Women with FA are also at increased risk for gynecologic cancers that include uterine, cervical, and vulvar. In one study, the median age of onset for leukemia in patients with FA was 11.3 years compared to 28.9 years for solid tumors [118]. The risk of cancer is higher, particularly at younger ages, for patients with the FANCD1/BRCA2 mutations [153]. Because of the inability to repair DNA well, patients with FA are particularly sensitive to chemotherapy and radiation. This necessitates modification of traditional chemotherapy regimens and leaves surgery alone as the preferred treatment modality when possible.

A complete history and physical exam are vital when determining the cause of pancytopenia. When present, classic dysmorphologic features such as thumb anomalies can be very helpful, but as above, the absence of any abnormal physical exam findings does not preclude a diagnosis of FA. In addition to a thorough physical examination, it is also important to make use of a standardized growth curve to help objectively determine if short stature is present. A detailed family history can often be helpful, particularly when looking for inheritance patterns. Blood work should include a complete blood count with differential and a reticulocyte count. If this continues to support a possible diagnosis of an IBMFS, a bone marrow evaluation with bone marrow biopsy should be obtained. For FA, a marrow evaluation typically shows a hypocellular marrow; however cases of normocellular and hypercellular marrows are known to occur and do not exclude the possibility of FA.

To aid in the diagnosis of FA, a chromosome breakage study can be obtained. In patients with FA, this study should show an increased chromosome breakage to cross-linking agents such as mitomycin C or diepoxybutane (DEB) [51]. Keep in mind that these results can be skewed if there is mosaicism within the cells. When a family history of FA is known, particularly if the gene involved is known, testing with a targeted gene mutation can be diagnostic. If there is no known family history, it is often helpful to send a genetic panel that includes testing for the most common genes associated with FA [15].

Once a diagnosis of FA is confirmed, family members should be offered screening with chromosome breakage or targeted gene testing if the gene involved has been identified. Given the known complications associated with FA, regular involvement by an ophthalmologist, endocrinologist, gynecologist, otolaryngologist, and hematologist should be arranged. Screening tests should include hearing tests and renal ultrasounds. Some guidelines recommend complete blood counts every 6 months to a year with a yearly bone marrow evaluation that includes testing for MDS and leukemia.

If mild findings of bone marrow failure are found, frequency of future evaluations should increase. Once moderate findings of bone marrow failure are seen, consider hematopoietic stem cell transplant (HSCT) if a matched related donor is available. Otherwise androgen therapy and growth factor (GCSF or GM-CSF) can be used to support these patients. There is some controversy of the use of growth factor in these patients given malignant potential. Historically, patients with FA have poorer outcomes after transplant with a matched unrelated done; therefore, transplant with a matched unrelated donor is reserved for patients who are more severely affected by bone marrow failure or those who have developed MDS or AML. HSCT is considered curative for the marrow failure associated with FA, but due to the uniqueness of the patients and sensitivity to the preparative regimen, these transplants should be performed at an institution that is experienced with transplanting patients with FA. Reduced intensity preparative regimens typically include the use of fludarabine and exclude the use of radiation due to its decreased morbidity and mortality when compared to higher intensity regimens [44]. The use of gene therapy in FA is still under investigation.

Dyskeratosis Congenita

Dyskeratosis congenita (DC) is an inherited bone marrow failure syndrome that is classically described as a triad of clinical findings, including abnormal skin pigmentation, nail dystrophy, and oral leukoplakia [149]. Inheritance patterns for DC include autosomal recessive, autosomal dominant, and, most commonly, X-linked recessive [127, 149]. That being said, the majority of cases within the DC registry seem to be sporadic in nature [152]. The known genetic mutations involve genes products that play a role in telomere maintenance and/or protection which is involved in maintaining chromosomal integrity.

To understand the pathophysiology, it is important to know the function of a few key proteins, such as telomerase, shelterin, and CST complex. Telomerase, a ribonucleoprotein complex, functions as a reverse transcriptase by adding a DNA sequence, TTAGGG, to the end of chromosomes, allowing for stability. Shelterin is a complex that protects the telomere sequences and prevents the activation of cell cycle checkpoints [22]. The CST complex promotes telomere DNA synthesis and inhibits the extension of the telomere by telomerase [34]. With each cell cycle, telomeres shorten, and once they become too short, cell death occurs [152].

The core of the telomerase complex includes telomerase reverse transcriptase (TERT) and the telomerase RNA component (TERC). TERC also contains the H/ACA domain. This domain is responsible for binding four proteins: dyskerin, GAR1, NOP10, and NHP2 as seen in Fig. 4.8a [22, 24, 114]. Specific to telomeres, shelterin is made up of six proteins: telomeric repeat binding factor 1 and 2 (TRF1 and TRF2), protection of telomeres 1 (POT1), TRF2- and TRF1-interacting nuclear protein 2 (TIN2), Rap1, TPP1, and POT1. TRF1 and TRF2 bind the duplex part of telomeres and POT1 binds the 3′ end with the TTAGGG repeats. TIN2, Rap1, TPP1, and POT1 are bound to the telomeres via TRF1 and TRF2, Fig. 4.8b [22, 109].

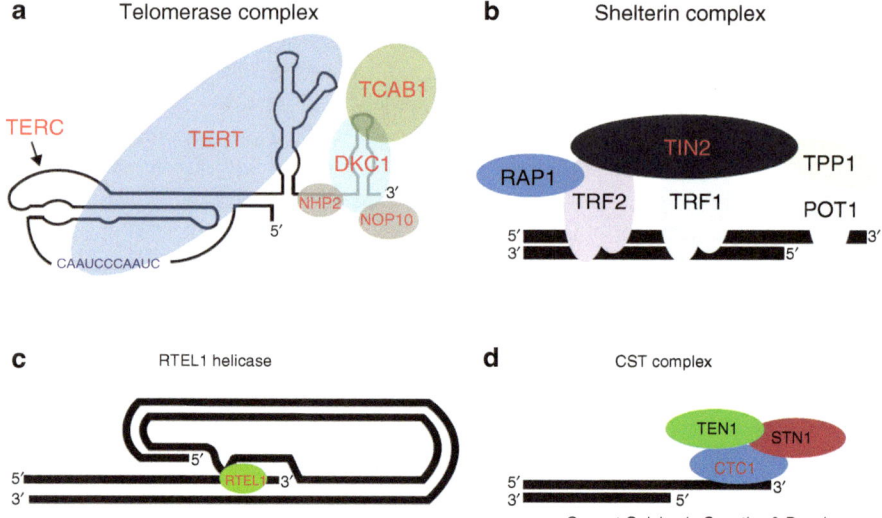

Fig. 4.8 (**a–d**) Depiction of the germline mutations in DC [22]. Used with permission

Regulator of telomere elongation 1 (RTEL1) is a DNA helicase that plays a role in telomere elongation, Fig. 4.8c [18, 22]. The CST complex is a trimeric complex that is made up of CTC1, STN1, and TEN1. This structure binds to ssDNA and allows for telomere DNA synthesis, Fig. 4.8d [22, 34].

The pathologic features of DC are secondary to shortened telomeres and thus decreased stability resulting in degradation resulting in premature cellular death. There are currently nine recognized germline mutations in the telomere pathway associated with DC; however, these are only found in 60–70% of patients with DC [128]. Currently, the genes known to be involved with DC are DKC1, TERT, TERC, TINF2, WRAP53, NOP10, NHP2, CTC1, and RTEL1 [152].

As above, an X-linked inheritance pattern is the most common pattern seen for patients with DC. Interesting, about half of these patients have a mutation in the dyskerin (DKC1) gene at Xq28, while no known mutation has been found for the other half of the families with an X-linked inheritance pattern [111]. TERC mutations are typically inherited in an autosomal dominant pattern with mutations found on chromosome 3q26 [151]. TERT mutations can be inherited in an autosomal dominant or recessive manner [22, 152]. TINF2 encodes for TIN2 and mutations are typically inherited in an autosomal dominant fashion. Mutations in CTC1 are associated with autosomal recessive DC. RTEL1 mutations are typically seen in autosomal recessive forms but have been reported in autosomal dominant inheritance patterns as well [128]. NOP10 mutations are inherited in an autosomal recessive fashion and have been reported in a consanguineous family [150].

DC is associated with a spectrum of clinical findings with variability seen to correspond to the exact mutation involved. The bone marrow failure associated with DC varies in onset and severity; however, greater than 90% of patients develop pancytopenia by the age 40 years [24, 52]. Many other clinical manifestations can be seen in DC as seen in Table 4.4 [127]. In the classic form of DC, the nail and skin findings are typically present in the first decade of life. Pulmonary complications such as pulmonary fibrosis are a known feature of DC and not only seen as a complication from hematopoietic stem cell transplant. There are atypical versions of DC where idiopathic pulmonary fibrosis is the only clinical finding and these are associated with TERC mutations [11, 24]. Due to family history of DC screening, telomere length can identify patients with germline mutations in TERT and TERC despite those with few symptoms [12].

Table 4.4 Clinical findings of dyskeratosis congenita [127]

System	Findings
Dermatologic	Lacey, reticular pigmentation, primarily of the neck and chest; may be subtle or diffuse hyper- or hypopigmentation Abnormal fingernails and toenails may be subtle, with ridging, flaking, or poor growth or more diffuse with nearly complete loss of nails Early gray hair or hair loss Hyperhidrosis
Growth and development	Short stature Intrauterine growth retardation Developmental delay
Ophthalmic	Epiphora due to stenosis of the lacrimal drainage system Blepheritis Sparse eyelashes, ectropion, entropion, trichiasis Exudative retinopathy (Revesz syndrome)
Dental	Dental caries, maybe less frequent now because of improved dental hygiene Periodontal disease Decreased root/crown ratio Taurodontism (enlarged pulp chambers of the teeth)
Ear, nose, throat	Oral leukoplakia Deafness (rare) Squamous cell head and neck cancer
Cardiovascular	Rare reported defects include atrial or ventricular septal defects, fibrosis, and dilated cardiomyopathy
Respiratory	Pulmonary fibrosis
Gastrointestinal	Esophageal stenosis Enteropathy Liver fibrosis
Genitourinary	Urethral stenosis in male patients Epithelial cancers
Musculoskeletal	Osteoporosis Avascular necrosis of the hips and shoulders
Neurologic	Developmental delay Microcephaly Cerebellar hypoplasia (Hoyeraal-Hreidarsson syndrome) Intracranial calcifications (Revesz syndrome)
Psychiatric	Schizophrenia (two case reports)
Endocrine	Hypogonadism
Hematologic	BMF a common presenting sign MDS Leukemia
Immunologic	Immunodeficiency

Mutations in the DKC1 gene have shown great variability in clinical symptoms between patients from minimal symptoms to a severe form called Hoyeraal-Hreidarsson syndrome (HHS) that develops very early in childhood and is associated with death during childhood. The characteristics of HHS are intrauterine growth retardation, microcephaly, cerebellar hypoplasia, mental retardation, progressive combined immunodeficiency, and aplastic anemia [140]. In contrast, with X-inactivation, affected female carriers of DKC1 mutation tend to present with the associated skin findings of DC but not the bone marrow failure [24].

Another severe form of DC is known as Revesz syndrome, which is characterized by bilateral exudative retinopathy, intrauterine growth retardation, fine hair, fine reticulate skin pigmentation, cerebellar hypoplasia, extensor hypertonia, psychomotor retardation, and progressive bone marrow failure. This syndrome is also associated with death during childhood [117]. TINF2 mutations have been found in patients with Revesz syndrome; however this mutation has not been found in all patients with Revesz syndrome [126].

Clinical presentation varies greatly and onset of symptoms does not follow a particular pattern in that clinical exam findings may occur before or after the laboratory changes associated with pancytopenia. As such, clinicians should have a low threshold to consider the diagnosis of DC. As with FA, a detailed family history has the potential to provide much insight and potentially reveal the opportunity for targeted genetic testing. Once suspected, testing telomere length is warranted. If hematologic abnormalities are present, a bone marrow evaluation should be undertaken. There are commercial genetic panels that test for the known genes involved in DC. If a genetic mutation is identified, screening family members with telomere testing, a complete blood count, and pulmonary function testing is warranted. Offering genetic counseling is also indicated.

The only curative treatment for the bone marrow failure associated with DC is a hematopoietic stem cell transplant; however, outcome data is fairly dismal. In one review, the overall survival at 5 years posttransplant was 50%; however that declined significantly and the 10-year overall survival was only 23%. Reported causes of death within the first year of transplant were infection, pulmonary disease, and failure to engraft; leading causes of death after the first year were pulmonary disease and liver disease. Improved short-term outcomes are seen among those transplanted younger than age 20 years with a reduced intensity preparative regimen and with a matched sibling donor; however, 10-year overall survival remains unchanged [21].

DC is also a cancer predisposition syndrome and includes increased incidence of MDS, AML, and solid tumors [8, 47, 127]. The most common types of solid tumors include head and neck squamous cell carcinomas, skin squamous cell carcinomas, and adenocarcinoma of the stomach, lung, and colon. By age 50, the risk of cancer in DC patients is approximately 40% [8]. Patients with a diagnosis of DC should undergo appropriate screening with particular involvement of a dermatologist, dentist (leukoplakia), otolaryngologist, and gynecologist for female patients.

References

1. Aase JM, Smith DW. Congenital anemia and triphalangeal thumbs: a new syndrome. J Pediatr. 1969;74(3):471–4.
2. Aggett PJ, Cavanagh NP, Matthew DJ, Pincott JR, Sutcliffe J, Harries JT. Shwachman's syndrome. A review of 21 cases. Arch Dis Child. 1980;55(5):331–47.
3. Al-Ahmari A, Ayas M, Al-Jefri A, Al-Mahr M, Rifai S, El Solh H. Allogeneic stem cell transplantation for patients with congenital amegakaryocytic thrombocytopenia (CAT). Bone Marrow Transplant. 2004;33:829–31.
4. Albers CA, Newbury-Ecob R, Ouwehand WH, Ghevaert C. New insights into the genetic basis of TAR (thrombocytopenia-absent radii) syndrome. Curr Opin Genet Dev. 2013;23:316–23.
5. Alter BP. Bone marrow failure syndromes in children. Pediatr Clin N Am. 2002;49:973–88.
6. Alter BP. Cancer in Fanconi Anemia. Blood. 2003;101(5):2072–3.
7. Alter BP. Inherited bone marrow failure syndromes: considerations pre- and posttransplant. Blood. 2017;130(21):2257–64. https://doi.org/10.1182/blood-2017-05-781799.
8. Alter BP, Girl N, Savage SA, Rosenberg PS. Cancer in dyskeratosis congenita. Blood. 2009;113(26):6549–57.
9. Alter BP, Girl N, Savage SA, Rosenberg PS. Cancer in the national Cancer institute inherited bone marrow failure syndrome cohort after fifteen years of follow-up. Haematologica. 2018;103(1):30–9. https://doi.org/10.3324/haematol.2017.178111.
10. Amanatiadou EP, Papadopoulos GL, Stouboulis J, Vizirianakis IS. GATA1 and PU.1 bind to ribosomal protein genes in erythroid cells: implications for ribosomopathis. PLoS One. 2015;10(10):e0140077. https://doi.org/10.1371/journal.pone.0140077.
11. Armanios M. Telomerase and idiopathic pulmonary fibrosis. Mutat Res. 2012;730(1–2):52–8. https://doi.org/10.1016/j.mrfmmm.2011.10.013.
12. Armanios MY, Chen JJ, Cogan JD, Alder JK, Ingersoll RG, Markin C, Lawson WE, Xie M, Vulto I, Phillips JA, Lansdorp PM, Greider CW, Loyd JE. Telomerase mutations in families with idiopathic pulmonary fibrosis. N Engl J Med. 2007;356:1317–26.
13. Ask K, Jasencakova Z, Menard P, Feng Y, Almouzni G, Groth A. Codanin-1, mutated in the anaemic disease CDA1, regulates Asf1 function in S-phase histone supply. EMBO J. 2012;31(8):2013–23. https://doi.org/10.1038/emboj.2012.55.
14. Atale A, Bonneau-Amati P, Rötig A, Fischer A, Perez-Martin S, de Lonlay P, Niaudet P, De Parscau L, Mousson C, Thauvin-Robinet C, Munnich A, Huet F, Faivre L. Tubulopathy and pancytopenia with normal pancreatic function: a variant of Pearson syndrome. Eur J Med Genet. 2009;52(1):23–6. https://doi.org/10.1016/j.ejmg.2008.10.003.
15. Auerbach A. Fanconi anemia and its diagnosis. Mutat Res. 2009;668:4–10. https://doi.org/10.1016/j.mrfmmm.2009.01.013.
16. Ayas M, al-Jefri A, Baothman A, al-Mahr M, Mustafa MM, Khalil S, Karaoui M, Solh H. Transfusion-dependent congenital dyserythropoietic anemia type I successfully treated with allogeneic stem cell transplantation. Bone Marrow Transplant. 2002;29(8):681–2.
17. Ball SE, McGuckin CP, Jenkins G, Gordon-Smith EC. Diamond-Blackfan anaemia in the U.K.: analysis of 80 cases from a 20-year birth cohort. Br J Haematol. 1996;94(4):645–53.
18. Ballew BJ, Yeager M, Jacobs K, Giri N, Boland J, Burdett L, Alter BP, Savage SA. Germline mutations in regulator of telomere elongation helicase 1, RTEL1, in dyskeratosis congenita. Hum Genet. 2013;132:473–80. https://doi.org/10.1007/s00439-013-1265-8.
19. Ballmaier M, Germeshausen M. Congenital amegakaryocytic thrombocytopenia: clinical presentation, diagnosis, and treatment. Semin Thromb Hemost. 2011;37(6):673–81. https://doi.org/10.1055/s-0031-1291377.
20. Ballmaier M, Schulze H, Straub G, Cherkaoui K, Wittner N, Lynen S, Wolters S, Bogenberger J, Welte K. Thrombopoietin in patients with congenital thrombocytopenia and absent radii: elevated serum levels, normal receptor expression, but defective reactivity to thrombopoietin. Blood. 1997;90(2):612–9.

21. Barbaro P, Vedi A. Survival after hematopoietic stem cell transplant in patients with dys-keratosis congenita: systematic review of the literature. Biol Blood Marrow Transplant. 2016;22(7):1152–8.
22. Batista L, Artandi SE. Understanding telomere diseases through analysis of patient-derived iPS cells. Curr Opin Genet Dev. 2013;23:526–33.
23. Ben Ami T, Batour M, Rakhtman D, et al. Iron deficiency anemia as a leading cause of severe anemia in children may be associated with unnecessary red bleed cells (RBCs) transfusion. Blood. 2015;126:4454.
24. Bessler M, Mason PJ, Link DC, Wilson DB. Inherited bone marrow failure syndromes. In: Orkin S, Nathan D, Ginsburg D, Look AT, Fisher D, Lux S, editors. Nathan and Oski's hematology of infancy and childhood. Philadelphia: Saunders; 2009. p. 307–95.
25. Bodian M, Sheldon W, Lightwood R. Congenital hypoplasia of the exocrine pancreas. Acta Paediatr. 1964;53:282–93.
26. Bonilla MA, Gillio AP, Ruggeiro M, Kernan NA, Brochstein JA, Abboud M, Fumagalli L, Vincent M, Gabrilove JL, Welte K, Souza LM, O'Reily RJ. Effects of recombinant human granulocyte colony-stimulating factor on neutropenia in patients with congenital agranulocytosis. N Engl J Med. 1989;320(24):1574–80.
27. Boogaerts MA, Verwilghen R. Variants of congenital dyserythropoietic anaemia: an update. Haematologia (Budap). 1982;15(2):211–9.
28. Boussaid I, Le Goff S, Floquet C, Raimbault A, Andrieu-Soler C, Gautier E, Kosmider O, Hatin I, Narla M, Soler E, Mayeux P, Fontenay M. Ribosome biogenesis controls erythroid differentiation via a p53-dependent transcriptional checkpoint and its limitation by RPS14 haploinsufficiency results in selective defects in translation. Blood. 2017;130:83.
29. Braun M, Wölfl M, Wiegering V, Winkler B, Ertan K, Bald R, Schwarz K, Heimpel H, Eyrich M, Schlegel PG. Successful treatment of an infant with CDA type II by intrauterine transfusions and postnatal stem cell transplantation. Pediatr Blood Cancer. 2014;61(4):743–5. https://doi.org/10.1002/pbc.24786.
30. Burroughs L, Woolfrey A, Shimamura A. Shwachman-Diamond syndrome: a review of the clinical presentation, molecular pathogenesis, diagnosis, and treatment. Hematol Oncol Clin North Am. 2009;23(2):233–48. https://doi.org/10.1016/j.hoc.2009.01.007.
31. Calis JC, Phiri KS, Faragher EB, Brabin BJ, Bates I, Cuevas LE, de Haan RJ, Phiri AI, Malange P, Khoka M, Hulshof PJ, van Lieshout L, Beld MG, Teo YY, Rockett KA, Richardson A, Kwiatkowski DP, Molyneux ME, van Hensbroek MB. Severe anemia in Malawian children. N Engl J Med. 2008;358(9):888–99. https://doi.org/10.1056/NEJMoa072727.
32. Camitta BM, Rock A. Acute lymphoidic leukemia in a patient with thrombocytopenia/absent radii (TAR) syndrome. Am J Pediatr Hematol Oncol. 1993;15(3):335–7.
33. Cathie IAB. Erythrogenesis Imperfecta. Arch Dis Child. 1950;25(124):313–24.
34. Chen LY, Majerska J, Lingner J. Molecular basis of telomere syndrome caused by CTC1 mutations. Genes Dev. 2013;27:2099–108.
35. Crookston JH, Godwin TF, Wightmann KJR, Dacie JV, Lewis SM, Patterson M. Congenital dyserythropoietic anemia. Sydney: Abstr XIth Congress Int Soc Hematol; 1966.
36. Da Costa L, O'Donohue MF, van Dooijeweert B, Albrecht K, Unal S, Ramenghi U, Leblanc T, Dianzani I, Tamary H, Bartels M, Gleizes PE, Wlodarkski M, MacInnes AW. Molecular approaches to diagnose Diamond-Blackfan anemia: the EuroDBA experience. Eur J Med Genet. 2017; pii:S1769-7212(17)30505-0. https://doi.org/10.1016/j.ejmg.2017.10.017.
37. Danks DM, Haslam R, Mayne V, Kaufmann HJ, Holtzapple PG. Metaphyseal chondrodysplasia, neutropenia, and pancreatic insufficiency presenting with respiratory distress in the neonatal period. Arch Dis Child. 1976;51(9):697–702.
38. Dauwerse JG, Dixon J, Seland S, Ruivenkamp CA, van Haeringen A, Hoefsloot LH, Peters DJ, Boers AC, Daumer-Haas C, Maiwald R, Zweier C, Kerr B, Cobo AM, Toral JF, Hoogeboom AJ, Lohmann DR, Hehr U, Dixon MJ, Breuning MH, Wieczorek D. Mutations in genes encoding subunits of RNA polymerase I and III cause Treacher Collins syndrome. Nat Genet. 2011;43:20–2. https://doi.org/10.1038/ng.724.

39. Dale DC. ELANE-Related Neutropenia In: GeneReviews. University of Washington. 2011. http://www.ncbi.nlm.nih.gov/books/NBK1116. Accessed 28 April 2018. / Bookshelf ID: NBK1533. PMID: 20301705.

40. Dale DC, Person RE, Bolyard AA, Aprikyan AG, Bos C, Bonilla MA, Boxer LA, Kannourakis G, Zeidler C, Welte K, Benson KF, Horwitz M. Mutations in the gene encoding neutrophil elastase in congenital and cyclic neutropenia. Blood. 2000;96(7):2317–22.

41. Denecke J, Marquardt T. Congenital dyerythropoietic anemia type II (CDAII/HEMPAS): where are we now? Biochim Biophys Acta. 2009;1792(9):915–20. https://doi.org/10.1016/j.bbadis.2008.12.005.

42. Dgany O, Avidan N, Delaunay J, Krasnov T, Shalmon L, Shalev H, Eidelitz-Markus T, Kapelushnik J, Cattan D, Pariente A, Tulliez M, Crétien A, Schischmanoff PO, Iolascon A, Fibach E, Koren A, Rössler J, Le Merrer M, Yaniv I, Zaizov R, Ben-Asher E, Olender T, Lancet D, Beckmann JS, Tamary H. Congenital dyserythropoietic anemia type I is caused by mutations in codanin-1. Am J Hum Genet. 2002;71(6):1467–74.

43. de Latour PR, Peters C, Gibson B, Strahm B, Lankester A, de Heredia CD, Longoni D, Fioredda F, Locatelli F, Yaniv I, Wachowiak J, Donadieu J, Lawitschka A, Bierings M, Wlodarski M, Corbacioglu S, Bonanomi S, Samarasinghe S, Leblanc T, Dufour C, Dalle JH, Pediatric Working Party of the European Group for Blood and Marrow Transplantation; Severe Aplastic Anemia Working Party of the European Group for Blood and Marrow Transplantation. Recommendations on hematopoietic stem cell transplantation for inherited bone marrow failure syndromes. Bone Marrow Transplant. 2015;50(9):1168–72. https://doi.org/10.1038/bmt.2015.117.

44. de Latour RP, Porcher R, Dalle JH, Aljurf M, Korthof ET, Svahn J, Willemze R, Barrenetxea C, Mialou V, Soulier J, Ayas M, Oneto R, Bacigalupo A, Marsh JCW, Peters C, Socie G, Dufour C. Allogeneic hematopoietic stem cell transplantation in fanconi anemia: the European group for blood and marrow transplantation experience. Blood. 2013;122(26):4279–86. https://doi.org/10.1182/blood-2013-01-479733.

45. Dhanraj S, Matveev A, Li H, Lauhasurayotin S, Jardine L, Cada M, Zlateska B, Tailor CS, Zhou J, Mendoza-Londono R, Vincent A, Durie PR, Scherer SW, Rommens JM, Heon E, Dror Y. Biallelic mutations in DNAJC21 cause Shwachman-Diamond syndrome. Blood. 2017;129(11):1557–62. https://doi.org/10.1182/blood-2016-08-735431.

46. Diamond LK, Blackfan KD. Hypoplastic anemia. Am J Dis Child. 1938;56:464–7.

47. Dokal I. Dyskeratosis congenita in all its forms. Br J Haematol. 2000;110(4):768–79.

48. Donadieu J, Fenneteau O, Beaupain B, Mahlaoui N, Chantelot CB. Congenital neutropenia: diagnosis, molecular bases and patient management. Orphanet J Rare Dis. 2011;6:26. https://doi.org/10.1186/1750-1172-6-26.

49. Donadieu J, Leblanc T, Bader Meunier B, Barkaoui M, Fenneteau O, Bertrand Y, Maier-Redelsperger M, Micheau M, Stephan JL, Phillipe N, Bordigoni P, Babin-Boilletot A, Bensaid P, Manel AM, Vilmer E, Thuret I, Blanche S, Gluckman E, Fischer A, Mechinaud F, Joly B, Lamy T, Hermine O, Cassinat B, Bellanné-Chantelot C, Chomienne C, French Severe Chronic Neutropenia Study Group. Analysis of risk factors for myelodysplasia, leukemia, and death from infection among patients with congenital neutropenia. Experience of the French Severe Chronic Neutropenia Study Group. Haematologica. 2005;90(1):45–53.

50. Farruggia P, Di Cataldo A, Pinto RM, Palmisani E, Macaluso A, Valvo LL, Cantarini ME, Tornesello A, Corti P, Fioredda F, Varotto S, Martire B, Moroni I, Puccio G, Russo G, Dufour C, Pillon M. Pearson syndrome: a retrospective cohort study from the marrow failure study group of A.I.E.O.P. (Associazione Italiana Emato-Oncologia Pediatrica). JIMD Rep. 2015;26:37–43. https://doi.org/10.1007/8904_2015_470.

51. Federman N, Sakamoto K. The genetic basis of bone marrow failure syndromes in children. Mol Genet Metab. 2005;86:100–9. https://doi.org/10.1016/j.ymgme.2005.07.006.

52. Fernandez Garcia MS, Teruya-Feldstein J. The diagnosis and treatment of dyskeratosis congenita: a review. 2014;5:157–67.

53. Ferreira R, Ohneda K, Yamamoto M, Philipsen S. GATA1 function, a paradigm for transcription factors in hematopoiesis. Mol Cell Biol. 2005;25(4):1215–27. https://doi.org/10.1128/MCB.25.4.1215-1227.2005.
54. Fleischman RA, Letestu R, Mi X, Stevens D, Winters J, Debili N, Vainchenker W. Absence of mutations in the HoxA10, HoxA11 and HoxD11 nucleotide coding sequences in thrombocytopenia with absent radius syndrome. Br J Haematol. 2002;116:367–75.
55. Flygare J, Aspesi A, Bailey JC, Miyake K, Caffrey JM, Karlsson S, Ellis SR. Human RPS19, the gene mutated in Diamond-Blackfan anemia, encodes a ribosomal protein required for the maturation of 40S ribosomal subunits. Blood. 2007;109:980–6.
56. Frimmel S, Kniestedt C. Angioid Streaks in Types I and II Congenital Dyserythropoietic Anaemia (CDA). Klin Monatsbl Augenheilkd. 2016;233(4):482–7. https://doi.org/10.1055/s-0042-102999.
57. Fukuda MNHEMPAS. Hereditary erythroblastic multinuclearity with positive acidified serum lysis test. Biochim Biophys Acta. 1999;1455(2–3):231–9.
58. Gagne KE, Ghazvinian R, Yuan D, Zon RL, Storm K, Mazur-Popinska M, Andolina L, Bubala H, Golebiowska S, Higman MA, Kalwak K, Kurre P, Matysiak M, Niewiadomska E, Pels S, Petruzzi MJ, Pobudejska-Pieniazek A, Szczepanski T, Fleming MD, Gazda HT, Agarwal S. Pearson marrow pancreas syndrome in patients suspected to have Diamond-Blackfan anemia. Blood. 2014;124(3):437–40. https://doi.org/10.1182/blood-2014-01-545830.
59. Geddis AE. Congenital amegakaryocytic thrombocytopenia and thrombocytopenia with absent radii. Hematol Oncol Clin North Am. 2009;23(2):321–31. https://doi.org/10.1016/j.hoc.2009.01.012.
60. Geddis AE. Congenital amegakaryocytic thrombocytopenia. Pediatr Blood Cancer. 2011;57:199–203. https://doi.org/10.1002/pbc.22927.
61. Germeshausen M, Ballmaier M, Welte K. MPL mutations in 23 patients suffering from congenital amegakaryocytic thrombocytopenia: the type of mutation predicts the course of the disease. Hum Mutat. 2006;886. https://doi.org/10.1002/humu.9415.
62. Ginzberg H, Shin J, Ellis L, Morrison J, Ip W, Dror Y, Freedman M, Heitlinger LA, Belt MA, Corey M, Rommens JM, Durie PR. Shwachman syndrome: phenotypic manifestations of sibling sets and isolated cases in a large patient cohort are similar. J Pediatr. 1999;135(1):81–8.
63. Goobie S, Popovic M, Morrison J, Ellis L, Ginzberg H, Boocock GR, Ehtesham N, Bétard C, Brewer CG, Roslin NM, Hudson TJ, Morgan K, Fujiwara TM, Durie PR, Rommens JM. Shwachman-Diamond syndrome with exocrine pancreatic dysfunction and bone marrow failure maps to the centromeric region of chromosome 7. Am J Hum Genet. 2001;68(4):1048–54. Epub 2001 Mar 15
64. Go RS, Johnston KL. Acute myelogenous leukemia in an adult with thrombocytopenia with absent radii syndrome. Eur J Haematol. 2003;70:246–8.
65. Gripp KW, Curry C, Olney AH, Sandoval C, Fisher J, Chong JX, UW Center for Mendelian Genomics, Pilchman L, Sahraoui R, Stabley DL, Sol-Church K. Diamond-Blackfan anemia with mandibulofacial dysostosis is heterogeneous, including the novel DBA genes TSR2 and RPS28. Am J Med Genet A. 2014;164A(9):2240–9. https://doi.org/10.1002/ajmg.a.36633.
66. Gorlin RJ, Gelb B, Diaz GA, Lofsness KG, Pittelkow MR, Fenyk JR Jr. WHIM syndrome, an autosomal dominant disorder: clinical, hematological, and molecular studies. Am J Med Genet. 2000;91(5):368–76.
67. Gustavsson P, Willing TN, van Haeringen A, Tchernia G, Dianzani I, Donnér M, Elinder G, Henter JI, Nilsson PG, Gordon L, Skeppner G, van't Veer-Korthof L, Kreuger A, Dahl N. Diamond-Blakfan Anemia: genetic homogeneity for a gene on chromosome 19q13 restricted to 1.8 Mb28. Nat Genet. 1997;16:368–71. https://doi.org/10.1038/ng0897-368.
68. Hall GW, Dale P, Dodge JA. Shwachman-Diamond syndrome: UK perspective. Arch Dis Child. 2006;91(6):521–4.
69. Hedberg VA, Lipton JM. Thrombocytopenia with absent radii. Am J Pediatr Hematol Oncol. 1988;10(1):51–64.

70. Heimpel H. Congenital dyserythropoietic anemias: epidemiology, clinical significance, and progress in understanding their pathogenesis. Ann Hematol. 2004;83(10):613–21.
71. Heimpel H, Dührsen U, Hofbauer P, Rigamonti-Wermlinger V, Kreuser ED, Schwarz K, Solenthaler M, Pauls S. Bulky extramedullary hematopoiesis is not a rare complication of congenital dyserythropoietic anemia. Ann Hematol. 2009;88(10):937–41. https://doi.org/10.1007/s00277-009-0735-5.
72. Heimpel H, Schwarz K, Ebnöther M, Goede JS, Heydrich D, Kamp T, Plaumann L, Rath B, Roessler J, Schildknecht O, Schmid M, Wuillemin W, Einsiedler B, Leichtle R, Tamary H, Kohne E. Congenital dyserythropoietic anemia type I (CDA I): molecular genetics, clinical appearance, and prognosis based on long-term observation. Blood. 2006;107(1):334–40.
73. Heimpel H, Wendt F. Congenital dyserythropoietic anemia with karyorrhexis and multinuclearity of erythroblasts. Helv Med Acta. 1968;34(2):103–15.
74. Horwitz M, Benson KF, Person RE, Aprikyan AG, Dale DC. Mutations in ELA2, encoding neutrophil elastase, define a 21-day biological clock in cyclic haematopoiesis. Nat Genet. 1999;23(4):433–6.
75. Huang J, Shimamura A. Clinical spectrum and molecular pathophysiology of Shwachman-Diamond syndrome. Curr Opin Hematol. 2011;18(1):30–5. https://doi.org/10.1097/MOH.0b013e32834114a5.
76. Hughes DW. Hypoplastic anaemia in infancy and childhood: erythroid hypoplasia. Arch Dis Child. 1961;36:349–61.
77. Hsu AP, McReynolds LJ, Holland SM. GATA2 deficiency. Curr Opin Allergy Clin Immunol 2015. 2016;15(1):104–9. https://doi.org/10.1097/ACI.0000000000000126.
78. Iolascon A, Esposito MR, Russo R. Clinical aspects and pathogenesis of congenital dyserythropoietic anemias: from morphology to molecular approach. Haematologica. 2012;97(12):1786–94. https://doi.org/10.3324/haematol.2012.072207.
79. Iolascon A, Andolfo I, Barcellini W, Corcione F, Garçon L, De Franceschi L, Pignata C, Graziadei G, Pospisilova D, Rees DC, de Montalembert M, Rivella S, Gambale A, Russo R, Ribeiro L, Vives-Corrons J, Martinez PA, Kattamis A, Gulbis B, Cappellini MD, Roberts I, Tamary H, Working Study Group on Red Cells. Recommendations regarding splenectomy in hereditary hemolytic anemias. Haematologica. 2017;102(8):1304–13. https://doi.org/10.3324/haematol.2016.161166.
80. Ishiai M, Kitao H, Smogorzewska A, Tomida J, Kinomura A, Uchida E, Saberi A, Kinoshita E, Kinoshita-Kikuta E, Koike T, Tashiro S, Elledge SJ, Takata M. FANCI phosphorylation functions as a molecular switch to turn on the fanconi anemia pathway. Nat Struct Mol Biol. 2008;15(11):1138–46. https://doi.org/10.1038/nsmb.1504.
81. Jameson-Lee M, Chen K, Ritchie E, Shore T, Al-Khattab O, Gergis U. Acute myeloid leukemia in a patient with thrombocytopenia with absent radii: a case report and review of the literature. Hematol Oncol Stem Cell Ther. 2017; https://doi.org/10.1016/j.hemonc.2017.02.001.
82. Josephs HW. Anemia of infancy and early childhood. Medicine. 1936;15:307–451.
83. Keogh SJ, McKee S, Smithson SF, Grier D, Steward CG. Shwachman-Diamond syndrome: a complex case demonstrating the potential for misdiagnosis as asphyxiating thoracic dystrophy (Jeune syndrome). BMC Pediatr. 2012;12:48.
84. Khincha PP, Savage SA. Neonatal manifestations of inherited bone marrow failure syndromes. Semin Fetal Neonatal Med. 2016;21(1):57–65. https://doi.org/10.1016/j.siny.2015.12.003.
85. King S, Germeshausen M, Strauss G, Welte K, Ballmaier M. Congenital amegakaryocytic thrombocytopenia: a retrospective clinical analysis of 20 patients. Br J Haematol. 2005;131:636–44. https://doi.org/10.1111/j.1365-2141.2005.05819.x.
86. Kitano T, Yoshida S. Pearson syndrome as a rare cause of failure to thrive, anemia, and exocrine pancreatic insufficiency: a case report. Pediatr Ther. 2018;8(1):341. https://doi.org/10.4172/2161-0665.1000341.
87. Klein C, Grudzien M, Appaswamy G, Germeshausen M, Sandrock I, Schäffer AA, Rathinam C, Boztug K, Schwinzer B, Rezaei N, Bohn G, Melin M, Carlsson G, Fadeel B, Dahl N,

76 J. D. Hamm and C. E. Sorge

Palmblad J, Henter JI, Zeidler C, Grimbacher B, Welte K. HAX1 deficiency causes autosomal recessive severe congenital neutropenia (Kostmann disease). Nat Genet. 2007;39(1):86–92.
88. Kostmann R. Hereditär reticulos – en ny systemsjukdom. Svenska Läkartideningen. 1950;47:2861–8.
89. Kostmann R. Infantile genetic agranulocytosis; agranulocytosis infantilis hereditaria. Acta Paediatr Suppl. 1956;45(Suppl 105):1–78.
90. Kristiansen JD, Rasmussen LN, Vetner M. Congenital dyserythropoietic anaemia (CDA) with intrauterine symptoms and early lethal outcome. Eur J Haematol. 1990;45(2):113–4.
91. Kudo K, Kato K, Matsuyama T, Kojima S. Successful engraftment of unrelated donor stem cells in two children with congenital amegakaryocytic thrombocytopenia. J Pediatr Hematol Oncol. 2002;24(1):78–80.
92. Lackner A, Basu O, Bierings M, Lassay L, Schaefer UW, Revesz T, Havers W, Kremens B. Haematopoietic stem cell transplantation for amegakaryocytic thrombocytopenia. Br J Haematol. 2000;109:773–5.
93. Lee HF, Lee HJ, Chi CS, Tsai CR, Chang TK, Wang CJ. The neurological evolution of Pearson syndrome: case report and literature review. Eur J Paediatr Neurol. 2007;11(4):208–14.
94. Leguit RJ, van den Tweel JG. The pathology of bone marrow failure. Histopathology. 2010;57(5):655–70. https://doi.org/10.1111/j.1365-2559.2010.03612.x.
95. Liljeholm M, Irvine AF, Vikberg AL, Norberg A, Month S, Sandström H, Wahlin A, Mishima M, Golovleva I. Congenital dyserythropoietic anemia type III (CDA III) is caused by a mutation in the kinesin family member, KIF23. Blood. 2013;121(23):4791–9. https://doi.org/10.1182/blood-2012-10-461392.
96. Lipton JM, Atsidaftos E, Zyskind I, Vlachos A. Improving clinical care and elucidating the pathophysiology of Diamond Blackfan anemia: an update from the Diamond Blackfan Anemia Registry. Pediatr Blood Cancer. 2006;46(5):558–64.
97. Lipton JM, Ellis SR. Diamond Blackfan anemia: diagnosis, treatment and molecular pathogenesis. Hematol Oncol Clin North Am. 2009;23(2):261–82. https://doi.org/10.1016/j.hoc.2009.01.004.
98. MacMillan ML, Davies SM, Wagner JE, Ramsay NKC. Engraftment of unrelated donor stem cells in children with familial amegakaryocytic thrombocytopenia. Bone Marrow Transplant. 1998;21:735–7.
99. McShane MA1, Hammans SR, Sweeney M, Holt IJ, Beattie TJ, Brett EM, Harding AE. Pearson syndrome and mitochondrial encephalomyopathy in a patient with a deletion of mtDNA. Am J Hum Genet. 1991;48(1):39–42.
100. Means RT Jr. Pure red cell aplasia. Blood. 2016;128(21):2504–9.
101. Mills EW, Green R. Ribosomopathies: There's strength in numbers. Science. 2017;358(6363):eaan2755. https://doi.org/10.1126/science.aan2755.
102. Modi G, Shah S, Madabhavi I, Panchal H, Patel A, Uparkar U, Anand A, Parikh S, Patel K, Shah K, Revannasiddaiah S. Successful allogeneic hematopoietic stem cell transplantation of a patient suffering from type II congenital dyserythropoietic anemia a rare case report from Western India. Case Rep Hematol. 2015;2015:792485. https://doi.org/10.1155/2015/792485.
103. Muraki K1, Nishimura S, Goto Y, Nonaka I, Sakura N, Ueda K. The association between haematological manifestation and mtDNA deletions in Pearson syndrome. J Inherit Metab Dis. 1997;20(5):697–703.
104. Muraoka K, ishii E, Ihara K, Imayoshi M, Miyazaki S, Hara T, Hamasaki Y. Successful bone marrow transplantation in a patient with c-mpl-mutated congenital amegakaryocytic thrombocytopenia from a carrier donor. Pediatr Transplant. 2005;9:101–3. https://doi.org/10.1111/j.1399-3046.2005.00247.x.
105. Nathan DG, Clarke BJ, Hillman DG, Alter BP, Housman DE. Erythroid precursors in congenital hypoplastic (Diamond-Blackfan) anemia. J Clin Invest. 1978;61(2):489–98.
106. Noy-Lotan S, Dgany O, Lahmi R, Marcoux N, Krasnov T, Yissachar N, Ginsberg D, Motro B, Resnitzky P, Yaniv I, Kupfer GM, Tamary H. Codanin-1, the protein encoded by the gene

mutated in congenital dyserythropoietic anemia type I (CDAN1), is cell cycle-regulated. Haematologica. 2009;94(5):629–37. https://doi.org/10.3324/haematol.2008.003327.

107. Ohene-Abuakwa Y, Orfali KA, Marius C, Ball SE. Two-phase culture in Diamond Blackfan anemia: localization of the erythroid defect. Blood. 2005;105(2):838–46.

108. Ohisalo JJ, Vitala J, Lintula R, Ruutu T. A new congenital dyserythropoietic anaemia. Br J Haematol. 1988;68(1):111–4.

109. Palm W, de Lange T. How shelterin protects mammalian telomeres. Annu Rev Genet. 2008;42:301–34. https://doi.org/10.1146/annurev.genet.41.110306.130350.

110. Parrella S, Aspesi A, Quarello P, Garelli E, Pavesi E, Carando A, Nardi M, Ellis SR, Ramenghi U, Dianzani I. Loss of GATA-1 full length as a cause of Diamond-Blakfan anemia phenotype. Pediatr Blood Cancer. 2014;61(7):1319–21. https://doi.org/10.1002/pbc.24944.

111. Parry EM, Alder JK, Lee SS, Phillips JA, Loyd JE, Duggal P, Armanios M. Decreased dyskerin levels as a mechanism of telomere shortening in X-linked dyskeratosis congenita. J Med Genet. 2011;48:327–33. https://doi.org/10.1136/jmg.2010.085100.

112. Pearson HA, Lobel JS, Kocoshis SA, Naiman JL, Windmiller J, Lammi AT, Hoffman R, Marsh JC. A new syndrome of refractory sideroblastic anemia with vacuolization of marrow precursors and exocrine pancreatic dysfunction. J Pediatr. 1979;95(6):976–84.

113. Person RE, Li FQ, Duan Z, Benson KF, Wechsler J, Papadaki HA, Eliopoulos G, Kaufman C, Bertolone SJ, Nakamoto B, Papayannopoulou T, Grimes HL, Horwitz M. Mutations in proto-oncogene GFI1 cause human neutropenia and target ELA2. Nat Genet. 2003;34(3):308–12.

114. Podlevsky JD, Chen JJL. It all comes together at the ends: telomerase structure, function, and biogenesis. Mutat Res. 2012;730:3–11. https://doi.org/10.1016/j.mrfmmm.2011.11.002.

115. Ramachandran S, Alessandri A, Price J, Balasubramaniam S. Breath-holding spell and macrocytic anaemia in a toddler. Br J Haematol. 2014;166(2):156. https://doi.org/10.1111/bjh.12927.

116. Renella R, Wood WG. The congenital dyserythropoietic anemias. Hematol Oncol Clin North Am. 2009;23(2):283–306. https://doi.org/10.1016/j.hoc.2009.01.010.

117. Riyaz A, Riyaz N, Jayakrishnan MP, Mohamed Shiras PT, Ajith Kumar VT, Ajuth BS. Revesz syndrome. Indian J Pediatr. 2007;74(9):862–3.

118. Rosenberg PS, Greene MH, Alter BP. Cancer incidence in persons with fanconi anemia. Blood. 2003;101(3):822–6. https://doi.org/10.1182/blood-2002-05-1498.

119. Rössler J, Havers W. Diagnosis and genetics of congenital dyserythropoietic anemias. Klin Padiatr. 2000;212(4):153–8.

120. Rothbaum R, Perrault J, Vlachos A, Cipolli M, Alter BP, Burroughs S, Durie P, Elghetany MT, Grand R, Hubbard V, Rommens J, Rossi T. Shwachman-Diamon syndrome: report from an international conference. J Pediatr. 2002;141(2):266–70.

121. Rötig A, Bourgeron T, Chretien D, Rustin P, Munnich A. Spectrum of mitochondrial DNA rearrangements in the Pearson marrow-pancreas syndrome. Hum Mol Genet. 1995;4(8):1327–30.

122. Rötig A, Cormier V, Blanche S, Bonnefont JP, Ledeist F, Romero N, Schmitz J, Rustin P, Fischer A, Saudubray JM. Pearson's marrow-pancreas syndrome. A multisystem mitochondrial disorder of infancy. J Clin Invest. 1990;86(5):1601–8.

123. Ru YX, Zhu XF, Yan WW, Gao JT, Schwarz K, Heimpel H. Congenital dyserythropoietic anemia in a Chinese family with a mutation of the CDAN1-gene. Ann Hematol. 2008;87(9):751–4. https://doi.org/10.1007/s00277-008-0519-3.

124. Sankaran VG1, Ghazvinian R, Do R, Thiru P, Vergilio JA, Beggs AH, Sieff CA, Orkin SH, Nathan DG, Lander ES, Gazda HT. Exome sequencing identifies GATA1 mutations resulting in Diamond-Blackfan anemia. J Clin Invest. 2012;122(7):2439–43. https://doi.org/10.1172/JCI63597.

125. Santorelli FM, Barmada MA, Pons R, Zhang LL, MeMauro S. Leigh-type neuropathology in Pearson syndrome associated with impaired ATP production and a novel mtDNA deletion. Neurology. 1996;47(5):1320–3.

126. Sasa GS, Ribes-Zamora A, Nelson ND, bertuch AA. Three novel truncating TINF2 mutations causing severe dyskeratosis congenita in early childhood. Clin Genet. 2012;81:470–8. https://doi.org/10.1111/j.1399-0004.2011.01658.x.
127. Savage SA, Alter BP. Dyskeratosis congenita. Hematol Oncol Clin North Am. 2009;23:215–31. https://doi.org/10.1016/j.hoc.2009.01.003.
128. Savage SA, Vulliamy TJ. The genetics of dyskeratosis congenita. In: Savage SA, Cook EF, editors. Dyskeratosis congenita and telomere biology disorders: diagnosis and management guidelines. New York: Dyskeratosis Congenita Outreach, Inc; 2015. p. 68–81.
129. Schwarz K, Iolascon A, Verissimo F, Trede NS, Horsley W, Chen W, Paw BH, Hopfner KP, Holzmann K, Russo R, Esposito MR, Spano D, De Falco L, Heinrich K, Joggerst B, Rojewski MT, Perrotta S, Denecke J, Pannicke U, Delaunay J, Pepperkok R, Heimpel H. Mutations affecting the secretory COPII coat component SEC23B cause congenital dyserythropoietic anemia type II. Nat Genet. 2009;41(8):936–40. https://doi.org/10.1038/ng.405.
130. Shalev H, Al-Athamen K, Levi I, Levitas A, Tamary H. Morbidity and mortality of adult patients with congenital dyserythropoietic anemia type I. Eur J Haematol. 2017;98(1):13–8. https://doi.org/10.1111/ejh.12778.
131. Shalev H, Kapelushnik J, Moser A, Dgany O, Krasnov T, Tamary H. A comprehensive study of the neonatal manifestations of congenital dyserythropoietic anemia type I. J Pediatr Hematol Oncol. 2004;26(11):746–8.
132. Shwachman H, Diamond LK, Oski FA, Khaw KT. The syndrome of pancreatic insufficiency and bone marrow dysfunction. J Pediatr. 1964;65:645–63.
133. Sieff CA, Yang J, Merida-Long LB, Lodish HF. Pathogenesis of the erythroid failure in Diamond Blackman anemia. Br J Haematol. 2010;148(4):611–22. https://doi.org/10.1111/j.1365-2141.2009.07993.x.
134. Souka AP, Bower S, Geerts L, Huggon I, Nicolaides KH. Blackfan-Diamond anemia and dyserythopoietic anemia presenting with increased nuchal translucency at 12 weeks of gestation. Ultrasound Obstet Gynecol. 2002;20(2):197–9.
135. Soulier J. Fanconi anemia. Hematology. 2011:492–7.
136. Stark AR, Carlo WA, Tyson JE, Papile LA, Wright LL, Shankaran S, Donovan EF, Oh W, Bauer CR, Saha S, Poole WK, Stoll BJ. National Institute of Child Health and Human Development Neonatal Research NetworkAdverse effects of early dexamethasone in extremely-low-birth-weight infants. National Institute of Child Health and Human Development Neonatal Research Network. N Engl J Med. 2001;344(2):95–101.
137. Steele JM, Sung L, Klaassen R, Fernandez CV, Yanofsky R, Wu J, Odame I, Silva M, Champagne J, Ali K, Brossard J, Samson Y, Abish S, Le D, Jardine L, Hand JP, Lipton JH, Charpentier K, Stephens D, Freedman M, Dror Y, Canadian Inherited Marrow Failure Registry. Disease progression in recently diagnosed patients with inherited marrow failure syndromes: a Canadian inherited marrow failure registry (CIMFR) report. Pediatr Blood Cancer. 2006;47(7):918–25.
138. Stepanovic V, Wessels D, Goldman FD, Geiger J, Soll DR. The chemotaxis defect of Shwachman-Diamond Syndrome leukocytes. Cell Motil Cytoskeleton. 2004;57:158–74.
139. Stepensky P, Chacón-Flores M, Kim KH, Abuzaitoun O, Bautista-Santos A, Simanovsky N, Siliqi D, Altamura D, Méndez-Godoy A, Gijsbers A, Naser Eddin A, Dor T, Charrow J, Sánchez-Puig N, Elpeleg O. Mutations in EFL1, an SBDS partner, are associated with infantile pancytopenia, exocrine pancreatic insufficiency and skeletal anomalies in a Shwachman-Diamond like syndrome. J Med Genet. 2017;54(8):558–66. https://doi.org/10.1136/jmedgenet-2016-104366.3.
140. Sznajer Y, Baumann C, David A, Journel H, Lacombe D, Perel Y, Blouin P, Segura JF, Cezard JP, Peuchmaur M, Vulliamy T, Dokal I, Verloes A. Further delineation of the congenital form of X-linked dyskeratosis congenita (Hoyeraal-Hreidarsson syndrome). Eur J Pediatr. 2003;162:863–7. https://doi.org/10.1007/s00431-003-1317-5.
141. Tadiotto E, Maines E, Degani D, Balter R, Bordugo A, Cesaro S. Bone marrow features in Pearson syndrome with neonatal onset: a case report and review of the literature. Pediatr Blood Cancer. 2018;65(4). https://doi.org/10.1002/pbc.26939.

142. Toiviainen-Salo S, Pitkänen O, Holmström M, Koikkalainen J, Lötjönen J, Lauerma K, Taskinen M, Savilahti E, Smallhorn J, Mäkitie O, Kivistö S. Myocardial function in patients with Shwachman-Diamond syndrome: aspects to consider before stem cell transplantation. Pediatr Blood Cancer. 2008;51(4):461–7. https://doi.org/10.1002/pbc.21686.

143. Toiviainen-Salo S, Raade M, Durie PR, Ip W, Marttinen E, Savilahti E, Mäkitie O. Magnetic resonance imaging findings of the pancreas in patients with Shwachman-Diamond syndrome and mutations in the SBDS gene. J Pediatr. 2007;152(3):434–6. https://doi.org/10.1016/j.jpeds.2007.12.013.

144. Toriello HV. Thrombocytopenia-absent radius syndrome. Semin Thromb Hemost. 2011;37(6):707–12. https://doi.org/10.1055/s-0031-1291381.

145. Tummala H, Walne AJ, Williams M, Bockett N, Collopy L, Cardoso S, Ellison A, Wynn R, Leblanc T, Fitzgibbon J, Kelsell DP, van Heel DA, Payne E, Plagnol V, Dokal I, Vulliamy T. DNAJC21 mutations link a cancer-prone bone marrow failure syndrome to corruption in 60S ribosome subunit maturation. Am J Hum Genet. 2016;99(1):115–24. https://doi.org/10.1016/j.ajhg.2016.05.002. Epub 2016 Jun 23.

146. Unal S, Russo R, Gumruk F, Kuskonmaz B, Cetin M, Sayli T, Tavil B, Langella C, Iolascon A, Uckan Cetinkaya D. Successful hematopoietic stem cell transplantation in a patient with congenital dyserythropoietic anemia type II. Pediatr Transplant. 2014;18(4):E130–3. https://doi.org/10.1111/petr.12254.

147. Vlachos A, Ball S, Dahl N, Alter BP, Sheth S, Ramenghi U, Meerpohl J, Karlsson S, Liu JM, Leblanc T, Paley C, Kang EM, Leder EJ, Atsidaftos E, Shimamura A, Bessler M, Glader B, Lipton JM. Participants of sixth annual Daniella Maria Arturi international consensus conference. Diagnosing and treating Diamond Blackfan anaemia: results of an international clinical consensus conference. Br J Haematol. 2008;142(6):859–76. https://doi.org/10.1111/j.1365-2141.2008.07269.x.

148. Vlachos A, Muir E. How I treat Diamond-Blackfan anemia. Blood. 2010;116(19):3715–23. https://doi.org/10.1182/blood-2010-02-251090.

149. Vulliamy TJ, Dokal I. Dyskeratosis congenita: the diverse clinical presentation of mutations in telomerase complex. Biochimie. 2008;90:122–30. https://doi.org/10.1016/j.biochi.2007.07.017.

150. Vulliamy T, Beswick R, Kirwan M, Marrone A, Digweed M, Walne A, Dokal I. Mutations in the telomerase component NHP2 cause the premature ageing syndrome dyskeratosis congenita. Proc Natl Acad Sci U S A. 2008;105(23):8073–8.

151. Vulliamy T, Marrone A, Goldman F, Dearlove A, Bessler M, Mason PJ, Dokal I. The RNA component of telomerase is mutated in autosomal dominant dyskeratosis congenita. Nature. 2001;413:432–5.

152. Vulliamy TJ, Marrone A, Knight SW, Walne A, Mason PJ, Dokal I. Mutations in dyskeratosis congenita: their impact on telomere length and the diversity of clinical presentation. Blood. 2006;107:2680–5. https://doi.org/10.1182/blood-2005-07-2622.

153. Walden H, Deans AJ. The fanconi anemia DNA repair pathway: structural and functional insights into a complex disorder. Annu Rev Biophys. 2014;43:257–78. https://doi.org/10.1146/annurev-biophys-051013-022737.

154. Warren AJ. Molecular basis of the human ribosomopathy Shwachman-Diamond syndrome. Adv Biol Regul. 2018;67:109–27. https://doi.org/10.1016/j.jbior.2017.09.002.

155. Wickramasinghe SN, Wood WG. Advances in the understanding of the congenital dyserythropoietic anaemias. Br J Haematol. 2005;131(4):431–46.

156. Yeh TF, Lin YJ, Huang CC, Chen YJ, Lin CH, Lin HC, Hsieh WS, Lien YJ. Early dexamethasone therapy in preterm infants: a follow-up study. Pediatrics. 1998;101(5):E7.

Chapter 5
Iron-Deficiency Anemia During Childhood

Yara Perez, Kendall Presti, Alvin N. Eden, and Claudio Sandoval

Introduction

Iron-deficiency anemia is a global public health challenge. Indeed, it is the most common micronutrient deficiency, and approximately 35% of the world's population is so affected [1]. No population or socioeconomic group is immune to iron deficiency, and children so affected may suffer long-lasting neurocognitive deficits. Iron deficiency occurs either because not enough iron traverses the intestinal epithelium or too much iron is loss through occult or clinically apparent bleeding. Identifying the cause of iron deficiency is paramount for appropriate therapy. For example, not diagnosing von Willebrand disease in a patient with epistaxis or menorrhagia will result in continued blood loss and iron deficiency. Indeed, iron deficiency should never be the final diagnosis – it always has a cause. Our review will focus on iron metabolism and the epidemiology, clinical features, diagnosis, prevention, and treatment of iron deficiency.

Iron Homeostasis and Molecular Regulation

Iron is indispensable in a variety of critical biological processes including oxygen transport (as heme in hemoglobin), DNA biosynthesis (as a cofactor of ribonucleotide reductase), and ATP generation (as a cofactor for many proteins in the citric acid cycle and electron transport chain) [2]. Therefore, to maintain physiologic amounts of iron, cells require the coordination of a wide variety of proteins, which tightly regulate both cellular and systemic iron homeostasis [3]. The majority of

Y. Perez, MD · K. Presti, BS · A. N. Eden, MD · C. Sandoval, MD (✉)
Department of Pediatrics, New York Medical College, Valhalla, NY, USA
e-mail: claudio_sandoval@nymc.edu

© Springer Nature Switzerland AG 2019   81
R. T. Means Jr. (ed.), *Anemia in the Young and Old*,
https://doi.org/10.1007/978-3-319-96487-4_5

iron flux in the body is a result of reutilization of iron recycled from damaged erythrocytes by macrophages. These damaged erythrocytes are phagocytosed, and the hemoglobin is degraded to release heme. Iron is further extracted by heme oxygenase and finally recycled to extracellular fluid and plasma. Iron is toxic and catalyzes reactive oxygen species that result in apoptosis and tissue injury. Therefore, it is imperative that iron is effectively distributed, stored, and regulated [4].

Approximately 10% of dietary iron is absorbed through the duodenum, and iron absorption may increase 20-fold during periods of blood loss. The primary importer of iron across the apical membrane of the intestinal epithelial cell is divalent metal transporter 1 (DMT1). This transporter is responsible for uptake of ferrous iron and is strongly regulated by iron status. Once internalized by the enterocyte, iron is transported across the cell, through tightly regulated cellular and intracellular trafficking mechanisms of which the best understood is transferrin-mediated iron uptake. Transferrin is an iron-binding glycoprotein found in the plasma. Cell membrane transferrin receptors (TfR1) endocytose and then internalize iron-transferrin into endosomal recycling vesicles. Through a process of acidification, the ferric iron-transferrin and iron-free transferrin-TfR1 complex are released and subsequently able to return to the cell membrane to restart the cycle. The iron that remains in the vesicles is transported to the mitochondria for integration into protoporphyrin IX to form heme. In addition, iron in vesicles can be transported into the cytoplasm for integration into cytoplasmic ferroproteins or stored in cytoplasmic ferritin. Ferritin is a protein-ferric iron complex with hydroxide and phosphate anions. Over time, iron bound to ferritin will either be mobilized for further transport or lost by normal sloughing of epithelial cells [4, 5].

Iron translocated across the cell is exported by ferroportin located in the basolateral membrane. Ferrous iron is oxidized by hephaestin, a copper-containing membrane-bound ferroxidase that co-localizes with FPN in the basolateral membrane. Following export of iron by ferroportin, iron in ferric form is transported to the liver bound to transferrin and utilized by the reticuloendothelial system for hemoglobin synthesis or deposited in iron stores [4]. The communication between the iron stores in the liver and the intestinal epithelial cell is mediated by hepcidin. Hepcidin (hepatic bactericidal protein) is an endocrine regulator of iron metabolism that covalently binds to ferroportin and causes ferroportin internalization and breakdown [6]. Iron subsequently accumulates in the intestinal cell and downregulates the expression of DMT1. This process allows effective downregulation of iron absorption which results in balanced iron homeostasis in all cells [3, 4]. Hepcidin synthesis is increased by plasma iron-transferrin and stored iron in hepatocytes, decreased in response to increased iron requirements, and potently stimulated by inflammation.

Phases of Iron Depletion

Since the majority of the body's iron is directed toward synthesis of hemoglobin, erythrocyte production is among the first casualties of iron deficiency to become clinically apparent in usual laboratory evaluations. However, the drop in hemoglobin concentration represents a late stage of iron depletion [2]. The first discernible phase, prelatent iron deficiency, occurs when tissue stores are depleted, without a change in hematocrit or serum iron levels. This stage of iron deficiency is represented by hypoferritinemia. The second phase, latent iron deficiency, occurs when reticuloendothelial macrophage iron stores are completely depleted. The serum iron level decreases and the total iron-binding capacity (TIBC) increases without a change in the hematocrit. Erythropoiesis decreases because of a lack of available iron and soluble transferrin receptor levels increase. The reticulocyte hemoglobin content (CHr) decreases because newly produced erythrocytes are iron deficient. This stage of iron deficiency is clinically occult because the majority of erythrocytes are iron replete. The final phase, clinically overt iron-deficiency anemia, is detected when iron deficiency has persisted long enough that a large proportion of the circulating erythrocytes were produced after iron became limiting. This is associated with erythrocyte microcytosis, hypochromia, increased red cell distribution width (RDW), and elevated levels of free erythrocyte protoporphyrin (FEP) [7].

Etiology of Iron-Deficiency Anemia

At birth, hemoglobin concentration is high as a result of fetal adaptation to the hypoxic environment of the uterus. Between birth and 4 months of age, abundant stores are mobilized to meet the infant's iron requirements. Additional iron from hemoglobin breakdown is also made available to meet the iron needs as the concentration of hemoglobin physiologically declines from a mean of 17.0 g/dl at birth to a nadir of 11.0 g/dl by 2 months of age. In term infants, iron requirement is approximately 1 mg/kg/day [3]. However, in low-birth-weight infants, infants with low initial hemoglobin values and those who have experienced significant blood loss, 2 mg/kg/day is required. Most infants are fed either breast milk or iron-fortified formula; therefore, understanding the difference in the bioavailability of iron is important. Even though cow milk and breast milk are equally poor in iron, breast-fed infants absorb 20–80% of the iron, in contrast to about 10% absorbed from cow milk. Therefore, after 6 months of age breast-feeding does not protect against iron deficiency, and a supplemental source of dietary or prescribed elemental iron is required for optimal iron nutrition [3, 7].

During the rapidly growing years, in particular between 6 and 23 months of age, there is an increased requirement for iron that is often not sufficiently maintained by diet and body stores. By 12 months of age, most children have tripled their birth weight with an increase of approximately 35–45 mg body iron required for each kilogram gain in weight. In addition, there is a doubling of circulating hemoglobin mass which also contributes to the increased iron requirement during this rapid growth period [7]. Iron-deficiency anemia can be more profound in infants or children with conditions that impair iron absorption such as celiac disease, severe prolonged diarrhea, and inflammatory bowel disease [8, 9].

Another common cause of iron-deficiency anemia is gastrointestinal blood loss which can be either occult or apparent. Irrespective of the underlying cause, iron deficiency by itself may result in occult blood loss from the gut. This blood loss is due to the effects of iron deficiency on the mucosal lining (e.g., deficiency of iron-containing enzymes in the gut), leading to mucosal blood loss. It can also induce an enteropathy, in which a number of blood constituents (e.g., plasma protein, albumin, immune globulins), in addition to red cells, are lost in the gut. Moreover, cow milk can result in an exudative enteropathy associated with chronic gastrointestinal blood loss resulting in iron deficiency. Therefore, several fecal occult blood tests should be performed in order to exclude intermittent occult GI bleeding. Less common, anatomic lesions such as hiatal hernia, Meckel's diverticulum, polyps, intestinal duplication, gastric/colorectal cancers, or peptic ulcers can be the cause of iron deficiency [7–11].

Clinical Features

Iron-deficiency anemia is classified as a microcytic and hypochromic anemia. The differential diagnosis for microcytosis comprises hemoglobinopathies such as thalassemias, lead toxicity, anemia of chronic inflammation, Wilson disease, sideroblastic anemia, and atransferrinemia.

Clinically, iron-deficiency anemia is often asymptomatic. However, patients may present with generalized symptoms of anemia such as fatigue, irritability, headache, vertigo, dyspnea, and tachycardia. These patients may also display symptoms that are more unique to the diagnosis including:

- Pica (originates from the Latin for magpie – a bird that will eat almost anything): The craving for substances not considered to be food. The pathogenesis of pica is insufficiently understood but expected to be a subconscious nutrient-seeking behavior in deficient individuals. Commonly sought substances are soil and rocks, paper, and paint chips; however many more have been documented. Pica is also observed in zinc deficiency [12]. Pagophagia, craving and eating ice, is uniquely observed in iron-deficiency anemia.
- Koilonychia: Spooning of the nails.
- Plummer-Vinson or Paterson-Kelly syndrome: A triad of iron-deficiency anemia, dysphagia, and esophageal webbing, most often described in middle-aged women [13].
- Beeturia: A phenomenon where individuals with iron deficiency will have red urine after consuming beets [14].
- Restless legs syndrome (Willis-Ekbom disease): Iron deficiency in the central nervous system may cause Willis-Ekbom disease; however the presence of this disease does not necessarily indicate iron deficiency [15, 16].
- Protein-losing enteropathy: A condition where protein is excessively lost by the gastrointestinal tract [17].

- Atrophic glossitis: The papilla of the tongue degrades. It is associated with oral pain and dryness.
- Angular cheilitis: Inflammation and irritation of the corners of the mouth.
- Alopecia (telogen effluvium): Loss of bodily hair. A rare occurrence in iron-deficiency anemia.
- Chlorosis: Development of a green hue to the skin that is thought to correspond with the hypochromia of erythrocytes. A rare occurrence in iron-deficiency anemia today.

During the early phase of iron deficiency, the physical examination is entirely normal. Symptoms and physical examination findings occur insidiously. The most common finding on examination is pallor of the skin and mucous membranes. Children with more severe anemia may exhibit listlessness and irritability, and a flow/hemic murmur may be appreciated. In unique clinical scenarios, the evaluating physician may encounter the following: periorbital edema due to hypoalbuminemia, bowel sounds in the thorax due to hiatal hernia, Castell's sign (dullness to percussion over Traube's space) due to gastric B cell lymphoma, and papilledema due to iron deficiency-associated pseudotumor cerebri.

Diagnosis of Iron-Deficiency Anemia

Early diagnosis of iron-deficiency anemia is imperative to prevent complications such as irreversible neurocognitive deficits, high-output heart failure, and stroke. The American Academy of Pediatrics (AAP) recommends universal screening for anemia at age 9 and 12 months with selective screening at any age if risk factors are present. In addition, the AAP, Centers for Disease Control and Prevention, and a Cochrane systematic review from 2001 recommend clinical management in young children ages 1–3 whose hemoglobin level is less 11.0 mg/dL (2 standard deviations below the mean for age and gender). Although measurement of the hemoglobin concentration is the primary screening test used for IDA, iron depletion progresses through several phases, with clinically significant anemia manifested only after erythropoiesis has become markedly impaired. Therefore, relying solely on hemoglobin concentration to screen for iron deficiency misses many children who are, in fact, iron deficient and in whom adverse consequences, such as potentially irreversible neurocognitive impairment, may have already occurred [18, 19].

Currently, there is no single measurement that correctly characterizes the iron status in a child. Therefore, in order to establish the correct diagnosis of IDA, all of the clinical information, laboratory data, and classic findings on peripheral blood smear must be taken into account [8]. However, the most convincing evidence of IDA is a response to a therapeutic trial of elemental ferrous sulfate [18, 20]. An adequate response involves a reticulocytosis with a peak occurring between the fifth and tenth days followed by a significant rise in hemoglobin level, 1 g/dl in 1 month. In patients with limited response to iron therapy and/or some normal iron measurements, other causes should be considered, such as lead poisoning, thalassemia trait, other hemoglobinopathy, or anemia of chronic inflammation [9, 21].

The findings on a complete blood cell count offers supporting evidence for the diagnosis of IDA. In general, there is a decrease in red cell indices which parallels the decrease in hemoglobin concentration: the mean corpuscular volume (MCV) is lower than the normal mean for age; mean corpuscular hemoglobin (MCH) is less than 27.0 pg, and mean corpuscular hemoglobin concentration (MCHC) is less than 30%. However, the RDW is higher than normal, usually 14.5%, but it is normal in thalassemia, usually <13%. The relative number of reticulocytes is often increased as well, but when corrected for anemia, the reticulocyte count is usually normal. In severe cases due to blood loss, the reticulocyte count can be as high as 4%. The platelet count varies from thrombocytopenia to thrombocytosis. Thrombocytopenia is more common in severe IDA, while thrombocytosis is associated with bleeding. On peripheral blood smear, the erythrocytes are hypochromic and microcytic with anisocytosis and poikilocytosis. Evaluation of the bone marrow is rarely indicated for the diagnosis of iron-deficiency anemia. Indications include abnormal clinical presentation, inconclusive laboratory results, lack of response to conventional treatment, and concern for concurrent malignancy. If performed, the bone marrow will reveal hypocellularity of red cell precursors and distortion of normoblast nuclei. Prussian blue staining will demonstrate little or no iron in normoblasts and reticular cells [7, 9].

The iron status of children can be assessed with iron-specific biomarkers (i.e., serum ferritin concentration, serum iron, TIBC, transferrin saturation, and erythrocyte protoporphyrin concentration). The level of serum ferritin reflects the level of body iron stores; however, it has to be interpreted with caution because ferritin is an acute-phase reactant which increases in acute/chronic infection or inflammation. A concentration of less than 12 ng/ml is considered diagnostic of iron deficiency [22]. Serum iron is difficult to interpret because of several limitations: wide range of normal, subject to error from dietary ingestion, and decreases with mild or transient infections. Free erythrocyte protoporphyrin, however, is an excellent diagnostic tool. The final stage in the biosynthetic pathway of heme involves the incorporation of iron into protoporphyrin. Therefore, inadequate iron supply results in an accumulation of free protoporphyrin not incorporated into heme synthesis in the normoblast and the release of erythrocytes into the circulation with high FEP levels. Most laboratories reference a normal FEP level of 15.5 +/− 8.3 mg/dl. FEP elevation occurs as soon as the body stores of iron are depleted, before microcytic anemia develops. Hence, an elevated FEP level is seen with both IDA and lead poisoning. Lead inhibits the mitochondrial enzyme ferrochelatase, which catalyzes the terminal step, by inserting ferrous iron into protoporphyrin IX, in the biosynthesis of heme. Therefore, the substrate protoporphyrin increases in blood. However, values are normal in α - and β -thalassemia minor. There are a few other tests for iron deficiency that are not discussed in this section because they are not used in the routine clinical evaluation of anemia, serum transferrin receptor levels (STfR), STfR/log ferritin ratio, red blood cell zinc protoporphyrin/heme ratio, and serum hepcidin levels [7, 9].

Table 5.1 summarizes the key clinically significant diagnostic test for iron-deficiency anemia, thalassemia, and anemia of chronic disease.

Prevalence and Prevention of Iron Deficiency

Iron-deficiency anemia remains the leading cause of anemia worldwide. Both iron deficiency and iron-deficiency anemia in early life are associated with impaired cognitive, motor, and social-emotional development. During the past 40 years, improvements in infant nutrition in the United States and other developed countries have resulted in a dramatic decline in the prevalence of iron-deficiency anemia during the first year of life. The active promotion of breast-feeding, the use of iron-fortified formulas and iron-fortified infant cereals, and the withholding of cow milk until age 1 are mainly responsible.

However, this success story does not appear to hold true for many toddlers (1–3 years of age). Prevalence rates for toddler iron deficiency vary considerably from study to study. The widely quoted Third Nutrition Health and Nutrition Survey (NAHNES) [23] conducted between 1988 and 1994 reported a 3% prevalence of iron-deficiency anemia and a 9% prevalence of iron deficiency in toddlers 1–2-years of age. It also stated that the daily intake of in 1–2-year-olds was lower than any other age group throughout life. Other more recent studies [24–26] showed higher prevalence rates of 10% iron-deficiency anemia and 30% iron deficiency. This high prevalence of iron deficiency and iron-deficiency anemia in toddlers, especially those from lower socioeconomic groups, comes as no great surprise. Many 1–3-year-olds are picky and finicky eaters, often consuming large quantities of cow milk and apple juice, neither containing iron, and eating small amounts of iron-rich foods. It is important to point out that in the developing world, the prevalence of iron-deficiency anemia and iron deficiency is much higher due to both poor nutrition and increased blood loss from parasitic (hematophagous) infections.

The threat of long-lasting and perhaps permanent developmental delay due to iron deficiency during the first 3 years of life is well established. Many studies have concluded that during this period of rapid brain growth, iron deficiency and iron-deficiency anemia resulted in impaired psychomotor and mental development [27–36]. There is yet another reason to be concerned about the continuing high prevalence

Table 5.1 Differentiating laboratory features for iron-deficiency anemia, thalassemia, and anemia of chronic disease

	Hgb	MCV	RDW	Ferritin	TIBC	Transferrin saturation
IDA	↓	↓ or ⇔	↑	↓	↑	↓
α- and β-Thalassemia	↓	↓	↓	⇔	⇔	⇔
Anemia of chronic disease	↓	⇔ to ↓	⇔ to ↑	↑	↓	↓

Decreased: ↓ increased: ↑ normal: ⇔

of iron deficiency and iron-deficiency anemia in toddlers. In recent years, studies have demonstrated a clear relationship between iron deficiency and lead absorption [37, 38]. Iron deficiency has been shown to increase the gastrointestinal absorption of lead. An iron-deficient infant and toddler absorb more lead from the environment than an iron-sufficient child. Of particular interest is the fact that we have learned that even a very low lead level, below 10ug per deciliter, a level previously thought to be harmless is in fact neurotoxic, resulting in cognitive damage [39–41]. Because of these findings, both the CDC and WHO now state that no level of lead in the blood is safe in young children. Tremendous strides have been made in lowering the average lead levels in children, primarily due to the elimination of leaded gasoline and lead-based paint. However, lead levels, especially in toddlers, remain too high. Lead exposure remains a problem, and every effort must be made to not only reduce exposure but also to reduce the absorption of lead. One simple way is preventing iron deficiency, especially during the first 3 years of life. The prevention of iron deficiency and iron-deficiency anemia remains a major public health problem. The authors believe that the current high prevalence of toddler iron deficiency and iron-deficiency anemia is unacceptable and hazardous to the health and well-being of thousands of young children, especially the socioeconomically deprived.

The 2010 report of the Committee on Nutrition (CON) of the AAP [42] revisited the ongoing problem of iron deficiency and iron-deficiency anemia in infants and toddlers. The report stated that iron deficiency alone can adversely affect long-term neurodevelopment and behavior, and the damage may be irreversible. The report continued to advise universal screening for iron-deficiency anemia at 12 months of age. It also stated that for "high-risk" toddlers, including those from low socioeconomic families, preterm infants, and those exclusively breast-fed beyond 4 months without iron supplementation and those exposed to lead (constituting over 1/2 of all toddlers) as well as those toddlers who do not consume 7 mg of elemental iron each day be tested for iron deficiency via a blood ferratin level. In our opinion, these recommendations are impractical, difficult to accomplish, as well as expensive. A normal hematocrit at 1 year of age does not allow for the development of iron-deficiency anemia or iron deficiency during the second year of life, as demonstrated by Moser [43] in 10% of the children tested.

Current efforts to prevent iron deficiency and iron-deficiency anemia have not been successful. The authors believe that a more proactive approach is necessary. The solution to the problem is universal iron supplementation for all toddlers. The "tragedy" of iron deficiency affecting our nation's infants and toddlers described by Buchanan [44] can be overcome. While it is true that no studies to date have demonstrated that iron supplementation given to infants and toddlers with iron deficiency and iron-deficiency anemia improves their cognitive development [45], there is clear and convincing evidence that infant and toddler iron deficiency adversely affects mental and psychomotor development. It therefore makes intuitive good sense to prevent it from ever happening in the first place.

In an attempt to reduce the high prevalence rate of iron deficiency and iron-deficiency anemia, the New York District II chapter of the CON of the AAP in 2007 endorsed the following recommendation: "In order to prevent iron deficiency and reduce lead absorption, all toddlers should be placed on daily supplemental iron (10 mg of elemental iron) when switched to regular cow's milk, via a standard iron fortified vitamin until age 3." This recommendation is simple, safe, and effective and has no downside risks. The National CON of the AAP has not as yet adopted this recommendation. Therefore, Women, Infants, Children (WIC) support program-eligible toddlers, the "high-risk" group most in need, do not receive an iron-fortified vitamin as part of their WIC package. They remain at risk for both iron deficiency and increased lead absorption.

It is the sincere hope of the authors that the National CON of AAP modifies and expands their current recommendations for the prevention of iron deficiency and iron-deficiency anemia in toddlers to include the universal use of an iron-fortified vitamin to be given at the time the toddler is switched to regular cow milk. These vulnerable young children cannot afford to continue to lose precious IQ points.

Management of Iron Deficiency

Iron-deficiency anemia is always caused by an imbalance of iron homeostasis-iron absorption, and a loss is essentially equivalent at 1 mg daily, and 30 mg of iron daily – available from the recycling of iron from senescent erythrocytes – is needed to meet erythropoietic requirements. Therefore, the etiology of iron-deficiency anemia is imperative for proper therapy and management. Common conditions in children and adolescents include sideropenic diet, malabsorption due to celiac disease or *Helicobacter pylori* infection, and blood loss via epistaxis and/or the gastrointestinal or genitourinary tracts. Failure to treat the underlying cause will result in therapy failure. Familiar clinical scenarios are an adolescent woman with menorrhagia or a "milkaholic" toddler whose appetite is satiated by cow milk exclusively. In the former scenario, tranexamic acid 1300 mg thrice daily during menstruation and in the latter weaning off cow milk and persistently offering iron-rich foods are essential adjuncts to iron therapy.

The standard of care is to treat iron-deficiency anemia with oral iron. However, there is a wide variability in how iron-deficiency anemia is diagnosed and treated and in duration of therapy. A 20-question survey in which 2 hypothetical iron-deficiency anemia cases was sent to active members of the American Society of Pediatric Hematology/Oncology (1217 physicians were surveyed and 476 responded) [46]. For the hypothetical toddler with nutritional iron-deficiency anemia, 15% responded that only a complete blood count is necessary. The remaining respondents would order additional testing with serum ferritin, iron, and total iron-binding capacity being the most common combination selected by 23%. Only five respondents selected stool guaiac testing. The vast majority of respondents used ferrous sulfate dosed at 6 mg/kg/day elemental iron in two divided doses. For the hypothetical adolescent woman with menorrhagia, most respondents would use ferrous sulfate dosed at two to three tablets daily and not a weight-based regimen. There was a wide range of therapy duration among the respondents. Longer time in practice, smaller practice size, and a lack of an institutional fellowship program were associated with no testing beyond a complete blood count but no other management features.

Powers et al. studied the effect of low-dose (3 mg/kg/day of elemental iron) ferrous sulfate versus iron polysaccharide complex in young children with nutritional iron-deficiency anemia [47]. Eighty children were randomized, and 59 completed the 12-week course of iron – 28 in the ferrous sulfate group and 31 in the iron polysaccharide complex group. At the end of 12 weeks, the hemoglobin concentration increased from 7.9 to 11.9 grams/dL in the ferrous sulfate group and from 7.7 to 11.1 grams/dL in the iron polysaccharide complex group. This resulted in a greater difference of 1.0 grams/dL in the group of children treated with ferrous sulfate. Moreover, the serum ferritin level increase was higher, and more children experienced complete resolution of iron-deficiency anemia in the ferrous sulfate group. The investigators concluded that once-daily low-dose ferrous sulfate should be considered in the therapy of children with nutritional iron-deficiency anemia.

Stoffel et al. prospectively studied the effects of consecutive versus alternate days and single versus twice-daily divided doses on iron absorption using ^{54}Fe-, ^{57}Fe-, or ^{58}Fe-labeled ferrous sulfate in iron-depleted women [48]. In the first trial, 21 women were prescribed 60 mg of iron on consecutive days for 14 days, and 19 were prescribed 60 mg of iron on alternate days for 28 days. Only four women were mildly anemic. At the end of therapy, the cumulative fractional iron absorptions were 16.3%, and cumulative total iron absorption was 131 mg in the consecutive day group and in the alternate day group, 21.8% and 175.3 mg, respectively. At the end of 14 days of therapy, serum hepcidin was higher in the consecutive day groups as compared to the alternate day group, which might explain the differences in iron absorption between the two groups. In the second trial, ten women each were randomized to receive either once-daily dosing (120 mg) or twice-daily divided dosing (two dose of 60 mg each). No differences were observed in fractional or total iron absorption, but higher serum hepcidin levels were detected in the twice-daily divided dosing group. The main limitations of these studies are the small number of women enrolled and the exclusion of severely anemic women. Therefore, study results and conclusions may not be generalizable to young children, men, or those with severe anemia.

Due to its unpalatability and adverse gastrointestinal effects, tolerance of and compliance with oral ferrous sulfate is low. Moreover, children with diseases involving the small intestine – short gut syndrome and inflammatory bowel disease – may be refractory to oral iron supplementation. In these cases, intravenous iron is a suitable second-line therapy. Several intravenous iron preparations can be used in children with iron sucrose requiring multiple infusions and ferric carboxymaltose requiring just one infusion in the majority of patients. Crary et al. reviewed Children's Medical Center Dallas Pharmacy records to retrospectively study the efficacy and toxicity of intravenous iron sucrose [49]. From 2004 to 2009, 38 children younger than 18 years of age received a total of 510 infusions of intravenous iron sucrose. Thirteen children were refractory to oral iron, 13 had malabsorption, 7 had chronic gastrointestinal blood loss, and 5 had other indications. The median increase in hemoglobin level ranges from 1.9 to 3.1 grams/dL and was dependent on indication for intravenous iron sucrose. Only 1% of infusions were associated with an adverse reaction. Crary et al. concluded that intravenous iron sucrose is efficacious and safe in the therapy of children with iron deficiency. The Children's Medical Center Dallas investigators also retrospectively reviewed their experience with intravenous ferric carboxymaltose in children with iron-deficiency anemia [50]. Seventy-two children so affected received a total of 116 infusions of intravenous ferric carboxymaltose. The median hemoglobin increased from 9.1 grams/dl to 12.3 grams/dL. Transient complications were observed during or imme-diately after seven infusions. These investigators concluded that intravenous ferric carboxymaltose is efficacious and safe in children with iron deficiency refractory to oral iron therapy.

We recommend ferrous sulfate at 3 mg/kg/day of elemental iron once daily to treat iron-deficiency anemia. The dose should be given with juice preferably on an empty stomach. Response and compliance to oral iron are assessed after 1 month of therapy. If there is no response and compliance is not an issue, we recommend a more detailed gastrointestinal evaluation to rule out malabsorption or chronic blood loss. If compliance is an issue, we recommend intravenous iron sucrose – 100 mg of elemental iron weekly for 4 weeks in children weighing more than 30 kilograms and 50 mg of elemental iron weekly for 4 weeks in children weighing less than 30 kilo-grams. We reserve blood transfusions to those patients with cardiorespiratory dis-tress. To reiterate the underlying cause of iron deficiency must be sought in order for iron therapy to succeed.

References

1. Auerbach M, Schrier S. Treatment of iron deficiency is getting trendy. Lancet Haematol. 2017;4:e500–1.
2. Fleming MD. Nathan and Oski's hematology and oncology of infancy and childhood. In: Disorders of iron and copper metabolism, the sideroblastic anemias, and lead toxicity (Chapter 11). 8th ed. London: Elsevier Health Sciences; 2015.
3. Lonnerdal B, Georgieff MK, Hernell O. Developmental physiology of iron absorption, homeo-stasis, and metabolism in the healthy term infant. J Pediatr. 2015;167(4 Suppl):S8–14.
4. Ganz T, Nemeth E. Iron metabolism: interactions with normal and disordered erythropoiesis. Cold Spring Harb Perspect Med. 2012;2:a011668.
5. Guo S, Frazer DM, Anderson GJ. Iron homeostasis: transport, metabolism, and regulation. Curr Opin Clin Nutr Metab Care. 2016;19(4):276–81.
6. Ganz T, Nemeth E. Hepcidin and iron homeostasis. Biochim Biophys Acta. 2012;1823:1434–43.
7. Lanzkowsky P. Lanzkowsky's manual of pediatric hematology and oncology. In: Iron-deficiency anemia (Chapter 6). 6th ed. London Wall, London: Academic Press; 2016.
8. Brugnara C, Oski FA, Nathan DG. Nathan and Oski's hematology and oncology of infancy and childhood. In: Diagnostic approach to the anemic patient (Chapter 9). 8th ed. London: Elsevier Health Sciences; 2015.
9. Lanzkowsky P. Lanzkowsky's Manual of pediatric hematology and oncology. In: Classification and diagnosis of anemia in children (Chapter 3). 6th ed. London Wall, London: Academic Press; 2016.

10. Sinaki B, Jayabose S, Sandoval C. Iron deficiency anemia associated with hiatal hernia: case reports and literature review. Clin Pediatr. 2010;49:984–5.
11. Keefe E, Eden AN, Pandya S, Islam H, Sandoval C. Burkitt lymphoma masquerading as iron deficiency anemia. Research. 2014;1:764.
12. Karayalcin G, Lanzkowskt P. Pica with zinc deficiency. Lancet. 1976;2:687.
13. Goel A, Bakshi SS, Soni N, Chhavi N. Iron deficiency anemia and Plummer-Vinson syndrome: current insights. J Blood Med. 2017;8:175–84.
14. Tunnessen WW, Smith C, Oski FA. Beeturia. A sign of iron deficiency. Am J Dis Child. 1969;117:424–6.
15. National Heart, Lung, and Blood Institute working group on restless legs syndrome. Restless legs syndrome: detection and management in primary are. Am Fam Physician. 2000;62:108–14.
16. Mehmood T, Auerbach M, Earley CJ, Allen RP. Response to intravenous iron in patients with iron deficiency anemia and restless leg syndrome (Willis-Ekbom disease). Sleep Med. 2014;15:1473–6.
17. Nickerson HJ, Silberman T, Park RW, DeVries EO, Broste SK. Treatment of iron deficiency anemia and associated protein-losing enteropathy in children. J Pediatr Hematol Oncol. 2000;22:50–4.
18. Baker RD, Greer FR, Committee on Nutrition American Academy of Pediatrics. Diagnosis and prevention of iron deficiency and iron-deficiency anemia in infants and young children (0-3 years of age). Pediatrics. 2010;126:1040–50.
19. McDonagh MS, Blazina I, Dana T, Cantor A, Bougatsos C. Screening and routine supplementation for iron deficiency anemia: a systematic review. Pediatrics. 2015;135(4):723–33.
20. Powers JM, Daniel CL, McCavit TL, Buchanan GR. Deficiencies in the management of iron deficiency anemia during childhood. Pediatr Blood Cancer. 2016;63(4):743–5.
21. Powers JM, Buchanan GR. Diagnosis and management of iron deficiency anemia. Hematol Oncol Clin N Am. 2014;28(4):729–45.
22. Abdullah K, Birken CS, Maguire JL, Fehlings D, Hanley AJ, Thorpe KE, Parkin PC. Re-evaluation of serum ferritin cut-off values for the diagnosis of iron deficiency in children aged 12–36 months. J Pediatr. 2017;188:287–90.
23. Looker AC, Dallman PR, Carrol MD, Gunter EW, Johnson CL. Prevalence of iron deficiency in the U.S. JAMA. 1997;277:973–6.
24. Eden AN, Mir MA. Iron deficiency in 1-3 year old children: a pediatric failure? Arch Pediatric Adolesc Med. 1997;151:986–8.
25. Brugnara C, Zurakowski D, Dicanzio J, Boyd T, Platt O. Reticulocyte hemoglobin content to diagnose iron deficiency anemia in children. JAMA. 1999;281:3225–30.
26. Bogan DL, Duggan AK, Dover GJ, Wilson MH. Screening for iron deficiency anemia by dietary history in a high risk population. Pediatrics. 2000;105:1254–9.
27. Oski FA, Honig AS, Helu B, Howanitz P. Effect of iron therapy on behavior performance in non-anemic iron deficient infants. Pediatrics. 1983;71:877–80.
28. Walter T, Kovalskys J, Sekel A. Effect of mild iron deficiency on infant mental developmental scores. J Pediatr. 1983;102:519–22.
29. Lozoff B, Brittenham GH, Wolf AW, McClish DK, Kuhnert PM, Jimenez E, Jimenez R, Mora LA, Gomez I, Krauskoph D. Iron deficiency anemia and iron therapy effects on infants developmental test performance. Pediatrics. 1987;79:981–95.
30. Aukett MA, Parks YA, Scott PH, Wharton PA. Treatment with iron increases weight gain and psychomotor development. Arch Dis Child. 1986;61:849–54.
31. Hurtado EK, Claussen AN, Scott KG. Early childhood anemia and mild or moderate mental retardation. Am J Clin Nutr. 1999;69:115–9.
32. Walter T, DeAndraca I, Chadud P, Perales CG. Iron deficiency anemia: adverse effect on infant psychomotor development. Pediatrics. 1989;84:7–11.
33. Lozoff B, Jimenez E, Wolf AW. Long term developmental outcome of infants with iron deficiency. N Engl J Med. 1991;325:687–94.

34. Lozoff B, Jimenez E, Hagen J, Mollen E, Wolf AW. Poorer behavioral and developmental outcome more than 10 years after treatment for iron deficiency in infancy. Pediatrics. 2000;105:e51.
35. Congdon EL, Westerlund A, Algarin CR, Peirano PD, Gregas M, Lozoff B, Nelson CA. Iron deficiency in infancy is associated with altered neural correlates of recognition memory at 10 years. J Pediatr. 2012;160:1027–33.
36. Idjradinata P, Pollitt E. Reversal of developmental delays in iron deficient anemic infants treated with iron. Lancet. 1993;341:1–4.
37. Wright RO, Tsaih SW, Schwartz J, Wright RJ, Hu H. Association between iron deficiency and blood lead level in a longitudinal analysis of children followed in an urban primary care clinic. J Pediatr. 2003;142:9–14.
38. Bradman A, Eskenazi B, Sutton P, Athanasoulis M, Goldman LR. Iron deficiency associated with higher blood lead in children living in contaminated environments. Environ Health Perspect. 2001;109:1979–84.
39. Canfield RL, Henderson CR, Cory-Slechta DA, Cox C, Jusko TA, Lanphear BP. Intellectual impairment in children with blood lead concentration below 10ug per deciliter. N Engl J Med. 2003;348:1517–26.
40. Bellinger DC, Stiles KM, Needleman HL. Low level lead exposure, intelligence and academic achievement: a long term follow up study. Pediatrics. 1992;90:855–61.
41. Schwartz J. Low level exposure and children's IQ: a meta-analysis and search for a threshold. Environ Res. 1994;65:42–55.
42. AAP CON. Diagnosis and prevention of iron deficiency anemia in infant and young children (0–3 years of age). Pediatrics. 2010;126:1040–50.
43. Moser AM, Urkin J, Shalev H. Normal hemoglobin at the age of 1 year does not protect infants from developing iron deficiency anemia in the second year of life. J Pediatr Hematol Oncol. 2011;33:467–9.
44. Buchanan GR. The tragedy of iron deficiency during infancy and early childhood. J Pediatr. 1999;135:413–5.
45. Thompson J, Biggs BA, Pasricha SR. Effects of daily iron supplementation in 2-5 year old children: systemic review and meta-analysis. Pediatrics. 2013;131:739–53.
46. Powers JM, McCavit TL, Buchanan GR. Management of iron deficiency anemia: a survey of pediatric hematology/oncology specialists. Pediatr Blood Cancer. 2015;62:842–6.
47. Powers JM, Buchanan GR, Adix L, Zhang S, Gao A, McCavit TL. Effect of low-dose ferrous sulfate versus iron polysaccharide complex on hemoglobin concentration in young children with nutritional iron deficiency anemia: a randomized clinical trial. JAMA. 2017;317:2297–304.
48. Stoffel NU, Cercamondi CI, Brittenham G, Zeder C, Geurts-Moespot AJ, Swinkels DW, Moretti D, Zimmermann MB. Iron absorption from oral iron supplements given on consecutive versus alternate days and as single morning doses versus twice-daily split dosing in iron depleted women: two open-label, randomised controlled trials. Lancet Haematol. 2017;4:e524e533.
49. Crary SE, Hall K, Buchanan GR. Intravenous iron sucrose for children with iron deficiency failing to respond to oral iron therapy. Pediatr Blood Cancer. 2011;56:615–9.
50. Powers JM, Shamoun M, McCavit TL, Adix L, Buchanan GR. Intravenous ferric carboxymaltose in children with iron deficiency anemia who respond poorly to oral iron. J Pediatr. 2017;180:212–6.

Chapter 6
Anemia at the Extremes of Life: Congenital Hemolytic Anemia

Ariel L. Reinish and Suzie A. Noronha

Overview

Anemia occurs across all age groups and is commonly encountered by pediatricians. Hemolytic anemia, characterized by increased red blood cell (RBC) destruction, occurs in the newborn period and throughout childhood. It is distinguished from other types of anemia by the presence of reticulocytosis, which marks the compensatory response to increased RBC turnover. In the neonatal period, hemolytic anemia produces unconjugated hyperbilirubinemia, resulting in jaundice and sometimes necessitating phototherapy or exchange transfusion to avoid neurologic damage. Later in childhood, the presentation ranges from mild, asymptomatic disease to severe disease that impairs growth and warrants chronic RBC transfusions. Hemolysis can be intravascular or extravascular and inherited or acquired (Table 6.1).

Congenital hemolytic anemia will be the focus of this chapter. These anemias are predominantly extravascular and may result from de novo or inherited genetic defects that affect the function, shape, or stability of the erythrocyte. The main classes of congenital hemolytic anemia include the hemoglobinopathies, membranopathies, and enzymopathies. The acquired forms of hemolysis which should be ruled out include various immune-mediated, mechanical, and infectious etiologies and occur either in the intravascular or extravascular space.

Intravascular hemolysis defines RBC destruction within the circulation. Circulating RBCs undergo lysis via damage to the membrane from shear vessel or mechanical stress, toxins, or complement fixation. Free hemoglobin is released from the lysed erythrocytes and irreversibly binds to haptoglobin circulating in the plasma, and the resultant hemoglobin-haptoglobin complex is cleared by the liver. When circulating haptoglobin exceeds its binding capacity, the excess free

A. L. Reinish, MD · S. A. Noronha, MD (✉)
Division of Pediatric Hematology/Oncology, Golisano Children's Hospital,
University of Rochester Medical Center, Rochester, NY, USA
e-mail: Suzie_Noronha@URMC.Rochester.edu

© Springer Nature Switzerland AG 2019   95
R. T. Means Jr. (ed.), *Anemia in the Young and Old*,
https://doi.org/10.1007/978-3-319-96487-4_6

Table 6.1 Overview of common pediatric congenital versus acquired hemolytic anemias

	Disease	Site of destruction
Congenital	Hemoglobinopathies	Extravascular
	Red blood cell membrane defects	Extravascular
	Red blood cell enzyme defects	Both
Acquired	Neonatal alloimmune disease	Extravascular
	Autoimmune hemolytic anemia	Both
	Microangiopathic hemolytic anemia	Intravascular

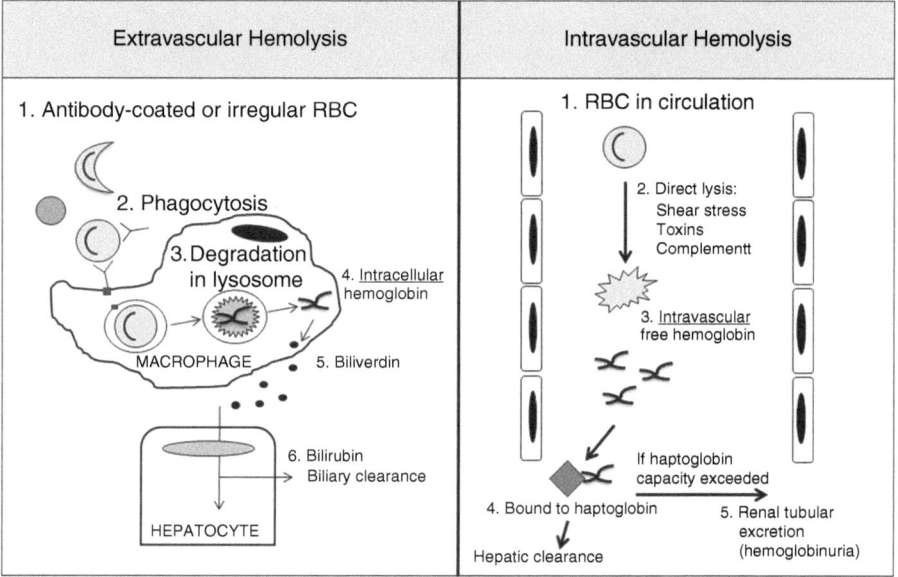

Fig. 6.1 Mechanism of intravascular versus extravascular hemolysis. (Reprinted from Noronha [1]. Copyright 2016, with permission from American Academy of Pediatrics)

hemoglobin continues to circulate in the blood; a fraction is reabsorbed by the proximal renal tubules, while the rest is excreted into the urine, causing hemoglobinuria (Fig. 6.1).

During extracellular hemolysis, splenic macrophages or hepatic Kupffer cells recognize RBCs that are either abnormally shaped or coated in antibody. The abnormal RBC structure impedes circulation through the 2-micron wide walls of the macrophage-rich splenic cords in the splenic sinusoids, leading to splenic sequestration and subsequent splenomegaly. Through these two effects, the splenic and hepatic macrophages phagocytose the abnormal RBCs. Heme is released and converted into biliverdin in the phagocyte and then into bilirubin in the hepatocyte, leading to the typical finding of hyperbilirubinemia [1, 2] (Fig. 6.1).

Immune-mediated etiologies of hemolytic anemia should be considered in the workup of a pediatric patient, particularly if unconjugated hyperbilirubinemia occurs in the newborn period. In neonatal alloimmune disease, which is extravascular, maternal antibodies to antigens on the fetal erythrocytes trigger hemolysis. Acquired newborn hemolytic disease may be due to ABO incompatibility, Rh isoimmunization, or minor antigen alloimmunization [1]. These patients will usually have a positive direct antiglobulin test (DAT), which detects IgG or complement coating the patient's RBCs [2]. If the DAT is negative, then an indirect antiglobulin test is done, which looks for maternal antibodies in the patient's serum. If the indirect test is also negative, then a congenital or nonimmune etiology is more likely. Later in childhood, primary or secondary autoimmune hemolytic anemia can occur, in which autoantibodies on the RBCs manifest in hemolysis under warm or cold conditions, which can be extravascular or intravascular. Secondary cases of autoimmune hemolytic anemia can result from acute infection, such as *Mycoplasma* or Epstein-Barr virus, primary immune disorder, drug exposure, or malignancy [1].

When considering congenital hemolytic anemia, the presentation can range from chronic to acute. Acute hemolysis should be considered when a patient presents suddenly with pallor, fatigue, dyspnea, chest pain, tachycardia, or other signs of anemia, with the acute onset of jaundice, dark urine, and abdominal or back pain further pointing toward the diagnosis [3]. In pediatric patients presenting with aplastic crisis in the setting of parvovirus infection, congenital hemolytic anemia should always be considered in the differential and workup [4]. Hemolytic anemia, either acquired or congenital, should also be considered in the newborn with jaundice or hyperbilirubinemia requiring intervention, especially within the first 24 h. Chronic hemolysis can lead to pigmented gallstones due to chronically elevated bilirubin. Other possible clinical findings include a flow murmur if the anemia is severe, leg ulcers, and evidence of extramedullary erythropoiesis, such as frontal bossing.

Initial laboratory evaluation for congenital hemolytic anemia should include a complete blood count (CBC), reticulocyte count, and complete metabolic panel (CMP), which would reveal normocytic or macrocytic anemia with indirect hyperbilirubinemia and reticulocytosis. The aspartate aminotransferase level might also be elevated, which can signify hemolysis. The next step in the workup should be a formal evaluation for hemolysis, including lactate dehydrogenase (LDH), haptoglobin, and peripheral blood smear. In most cases, the anemia is normocytic, but if the reticulocytosis is substantial, that can falsely elevate the MCV, causing an apparent macrocytic anemia [2]. Reticulocytosis usually exceeds 2%, but some patients can exhibit reticulocytopenia, such as during parvovirus infection or if a patient has bone marrow dysfunction or hemolysis affecting the reticulocytes [1]. Increased LDH and decreased haptoglobin may be seen. However, states of inflammation can elevate haptoglobin, an acute-phase reactant, whereas other conditions, such as malnutrition and liver disease, can cause haptoglobin to be low. Furthermore, LDH can be elevated in other scenarios besides hemolysis, including heart failure and malignancy [3]. Peripheral blood smear findings vary but can show abnormally shaped RBCs, with schistocytes being a hallmark of intravascular hemolysis. Spherocytes will be present in both immune-mediated hemolysis as well as hereditary spherocytosis. The smear will also show stigmata typical of other diseases, such as schistocytes, erythrocyte fragments, and thrombocytopenia in the setting of disseminated intravascular coagulation, or Heinz bodies in the setting of glucose-6-phosphate dehydrogenase deficiency [2, 3].

If hemolysis labs are unrevealing, then other etiologies of anemia should be considered. Once hemolysis has been confirmed or is highly suspected, direct antiglobulin testing, or DAT, is performed [2]. A negative DAT rules out most immune-mediated etiologies, but if autoimmune hemolytic anemia is still suspected, indirect antiglobulin testing might be needed [1]. Further workup depends on family history, infection or drug exposure, and RBC morphology, which will guide the clinician down different diagnostic pathways, possibly requiring hemoglobin electrophoresis, enzyme assays, or genetic testing. Subsequent treatment will depend on the etiology that is determined.

Hemoglobinopathies

Hemoglobin Structure is a four-unit protein, or tetramer, comprising four globin chain subunits bound to iron-containing heme, which carries oxygen. Fetal hemoglobin, or hemoglobin F ($\alpha2\gamma2$), consists of two alpha-globin units and two gamma-globin units, while the predominant adult hemoglobin, hemoglobin A ($\alpha2\beta2$), consists of two alpha-globin units and two beta-globin units. Over the first 6 months of life, a transcriptional shift in erythroid progenitors occurs, switching β-like globin chain production from gamma-globin to beta-globin, resulting in the observed shift from fetal hemoglobin to adult hemoglobin, which accounts for about 96–98% of the total hemoglobin in the normal individual [5, 6]. To a lesser degree, children and adults also express hemoglobin A2 ($\alpha2\delta2$), consisting of two alpha-globin units and two delta-globin units and making up about 2–3% of total hemoglobin [6]. The production of alpha-globins is governed by a set of genes in the alpha-globin gene locus on the short arm of chromosome 16. Four alpha-globin alleles exist in total, with two inherited on each copy of chromosome 16 [7, 8]. The β-like globin chains are encoded by a cluster of genes on the short arm of chromosome 11, with a single gene locus coding for beta-globin, such that two beta-globin alleles exist in total with one inherited on each copy of the chromosome [9]. If a genetic mutation causes impaired incorporation of the globin chain into the hemoglobin molecule, then the resultant destabilized hemoglobin can lead to hemolytic anemia in varying degrees [10].

Alpha-Thalassemias

Alpha-thalassemia is a frequent cause of unexplained hypochromic microcytic anemia. In one study in Turkey, 46.1% of patients with hypochromic microcytic anemia carried a mutation causing thalassemia [11]. The disease occurs worldwide with high frequencies in subtropical and tropical regions; the clinically significant forms occur most frequently in Southeast Asia, the Mediterranean region, and the Middle East [8, 12]. Alpha-thalassemia, like many of the other hemoglobinopathies to be discussed, has been shown to confer a protective effect against malaria [13]. In the Tharu people of Nepal, alpha-thalassemia occurs with a gene frequency of 80%; concurrently, the rate of malaria in that population is significantly less compared to other populations in that region [14]. Most patients with alpha-thalassemia in North America are of Asian descent, but mixed-race patients comprise an important and growing population as immigration patterns change [15, 16].

Alpha-thalassemia results from mutations that decrease the production of functional alpha-globin chains. Usually, the inherited mutation results in deletion of an alpha gene, although in some cases, non-deletional (e.g., point mutations) determinants are inherited that can result in less alpha-globin production than the deletion would [12]. An excellent example of genotype-phenotype correlation, the number of inherited mutated genes dictates disease severity (Table 6.2).

In the "silent carrier state," affected individuals inherit one deleted or inactivated alpha allele and demonstrate no phenotypic changes; these individuals are referred to as α^+ carriers [6]. When two deleted or inactivated alleles are inherited, affected individuals have α-thalassemia trait or minor. When both affected alleles reside on the same chromosome, the condition is referred to as *cis*-type α-thalassemia trait, with the affected individual being referred to as an α^0 carrier. When the two affected alelles are on different chromosomes, the condition is referred to as *trans*-type α-thalassemia trait. Individuals with α-thalassemia trait are generally asymptomatic without any growth impairment. These individuals are often diagnosed after the incidental finding of mild microcytic hypochromic anemia in the setting of normal iron studies. If clinically significant anemia arises in these patients, alternative diagnoses beyond α-thalassemia trait should be pursued [8, 12].

When three mutated alleles are inherited, affected individuals can exhibit clinically significant although variable hemoglobin H (HbH) disease. Affected individuals express 30% less than the normal amount of alpha-globin units, resulting in the

Table 6.2 Overview of alpha-thalassemia genetics and phenotype

	Genetics	Lab findings	Clinical course
Normal	$\alpha\alpha/\alpha\alpha$	n/a	n/a
Silent carrier state	$\alpha\alpha/-\alpha$	None	None
Alpha-thalassemia trait/ minor	$-\alpha/-\alpha$ or $\alpha\alpha/--$	Mild, microcytic hypochromic anemia	Usually asymptomatic
Hemoglobin H disease	$-\alpha/--$	Microcytic hypochromic anemia Hb Bart's peak on newborn screen Varying percentages of HbH	Variable
Hemoglobin Bart's hydrops fetalis syndrome	$--/--$	Severe in utero anemia	Heart failure, usually intrauterine death or soon after birth

formation of insoluble, unstable β-like globin chain tetramers with high oxygen affinity that cause oxidative damage, impair erythropoiesis, and predispose RBCs to hemolysis [8, 12, 15, 17]. During early infancy, the relative deficiency of alpha-globin chains leaves unpaired gamma-globin units to coprecipitate, forming Hb Barts (ɣ4). Likewise, after the transcriptional shift to adult hemoglobin, excess beta-globin units form the homotetramer HbH (β4). Blood work is notable for a microcytic, hypochromic anemia with MCV ranging from 62 to 67 fl, MCH below 20 pg, and hemoglobin between 8.8 and 11 g/dl [17, 18]. During newborn screening, high-performance liquid chromatography (HPLC) or capillary electrophoresis will detect an Hb Bart's peak. Later in childhood, these methods will show varying percentages of HbH [8].

Deletional forms of HbH disease are far more common but much less severe than non-deletional forms. Eighty percent of cases are deletional in nature, which is what this chapter will focus on [19–21]. Patients with HbH tend to express relatively high baseline levels of hemoglobin and do not require transfusion unless their hemoglobin level drops below 8–9 g/dl, which can be symptomatic [19]. Patients with classic HbH disease rarely have growth retardation, 15% have splenomegaly, and most do not require a blood transfusion until their early teenage years. Up to three-quarters of adult patients with HbH disease exhibit iron overload, independent of transfusion history. This consequence is thought to be related to the increased erythropoiesis that occurs in response to ongoing hemolysis, which then upregulates gastrointestinal absorption of iron [17, 22].

Treatment of HbH disease generally revolves around management of hemolytic episodes, during which hemoglobin can drop as low as 3 g/dl. Hemolytic episodes may be precipitated by fever, exposure to an oxidative drug, or acute infection [19, 21]. Recommended management of hemolytic episodes includes transfusing to levels between 8 and 9 g/dl to avoid cardiovascular compromise, providing adequate hydration, ensuring normal electrolyte status, and providing appropriate antibiotic treatment and infection control when indicated; in the case of a patient with splenic dysfunction, coverage of encapsulated bacteria must be considered. Patients with HbH disease may benefit from folic acid supplementation (2–5 mg/day) to support enhanced erythropoiesis [19]. Distinct from hemolytic crisis, patients can experience red cell aplasia secondary to parvovirus B19 infection. The virus preferentially infects erythrocyte precursors via binding to the erythrocyte P antigen and disrupts erythropoiesis. In patients with chronic hemolytic diseases such as HbH disease, which results in erythrocytes with shortened lifespan, interruptions in erythropoiesis can be life-threatening. In contrast to hemolytic crises, aplastic crises are characterized by reticulocytopenia in addition to severe anemia [19, 23]. Chelation therapy may be required for patients who develop iron overload.

When four mutated alleles are inherited, affected individuals cannot produce functional hemoglobin and develop the devastating Hb Bart's hydrops fetalis syndrome. Most fetuses with this condition will die in utero or soon after birth, with the pregnancy conferring life-threatening maternal health risks, such as preeclampsia and disseminated intravascular coagulation [21]. The affected fetus cannot effectively produce hemoglobin, resulting in massive extramedullary hematopoiesis and fetal hypoxia, which in turn cause massive hydrops and developmental anomalies

[15, 21]. Advances in recent years, including intrauterine and postnatal transfusions and even hematopoietic stem cell transplants, have resulted in some increased survival. However, these individuals still suffer multiple morbidities, including severe growth retardation, neurodevelopmental delay, and the need for lifelong transfusions [15, 24]. Management of Hb Bart's hydrops fetalis syndrome revolves around prevention and multidisciplinary prenatal care, including counseling and providing molecular diagnostic testing to at-risk couples and monitoring for severity of intrauterine anemia during an at-risk pregnancy [15].

Beta-Thalassemia

Beta-thalassemia occurs worldwide, affecting 1.5% of the global population with a notable prevalence in subtropical and tropical regions such as the Mediterranean, sub-Saharan Africa, and the Middle East. More than 200 beta-thalassemia mutations have been identified. Like alpha-thalassemia, beta-thalassemia confers a protective effect against malaria, thus explaining its high gene frequency in those areas [9, 25]. Shifting migration patterns have led to increasing prevalence of beta-thalassemia in other regions of the world [25, 26]. An increasing proportion of patients with beta-thalassemia in North America are now of Asian descent, in contrast to approximately 50 years ago, when most patients were of Italian or Greek descent. This change is attributed to shifting immigration patterns to North America [16].

   Beta-thalassemia is caused by one or more inherited mutations in the beta-globin gene (Table 6.3). Unlike alpha-thalassemia, these mutations are usually nondeletional. The insufficient production of beta units causes excess alpha chains to

Table 6.3 Overview of beta-thalassemia genetics and phenotype

	Possible genetics	Lab findings	Clinical course
Normal	β/β	n/a	n/a
Beta-thalassemia trait/ minor	β/β^0, β/β^+	Mild microcytic, hypochromic anemia Increased HbA2 Mildly increased HbF	Asymptomatic to mild
Beta-thalassemia intermedia	β^+/β^0, β^+/β^+	Microcytic, hypochromic anemia Increased HbA2 (>4%) Increased HbF (10–50%)	Variable
Beta-thalassemia major	β^0/β^0	Severe microcytic, hypochromic anemia Increased HbA2 Increased HbF Absence of HbA1 after 6 months of age	Severe, transfusion dependent

form an unstable hemoglobin tetramer, leading to ineffective erythropoiesis and hemolysis [27]. The β^0 designation indicates a mutation associated with no production of beta-globin, whereas β^+ refers to a mutation with some, albeit decreased, beta-globin production [9]. When individuals inherit one mutated allele, they have beta-thalassemia trait or minor, which is a benign condition characterized by mild microcytic hypochromic anemia. In addition, they express increased HbA2 and sometimes mildly increased fetal hemoglobin on hemoglobin electrophoresis [9]. Beta-thalassemia trait is the most common inherited hemoglobinopathy and is often confused for iron deficiency anemia on routine blood work. One study found the Mentzer index, or the ratio of MCV to RBC count, demonstrated the best reliability compared to other RBC indices for differentiating between the two disorders [28].

Homozygosity or compound heterozygosity of beta-globin mutations leads to clinically significant disease. Co-inheritance of two mild mutations or a mild and a severe mutation typically produces the beta-thalassemia intermedia phenotype [27]. The hallmarks of beta-thalassemia intermedia are ineffective erythropoiesis and non-transfusion-dependent hemolytic anemia. Patients may also experience iron overload, a consequence of intermittent transfusions and/or increased gastrointestinal iron absorption from enhanced erythropoiesis [26, 29]. Ineffective erythropoiesis induces extramedullary hematopoiesis, resulting in skull and facial deformities and the development of extramedullary pseudotumors in nearly all areas of the body; up to 20% of patients with beta-thalassemia intermedia develop extramedullary hematopoiesis by the third decade of life [26, 30, 31]. Physical examination of affected individuals may reveal hepatosplenomegaly and characteristic facial bone expansion known as frontal bossing with lower jaw protrusion [31]. These individuals may experience increased thrombotic events, some of which go unrecognized; one study showed that 37.5% of patients with beta-thalassemia intermedia had silent cerebral infarcts on MRI [31, 32]. Other complications, due to ongoing hemolysis, tissue hypoxia, and hypercoagulability, include growth retardation, gallstones, leg ulcers, pulmonary hypertension, and heart failure. Furthermore, complications of the aforementioned iron overload include endocrine abnormalities and bone disease [26, 31].

The overall presentation for beta-thalassemia intermedia varies, and diagnosis is typically made clinically. Blood work will reveal a microcytic, hypochromic anemia with hemoglobin in the 7–10 g/dl range, MCH in the 16–24 pg range, and MCV in the 50–80 range, with nucleated RBCs, target cells, teardrop cells, and RBC fragments on the peripheral smear. Hemoglobin electrophoresis will show greater than 4% HbA2 and 10–50% fetal hemoglobin [25, 31]. While not the current standard, increasing evidence supports a genetic approach to diagnosis. In particular, current research entails calculating predictive scores for disease severity based on underlying disease mutation in combination with other genetic modifiers, such as polymorphisms affecting adult levels of fetal hemoglobin [33–35].

Management of beta-thalassemia intermedia is multifaceted and based on consensus rather than robust clinical trials. Transfusion plays a large role in supportive care, but the risks of chronic transfusion need to be balanced with the clinical need. Indications for transfusion include growth failure in children, exercise intolerance in adults, upcoming surgery, severe infection, an acute drop in hemoglobin less than 5 g/dl, pregnancy, and treatment of complications such as pulmonary hypertension [26, 30]. Patients generally do not require a scheduled transfusion regimen, particularly in light of the risk of alloimmunization incurred by chronic transfusions in pediatric patients [31, 36]. Iron overload can be a significant problem independent of transfusion history; patients should initiate chelation therapy when serum ferritin levels exceed 800–1000 µg/l [22, 30]. Select patients may undergo splenectomy, especially if they have persistent poor growth, increasing need for transfusion, hypersplenism, or splenomegaly at risk for rupture. Splenectomy is avoided prior to the age of five due to the risk of fulminant sepsis with encapsulated bacteria [26, 31]. In addition, evidence suggests that splenectomy may increase the risk of thromboembolic events, so the decision to proceed with splenectomy should not be taken lightly [37–39]. Fetal hemoglobin inducers such as hydroxyurea may be considered. These agents increase the production of gamma-globins which then bind to the excess alpha-globins and increase the proportion of circulating stable hemoglobin tetramers. Hydroxyurea has been shown to raise baseline hemoglobin with generally minor side effects; evidence remains unclear regarding whether or not hydroxyurea actually reduces transfusion needs [26, 40–43]. Finally, as a curative option, patients can undergo stem cell transplantation, but the data regarding outcomes is limited [31].

Beta-thalassemia major manifests when patients inherit two severe beta-globin gene mutations, which express no to minimal adult hemoglobin. Laboratory work will show hemoglobin less than 7 g/dl, MCV ranging from 50 to 70 fl, and MCH in the 12–20 pg range; hemoglobin electrophoresis and HPLC will be notable for greater than 90% fetal hemoglobin and increased HbA2 [25]. The same red cell morphologic changes seen with beta-thalassemia minor will be seen with beta-thalassemia major. The absence of HbA1 after 6 months of age, due to deficient beta-globin expression, confirms the diagnosis.

Beta-thalassemia major is characterized by a more severe disease course than beta-thalassemia intermedia. Affected individuals often present after 6 months of age and generally by 2 years of age, once fetal hemoglobin expression declines. Markedly severe microcytic anemia as well as jaundice and hepatosplenomegaly can be seen, with undiagnosed infants exhibiting failure to thrive, irritability, and worsening pallor. Affected patients require chronic transfusions to survive. Clinical manifestations of note, especially in undertransfused patients, include growth retardation, skeletal deformities with craniofacial changes as described in beta-thalassemia intermedia, extramedullary hematopoietic pseudotumors, worsening hepatosplenomegaly, and iron overload as a result of both the disease and chronic transfusions [25]. High-output heart failure also occurs, with cardiac failure serving as a large cause of mortality in these patients [25, 44]. Thromboembolic events also occur, but they seem to be more prevalent in patients with beta-thalassemia intermedia than beta-thalassemia major [29, 37].

Treatment of beta-thalassemia major requires chronic transfusions in order to support growth and development, suppress ineffective erythropoiesis, and inhibit gastrointestinal absorption of iron. Current recommendations include transfusions every 2–5 weeks in order to maintain hemoglobin in the range of 9–10.5 g/dl; this range has been shown to optimize growth and minimize enhanced erythropoiesis. Iron overload develops at a slower rate than that observed in more aggressive transfusion regimens [25, 45]. Indications for splenectomy are similar to those for beta-thalassemia intermedia, including increasing transfusion requirements, hypersplenism, and splenomegaly with concern for rupture. The benefits of splenectomy must be weighed against the risk for sepsis, especially in young children, as well as the observed increase in thrombotic events [25, 37]. Iron overload inevitably develops, so chelation therapy should begin after individuals have received between 10 and 15 transfusions or when their ferritin level exceeds 1000 µg/l, usually by 2 years of age [46–48]. Inducers of fetal hemoglobin such as hydroxyurea may provide some benefit to patients and decrease the need for transfusions, but further evidence is needed to determine their efficacy [5, 25, 49]. Hematopoietic stem cell transplantation remains the only curative option for beta-thalassemia major, with the best outcomes seen in human leukocyte antigen (HLA)-matched sibling donor transplants [50]. Of note, one study in Italy found similar 30-year survival rates between patients treated with stem cell transplantation compared to conventional supportive therapy, perhaps reflecting the progress that has been made with current supportive therapy [25]. Lastly, many experimental therapies are currently being pursued for the treatment of beta-thalassemia major, including new conditioning regimens for stem cell transplantation and phase I clinical trials in gene therapy [51].

Sickle Cell Disease

Historical Context

The first description of sickle cell disease in English literature is credited to Dr. James B. Herrick, a Chicago physician who reported his experience treating a young dental student from Grenada in 1910. Remarking on the "large number of thin, elongated, sickle-shaped and crescent-shaped forms" on the patient's blood smear, Dr. Herrick was unable to diagnose the patient, who experienced recurrent episodes of pain, low-grade fever, and jaundice [52]. By 1949, the electrophoretic mobility and Mendelian inheritance pattern of sickle hemoglobin had been elucidated [53–55].

Epidemiology and Genetics

Sickle cell disease (SCD) is a heterogeneous inherited disease affecting 70,000–140,000 Americans. The sickle haplotype is prevalent in equatorial areas in Africa, Asia, and Central and South America, amounting to more than 300,000 infants born with homozygous disease worldwide in 2010. An estimated 75% of those infants were born in sub-Saharan Africa [56]. Co-inheritance of the sickle haplotype with other hemoglobin mutations results in sickle cell manifestations of variable severity.

One in 300–400 infants are diagnosed annually with SCD in the United States through universal newborn screening. Most infants (60–65%) have homozygous SS disease, 20–25% have hemoglobin SC disease, while 9% co-inherit hemoglobin S and beta-thalassemia trait [57].

Pathophysiology

Thought to confer protection from malaria, the central anomaly is a single point mutation changing glutamine to valine in the sixth position of the beta-globin molecule. This results in interactions between valine and the phenylalanine and leucine of adjoining tetramers, leading to abnormal polymerization of the beta-globin in the setting of deoxygenation [58]. This leads to reversible then irreversible deformation of the erythrocyte into the characteristic "sickle" shape, which moves poorly through the microvasculature (Fig. 6.2). While vaso-occlusion was long thought to be the sole physiologic change in SCD, it is now clear that multiple mechanisms contribute to the tissue ischemia and damage that are hallmarks of the disease. Chronic hemolysis resulting from membrane damage leads to release of erythrocyte arginase, which depletes arginine, a key substrate in the production of nitric oxide (NO). NO deficiency leads to vasomotor dysfunction (Fig. 6.3). Chronic hemolysis also releases free oxygen radicals which injure vascular endothelial cells, triggering cytokine release, upregulation of inflammatory mediators, recruitment and sequestration of neutrophils, and activation of platelets [59, 60]. This confluence of abnormalities ultimately leads to a chronic inflammatory and hypercoagulable state.

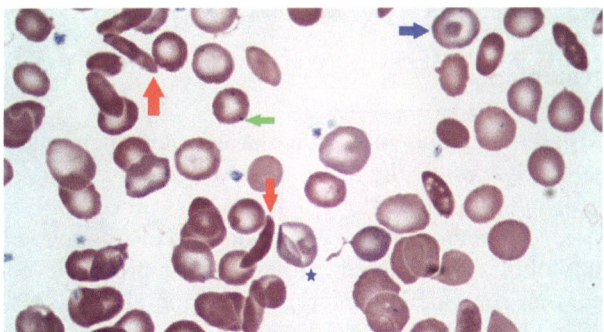

Fig. 6.2 Red blood cell morphology in sickle cell disease. The smear depicts blood from a patient on hydroxyurea, so the percentage of sickled cells relative to a patient not on treatment is substantially lower. Sickled erythrocytes (red arrows), target cells (blue arrow), and reticulocytes (star) are present. The green arrow denotes Howell-Jolly bodies, indicative of impaired splenic function

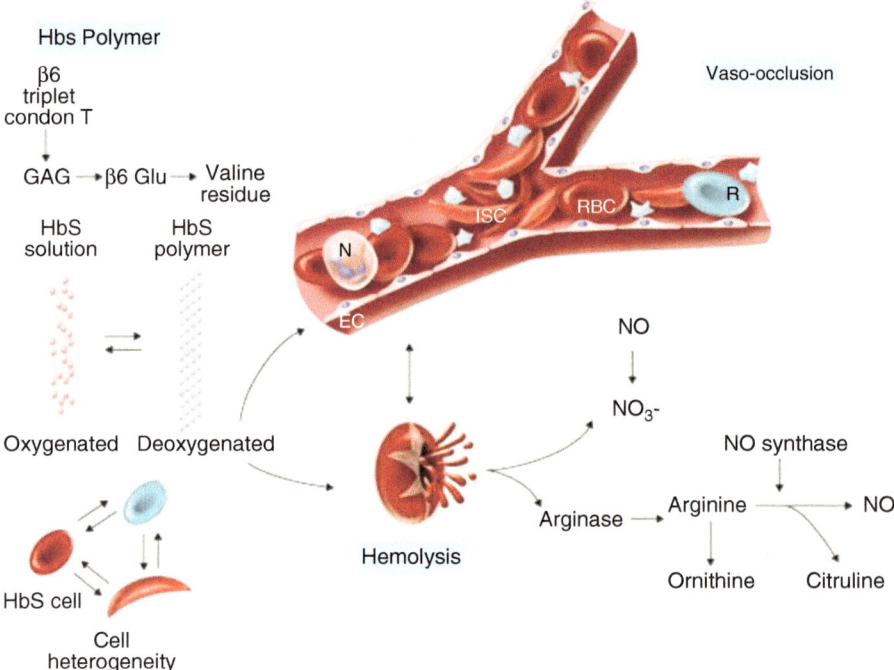

Fig. 6.3 Pathophysiology of sickle cell disease. A single point mutation leads to replacement of glutamine by valine in the beta-globin molecule. In deoxygenated state, the abnormal beta-globin protein undergoes reversible and then irreversible abnormal polymerization. The rigid protein forces the erythrocyte to take on a sickled shape, which is injurious to the cell. The resulting hemolysis depletes nitric oxide through the release of erythrocyte arginase. Within the vasculature, neutrophil recruitment, platelet activation, and endothelial cell injury contribute to the chronic inflammatory state of SCD. (Reprinted from Steinberg [248]. Copyright 2016 with permission from Elsevier)

Clinical Presentation

Individuals with homozygous inheritance of the sickle hemoglobin (i.e., hemoglobin SS) generally exhibit the most severe phenotype, although this may be attenuated by co-inheritance of alpha-thalassemia trait or a polymorphism associated with increased hemoglobin F expression [61]. Compound heterozygosity of sickle hemoglobin and a severe beta-thalassemia mutation (beta-zero-thalassemia) produces an equivalent phenotype to hemoglobin SS. Co-inheritance of hemoglobin S and hemoglobin C can be associated with vaso-occlusive complications to a lesser extent but is not associated with increased risk of stroke. They have increased rates of retinal disease [62]. By convention, the term "sickle cell anemia" connotes hemoglobin SS or hemoglobin S-beta-zero-thalassemia.

Pain Infants are generally asymptomatic due to predominance of hemoglobin F expression, but some may experience dactylitis, defined as painful swelling of the hands and feet. This may be a potential marker of severe disease, but there is no consensus on predictors of severity for SCD [63–66]. As hemoglobin F expression declines, children may begin to experience acute onset of mild to severe pain affecting various parts of the body, including long bones, joints, abdomen, back, and chest. Triggers of pain can include dehydration, illness, exposure to temperature extremes, hypoxia, and emotional stress [67]. These painful episodes, often called vaso-occlusive crises (VOC), may last 1 day to 2 weeks. Young children may present in obvious distress accompanied by rise in temperature, baseline heart rate, and/or blood pressure. As children age, changes in vital signs may be less marked. Older children and adolescents are often less demonstrative of pain as they acquire coping skills and apply distraction techniques. Physical examination findings may be unremarkable or include scleral icterus and jaundice if hemolysis has increased or localized swelling and tenderness to palpation of the affected area. Subtle changes in laboratory markers, such as leukocytosis, thrombocytosis, reticulocytosis, or increased nucleated RBCs, may be observed, but the absence of such changes does not preclude the presence of a crisis. Alternative diagnoses such as acute chest syndrome, pulmonary emboli, stroke, osteomyelitis, cholelithiasis, avascular necrosis, and delayed hemolytic transfusion reaction should be ruled out in the appropriate clinical context.

Management of painful crises usually includes application of heat to the affected area, judicious hydration, anti-inflammatory agents, and opioid medications. Mild pain is usually managed at home with oral medication. Adolescents and young adults with frequent severe pain crises benefit from standardized protocols that can be implemented quickly in the emergency room or ambulatory infusion center. If management in the ambulatory setting does not sufficiently control the pain within 3–4 h, admission is warranted. Severe pain is best managed by patient-controlled analgesia, which is associated with lower total doses of opioid and shorter length of stay compared with intermittent dosing [68, 69]. Supportive care while on narcotics should include a bowel regimen to prevent opioid-induced constipation and aggressive pulmonary toilet to prevent the development of acute chest syndrome.

As seen in other pain syndromes, some adult patients go on to develop central sensitization, whereby modification of nociceptors leads to hyperalgesia (increased sensitivity to painful stimuli), allodynia (pain due to non-noxious stimuli), and expanded receptor fields (pain felt beyond the injured area) [70]. Chronic pain is a significant challenge in these patients as they age, and there is little useful data on optimal management of this difficult complication.

The social consequences of VOC can be as complex and troubling as the physiologic complications. The nationwide surge in opioid misuse and related mortality prompted the CDC to issue guidelines for opioid prescribing practices [71]. These guidelines do not apply to children nor do they address the unique nuances of pain management for chronic disorders like SCD. Opioid prescribing practices for SCD patients has not been well studied and are not standardized. Misconceptions about opioid use by medical providers in the ED or clinic can lead to delays in appropriate care and compromise mutual trust among patients and medical staff [72–74]. School absenteeism and grade retention are major problems for these children and their caregivers [75–77]. Physician partnership with school officials can facilitate accommodations that will support academic performance.

Spleen/Immune System   Infants exhibit hyposplenism as early as 5 months of age [78]. The relatively slow flow rate of blood through the splenic matrix promotes deoxygenation and resultant deformation and adhesion of sickle erythrocytes. Recurrent obstruction of the splenic microvasculature leads to progressive fibrosis and eventual atrophy of the spleen by age 5. Prior to uniform institution of penicillin prophylaxis in infancy, bacteremia ranged from 3.7 to 8.3 cases per 100 person-years. Mortality rates from pneumococcal and *Haemophilus* infections were 14.5% and 20%, respectively [57]. The landmark PROPS study, which randomized infants with SCD to observation or penicillin prophylaxis, was halted early due to interim analysis showing an 84% reduction in sepsis in the penicillin arm [79]. Penicillin prophylaxis is now initiated in all infants diagnosed with SCD. Further reductions in morbidity and mortality were achieved after introduction of the pneumococcal and *Haemophilus influenzae* vaccines [80]. Nonetheless, breakthrough infections occur [81, 82], so families are educated to bring their children for evaluation of fever. Broad-spectrum antibiotics with antipneumococcal activity are given after collection of a blood culture. The decision to admit or discharge home while monitoring cultures appears to be institution-specific [83].

Some children are at increased risk for acute sequestration of erythrocytes within the spleen. This complication is defined by acute enlargement of the spleen accompanied by a drop in hemoglobin by 2 g/dl from baseline. Thrombocytopenia may be observed as well. Episodes may be mild and self-resolve, or they can be life-threatening with sequestration of a large percentage of blood volume within the spleen, causing cardiovascular collapse. Children experiencing splenic sequestration are at risk for recurrent episodes. There is no consensus on preventive measures which can include observation, chronic transfusion, or splenectomy [57, 84].

Neurologic Disease   The pathophysiology of stroke remains incompletely understood but is thought to result from increased red cell adherence to vascular endothelium, a chronic inflammatory and hypercoagulable state as a result of recurrent endothelial injury, and NO deficiency related to chronic hemolysis. Poor cerebrovascular reserve due to anemia may also play a role [85].

Prior to widespread transcranial Doppler screening, 11% of children with severe sickle cell disease (i.e., hemoglobin SS and S-beta-zero-thalassemia) experienced stroke by age 20 [86]. New-onset unilateral facial droop, slurred speech, unilateral weakness, seizures, and/or headache may be suggestive of stroke and should prompt emergent non-contrast head computed tomography and magnetic resonance imaging (MRI). Ischemic stroke is far more common in children than in adults, who experience greater rates of hemorrhagic stroke. MRI shows changes associated with acute infarction. Angiography may show stenosis or obstruction of cerebral arteries. Once stroke is diagnosed, the patient should undergo emergent exchange transfusion to rapidly reduce the sickle hemoglobin percentage to less than 30%. Recurrent stroke occurs in 47–66% [87, 88], but several groups demonstrated that lifelong, chronic transfusions to keep the hemoglobin S percentage ≤30% are effective secondary prevention [89, 90]. About 40% of patients after ischemic stroke may go on to develop moyamoya syndrome, in which chronic obstruction of cerebral arteries promotes neovascularization. These collateral vessels appear as a "puff of smoke" on angiography and confer an elevated risk of stroke in these patients, in spite of chronic transfusion. Revascularization procedures or bone marrow transplantation should be considered to ameliorate this risk [91–93].

Elevated cerebral arterial flow (>200 cm/s) on transcranial Doppler (TCD) ultrasounds can identify asymptomatic sickle cell patients with increased risk of stroke [94, 95]. The landmark, randomized controlled Stroke Prevention Trial in Sickle Cell Anemia (STOP) trial established that chronic transfusion can prevent stroke in sickle cell patients with abnormal TCDs aged 2–16 years. Compared with the observation arm, patients who were randomized to chronic transfusion to keep the hemoglobin S percentage ≤30% experienced a 92% reduction in risk of stroke [96]. Discontinuation of transfusions led to reversion to abnormal velocities and increased rate of stroke in a subsequent randomized controlled trial [97]. The multicenter TWITCH trial compared TCD velocities of 121 patients randomized to transfusions or hydroxyurea after at least 12 months of chronic transfusions. Hydroxyurea, at maximum tolerated dose, was shown to be non-inferior to transfusions in maintaining TCD velocities [98]. The decision to switch to hydroxyurea should be made cautiously and in partnership with the family, due to concerns about relatively short follow-up of the trial (2 years) and the critical importance of medication adherence.

Silent cerebral infarction (SCI) represents a more insidious and increasingly prevalent complication. Defined as white matter changes on MRI without associated overt neurologic deficit, SCI is more common in patients with HbSS or HbS-beta-zero-thalassemia patients but is also seen in the milder phenotypes. Prevalence rises with age, with 11% at 15 months of age and 27% by age 3.4 years in patients with HbSS [99, 100]. SCI are associated with impaired neurocognitive function and overt stroke [101, 102]. The multicenter SIT trial randomized patients with SCI and normal TCD to observation or transfusions over 3 years. Patients on the transfusion arm acquired fewer SCI and exhibited a decreased rate of overt stroke compared with patients on the observation arm [103]. Some authors recommend screening patients with MRI starting at 5 years of age or if they are having learning difficulties in school.

Ophthalmologic Disease Recurrent ischemic-reperfusion injury can lead to proliferative retinopathy in patients with SCD. Prevalence is greater in patients with HbSC disease for unknown reasons, reaching 45% by early adulthood, compared to 11% of patients with HbSS disease [104]. Retinal disease can progress to neovascularization and retinal detachment. Laser photocoagulation and vitrectomy may be treatment options in severe cases.

Respiratory Disease Acute chest syndrome (ACS) is the leading cause of death in patients with SCD and the second most common indication for hospitalization [80, 105]. Defined as a new infiltrate on chest radiography accompanied by at least one sign or symptom of lower respiratory tract disease (e.g., fever, cough, chest pain, dyspnea, tachypnea, hypoxia), ACS may present with variable severity and can progress to respiratory and multiorgan failure. ACS can develop for numerous reasons. Individuals with asthma are at higher risk for ACS. It may also develop as a complication of vaso-occlusive pain crisis. In a study conducted by the National ACS Study Group, 537 adults and children from 30 centers diagnosed with ACS underwent diagnostic testing, including sputum or nasopharyngeal sampling, serology, or bronchoscopy. Fourteen percent of cases were specifically attributable to *Chlamydia* or *Mycoplasma*, 9.2% due to bacterial or mixed infections, 8.8% revealed lipid-laden macrophages indicative of fat emboli, 6.4% were due to viral infection, 16% were attributed to lung infarction, and more than 45% did not have an identified etiology. Thirteen percent of all patients required mechanical ventilation [106]. Standard management of ACS does not typically include bronchoscopy, but initiating empiric antibiotics with antipneumococcal activity and coverage for atypical organisms like *Mycoplasma* is recommended. If a patient's respiratory status worsens, a simple transfusion of packed red cells to a hemoglobin of 10 g/dl or exchange transfusion in patients with higher baseline hemoglobin will improve oxygen-carrying capacity and ameliorate the ventilation-perfusion mismatch. Exchange transfusion should also be considered for patients with rapidly progressive or severe ACS.

The role of corticosteroids in ACS management has been examined in retrospective studies and placebo-controlled trials and has been associated with rebound VOC [107–109]. Strouse et al. reported an association with hemorrhagic stroke [108]. Steroids are generally limited to patients with evidence of asthma exacerbation.

Compared with age-matched, ethnic controls, children with HbSS disease displayed lower forced expiratory volume, forced vital capacity, and peak expiratory flow, suggesting mild restrictive defects. These defects were worse in older children [110]. In a longitudinal study, lung function declined with age in children with HbSS, also consistent with a restrictive pattern [111]. Patients with a history of frequent ACS may be at higher risk for developing restrictive lung disease as they age. Computed tomography of the chest in these individuals will demonstrate areas of fibrosis.

Mild obstructive sleep apnea (OSA) was seen in 41% of children, while 10% exhibited moderate to severe OSA in the Sleep and Asthma Cohort Study [112]. OSA is associated with hypoxemia, hypercapnia, and acidosis which may promote greater red cell sickling.

Cardiovascular Disease Pulmonary arterial and venous hypertension is prevalent in 6–10.4% of adult patients with SCD [113–115]. The development of pulmonary hypertension (PHTN) is likely a multifactorial process, which is comprehensively summarized by Gordeuk et al. [116]. As seen in other chronic hemolytic processes, free hemoglobin from injured sickle cells reacts with NO to form nitrate. Erythrocyte arginase depletes arginine, a substrate of NO. The resulting NO deficiency leads to vasomotor dysfunction. SCD is also a hypercoagulable state, with 12% of patients in one series exhibiting chronic pulmonary thromboembolic disease. These factors play a role in the development of precapillary pulmonary hypertension. Left ventricular (LV) diastolic dysfunction is often observed in adults with SCD, likely related to structural abnormalities like ventricular dilation and hypertrophy. LV dysfunction may contribute to postcapillary pulmonary hypertension.

Increased tricuspid regurgitant (TR) jet velocity (≥ 2.5 m/s) has been validated as a screening tool to identify patients who would benefit from right heart catheterization. Elevated TR jet is associated with increased mortality in adults with SCD [114, 117]. This has not been observed in children. However, pulmonary hypertension can lead to exercise intolerance and persistent hypoxemia, so these complaints should prompt a screening echocardiogram and subsequent consideration of cardiac catheterization if abnormal.

Gastrointestinal Disease Chronic hemolysis can lead to the development of pigment stones in 10–50% of children with SCD [118–121]. Cholelithiasis may be asymptomatic or may cause recurrent right upper quadrant pain and jaundice associated with direct hyperbilirubinemia. A right upper quadrant ultrasound is diagnostic. Patients with cholelithiasis should undergo cholecystectomy to avoid complications like cholecystitis, ascending cholangitis, or pancreatitis.

Intrahepatic cholestasis or sickle hepatopathy represents an uncommon clinical syndrome, characterized by severe direct hyperbilirubinemia ranging from 13 to 76 mg/dl, not attributable to infection or extrahepatic obstruction. The pathophysiology of sickle hepatopathy remains unclear but may be related to sickling within hepatic sinusoids causing injury to the liver parenchyma [122]. The clinical course may be mild or may lead to fulminant liver failure. Emergent exchange transfusion may be effective in severe cases [123, 124].

Genitourinary Disease Priapism, or unwanted painful erection, may occur in boys of any age and with any sickle variant. It may manifest in a stuttering (multiple short episodes lasting less than 2 h) or prolonged manner. Approaches for home management include increased hydration, pain medication, use of an oral alpha-adrenergic agonist (e.g., pseudoephedrine), ejaculation, urination, and warm baths. Episodes lasting more than 4 h require emergency intervention to prevent long-term development of fibrosis and impotence. In the ED, intravenous fluids and analgesia are offered. If unresponsive to standard treatment, urology consult is necessary for drainage and irrigation of the corpus cavernosum. Intrapenile injection of alpha-adrenergic agonists may be employed. Men with recurrent episodes may be at risk for erectile dysfunction. There is no consensus on preventive management.

Renal Disease Recurrent sickling within the renal vascular bed causes tubular and glomerular injury. Children with SCD often suffer from nocturnal enuresis due to hyposthenuria, or the inability to concentrate urine appropriately. Dehydration can develop quickly as a result. Microalbuminuria can develop in childhood, so screening should start as early as 10 years of age. If detected, referral to pediatric nephrology is warranted. Renal dysfunction may progress over time, leading to proteinuria, glomerular sclerosis, and chronic kidney disease. The latter has been reported in

8–26.5% of children. Angiotensin-converting enzyme inhibitors may be helpful. Hydroxyurea has been shown to improve concentrating ability and reduce hyperfiltration and glomerular hypertrophy [125, 126].

Preventive Care

Overall survival of sickle cell patients in the United States by 18 years of age has improved from 75% in the 1970s to 98% in the twenty-first century [80]. This is in large part due to advances in preventive care. The National Heart, Lung, and Blood Institute issued an updated evidence-based compilation of guidelines in 2014 that serves as the basis of the following recommendations [127] (Table 6.4).

Once identified through universal newborn screening, affected infants are referred to the regional hemoglobinopathy center, where preventive care and education about the disease begin. During regular appointments throughout childhood, the hematologist prepares the family for possible complications such as pain crises, acute chest syndrome, stroke, or priapism and provides guidance on home management as well as reasons for acute care. Families are taught how to palpate the spleen in order to detect possible enlargement and facilitate early evaluation. Starting at age 12, hematologists should start to introduce the concept of transition to adult care and prepare patients and families for that phase.

The most important initial discussion encompasses the risk of infection and the need for evaluation of all febrile episodes. Infants with SCD should be prescribed penicillin 125 mg twice daily. After age 3, the dose should be increased to 250 mg twice daily. In addition to standard childhood vaccinations, pneumococcal polysac-

Table 6.4 Recommended preventive care for SCD

Complication	Prophylaxis	Genotype	Schedule
Pneumococcal infection	Penicillin	All	Upon diagnosis, twice daily until at least 5 years old
	Prevnar-13		Per infant schedule
	Pneumovax-23		At 2 years old and then 3–5 years later
Meningococcal infection	Meningococcal A vaccine	All	Either infancy or after 2 years old depending on product and then every 5 years
	Meningococcal B vaccine		Starting at 10 years old
Stroke	Transcranial Doppler	SS, S-β^{0-} thalassemia	Annually from 2 to 16 years old
Retinopathy	Dilated retinal examination	All	Annually starting at 10 years old
Nephropathy	Urinalysis with microscopy	All	Annually starting at 10 years old

charide vaccine (Pneumovax-23) and meningococcal vaccine (Menactra) should be administered after age 2, followed by additional boosters as recommended by the Centers for Disease Control (CDC). Even if fully adherent to prophylactic measures, parents are educated on the importance of bringing their child in for evaluation of fever, since breakthrough infections occur.

Based on a study showing decreased rates of pneumococcal sepsis in older children with SCD independent of prophylaxis status, discontinuation of penicillin can be considered after age 5 provided the patient has received all antipneumococcal vaccines and has not undergone splenectomy nor experienced pneumococcal infection [128]. However, pneumococcal immunity may wane with time, so fevers should continue to be evaluated.

Transcranial Doppler ultrasound should be performed annually on children with HbSS or HbS-beta-0-thalassemia from ages 2 to 16. Children exhibiting elevated cerebral artery velocities (≥ 200 cm/s) require repeat TCD within 2 weeks and prompt institution of chronic transfusions with persistent elevated velocities. Children with conditional velocities (≥ 170–199 cm/s) require repeat TCD within 3 months to determine persistence or worsening of elevated velocities.

All patients with sickle cell disease should undergo annual dilated retinal examination to detect retinopathy starting at age 10. Annual urinalysis with microscopy starting at age 10 will facilitate detection of sickle nephropathy.

Treatment

Hydroxyurea. Hydroxycarbamide or hydroxyurea (HU) has changed the landscape of sickle cell disease. A ribonucleotide reductase inhibitor, HU increases fetal hemoglobin production and total hemoglobin. By increasing fetal hemoglobin, HU reduces hemolysis rate, which in turn may reduce free hemoglobin's consumption of nitric oxide (NO). Through its cytoreductive effects, HU also reduces neutrophil and platelet count, which decreases whole blood viscosity and cellular adhesion [129].

Since Platt et al. reported on the first two patients treated with hydroxyurea [130], multiple large randomized, controlled trials in children and adults have shown the benefits of this agent. The Multicenter Study of Hydroxyurea demonstrated that, compared with placebo, HU was associated with significantly fewer pain crises, episodes of acute chest syndrome, number of transfusions, and lower costs of hospitalization for pain [131]. HU was approved by the US Food and Drug Administration (FDA) for adults in 1998 as a result. Subsequent studies have shown reduction in mortality among adults using hydroxyurea after 9 and 17 years of follow-up, respectively [132–134]. The phase I/II HUG-KIDS trial demonstrated that HU was safe in children ages 5–15 years [135]. The phase III BABY HUG study randomized children as young as 9 months of age to either HU or placebo. HU was associated with fewer episodes of pain, acute chest syndrome, hospitalization, and dactylitis [136]. The reduction in hospitalization rate translated into 21% lower annual healthcare costs in patients treated with HU [137]. The FDA approved HU for use in children down to age 2 in 2017. The main side effects are infrequent and include cytopenias, rash, hair thinning, and nail changes. Regular monitoring of blood counts with appropriate dose adjustments for myelosuppression is recommended.

HU should be considered part of standard of care for patients with SCA. However, adherence remains a significant challenge especially for adolescent and young adult (AYA) patients. Survey studies of AYA patients show that although HU adherence is associated with better quality of life, poor adherence is common and associated with forgetfulness, negative beliefs about HU, cost, or inability to obtain timely refills [138–141]. Many misconceptions also still exist that are a barrier to acceptance of this medication [140, 142, 143].

L-Glutamine Oxidative damage likely plays a role in the pathophysiology of SCD. Studies have demonstrated altered glutamine metabolism and lower nicotinamide adenine dinucleotide (NAD) redox potential in sickle erythrocytes, suggesting an increased vulnerability to oxidant damage [144]. Supplementation with L-glutamine appeared to increase NAD redox potential and was associated with subjective improvement in chronic pain and energy in a pilot study [145]. The US Food and Drug Administration recently approved L-glutamine for use in sickle cell patients aged 5 years and older. The approval was based on a multicenter, double-blinded trial randomizing 230 patients with sickle cell anemia (SCA) to L-glutamine or placebo for a 48-week period followed by a 3-week tapering phase. Patients receiving L-glutamine experienced a median of three crises compared with four crises in the placebo arm. L-glutamine was also associated with fewer hospitalizations, fewer cumulative hospital days, and fewer episodes of acute chest syndrome. At the time of preparation of this manuscript, the results had not been formally published.

Crizanlizumab As greater understanding of the molecular processes underlying vaso-occlusive crises is achieved, targeted therapy becomes more feasible. P-selectin is a molecule normally stored in granules in resting endothelial cells and platelets. Upon activation of these cells, P-selectin is transferred to the cell surface, facilitating adherence of sickled RBCs to the vascular endothelium. P-selectin also mediates adherence between platelets and neutrophils, which may play a role in vaso-occlusion [146, 147]. Crizanlizumab is a humanized monoclonal p-selectin antagonist which significantly reduced the rate of VOC in a randomized, placebo-controlled, double-blinded phase II trial. Almost 200 patients aged 16–65 years of age with any sickle genotype were assigned to receive low- or high-dose crizanlizumab or placebo over a period of 12 months, followed by an observation period. Crizanlizumab was given as two loading doses and then every 4 weeks for a 50-week duration. Subjects receiving high-dose crizanlizumab experienced a 45.3% lower median rate of annual crises compared with subjects receiving placebo (1.63 versus 2.98). Median time to first crisis was also substantially longer in the high-dose crizanlizumab arm (4.07 versus 1.38 months) [148].

Hematopoietic Stem Cell Transplantation The only established cure for SCD is human leukocyte antigen (HLA)-matched sibling stem cell transplantation (SCT). Most centers use myeloablative conditioning, comprising busulfan, cyclophosphamide, and antithymocyte globulin or alemtuzumab. Overall survival at 3 years reaches greater than 90%, and event-free survival is nearly as good at 86%. There is a lack of consensus on indications for transplant, but most clinicians would offer it to patients who have experienced stroke or elevated TCD velocity. Some clinicians would consider SCT for patients with RBC alloimmunization, sickle nephropathy, or recurrent episodes of severe ACS or VOC. Despite excellent outcomes reported in both Europe and the United States, relatively few patients undergo transplant. Limiting factors include lack of awareness of this modality, lack of availability of an appropriate HLA-matched sibling donor, age, comorbidities, or sociocultural factors [149].

To expand the donor pool and eligibility of patients, alternative donor transplants are being examined. Outcomes after HLA-matched unrelated donor (MUD) SCT have thus far been discouraging. In a recent multicenter series of 29 children, MUD SCT following reduced-intensity conditioning was examined. Despite robust GVHD prophylaxis comprising methotrexate, methylprednisolone, and a calcineurin inhibitor, there was a 1-year incidence rate of chronic graft-versus-host disease (GVHD) of 62% and 7 GVHD-related deaths [150].

Haploidentical donors may prove to be more viable as a source of stem cells than matched unrelated donors. Several studies have demonstrated feasibility and safety of non-myeloablative conditioning. Using alemtuzumab, total body irradiation, and posttransplant sirolimus and cohort-specific escalating cyclophosphamide, Fitzhugh et al. recently reported 87% overall survival in a study of 23 patients. Cohort 1, which received no cyclophosphamide, had 0% disease-free survival (DFS) at 1 year. Cohort 3 received 100 mg/kg cyclophosphamide and exhibited 50% DFS. There were no patients with grade 2–4 GVHD [151]. The intensity of the conditioning and posttransplant immunosuppression continues to evolve to minimize rates of GVHD and graft failure [151–154].

Gene Therapy The use of gene replacement or editing technology to restore healthy erythropoiesis would be an ideal method to bypass the obstacles of stem cell transplantation. Hematopoietic stem cells would be mobilized and collected from eligible patients, genetically modified to correct the beta-globin gene defect and expanded in culture. After the appropriate myeloablative conditioning, the modified stem cells would be reinfused into the patient. Preclinical studies have most recently employed lentiviral vectors to introduce the corrective beta-globin elements. Clinical trials are ongoing. The current state of the technology and the challenges of clinical application to hemoglobinopathies have recently been reviewed [155].

Red Blood Cell Membrane Defects

Red Blood Cell Membrane Structure

The RBC membrane has a phospholipid bilayer that facilitates interaction with the cytoplasm and the surrounding plasma. The biconcave structure of the RBC allows it to squeeze through capillaries and maintain a high surface area to volume ratio. The structural proteins, including spectrin, ankyrin, protein 4.1, and actin, are interspersed throughout the lipid bilayer and give the RBC its biconcave shape and strength. Vertical protein interactions allow the membrane skeleton to communicate with the phospholipid bilayer and maintain erythrocyte cohesion and surface area; the important proteins in these interactions include α-spectrin, β-spectrin, band 3, ankyrin, and protein 4.2. Horizontal protein interactions maintain the erythrocyte's mechanical integrity; the critical proteins in these interactions include the spectrins, protein 4.1, and actin. Classically, defects in the horizontal interactions cause hereditary elliptocytosis (HE) and its variant, hereditary pyropoikilocytosis (HPP), while defects in the vertical interactions cause hereditary spherocytosis (HS) [156–158].

Hereditary Elliptocytosis

HE exists worldwide, affecting about 3–5 patients out of 10,000, with higher prevalence in malaria endemic regions [159, 160]. The classic genes affected encode the spectrins and protein 4.1. A variety of defects in the spectrin genes are associated with HE and HPP, including missense, deletion, insertion, and splice mutations [159, 161, 162]. It is typically inherited in an autosomal dominant fashion, but spontaneous cases have also been reported [159, 163].

The severity of HE depends on the degree of mechanical instability of the RBC membrane due to the underlying defect [159, 164, 165]. Most patients with HE are asymptomatic and diagnosed after the incidental discovery of elliptocytes on a peripheral blood smear, while about 10% of cases will have a moderate to severe anemia [159, 165]. Symptomatic patients can experience episodic hemolytic anemia with splenomegaly and jaundice [159]. In more severe cases, it can present at birth with severe hemolysis and hydrops fetalis [166, 167]. Some patients may present with transient pure red cell aplasia, precipitated by certain viral infections and drug exposures [163]. In the most severe variant of HE, hereditary elliptocytosis with pyropoikilocytosis, the RBC membrane exhibits fragmentation with resultant low MCV and decreased surface area [165, 168].

Diagnosis of HE depends on morphologic analysis. A peripheral blood smear will reveal normocytic, normochromic elliptocytes, involving some or all of the RBCs. The CBC will show variable anemia with elevated reticulocyte count, ranging from less than 5% to 30% in severe cases [163]. Most cases of HE are mild and do not require treatment. Patients with severe hemolysis in the neonatal period may require phototherapy or exchange transfusions. Patients with chronic ongoing hemolysis may need episodic red blood cell transfusions and should be supplemented with folic acid [163]. Splenectomy can be considered to reduce transfusion needs, but it should be deferred until after the age of 5 in order to avoid fulminant sepsis [159, 163].

Hereditary Spherocytosis

The most common red blood cell membrane defect disease, HS, has a prevalence of at least 1 in 2000–3000 individuals [159]. HS is the most common cause of congenital hemolytic anemia in Caucasian patients [165], although it has been observed in most ethnic and racial groups. Three-fourths of cases are inherited in an autosomal dominant fashion, usually related to mutations in the ankyrin, β-spectrin, or band 3 genes, while the remainder are sporadic or inherited in an autosomal recessive fashion and related to mutations in the alpha-spectrin or protein 4.2 genes [159, 169].

In affected erythrocytes, the weakened vertical interactions between the lipid bilayer and cytoskeleton lead to the release of lipid microvesicles, with resultant membrane loss and spherocyte formation due to membrane vesiculation. The resultant spherocytes have less surface area to volume ratio and thus cannot deform as easily as unaffected erythrocytes. This deformability is an important characteristic for erythrocytes entering the spleen when they pass from the splenic cords into the sinusoids, as the space between the endothelial cells is very tight. In HS, the erythrocytes lack the necessary flexibility and subsequently are retained in the spleen, where they are either further damaged or targeted for destruction by splenic macrophages resulting in hemolysis [170–172].

The typical presentation of HS includes hemolytic anemia, jaundice, gallstones, and splenomegaly, usually in the context of a positive family history [170, 173]. The peripheral smear shows varying numbers of dense, hyperchromic RBCs without the central pallor of normal erythrocytes (Fig. 6.4). Anemia is the most common presenting symptom in children, while the most severe cases can present with hydrops fetalis and stillbirth [170, 171]. Per criteria by Bolton-Maggs et al., HS represents a spectrum of disease, based on the severity of ongoing hemolysis and need for splenectomy. In the mild form, hemoglobin levels can be normal, ranging between 11 and 15 g/dl. Reticulocytosis ranges from 3% to 6%, with bilirubin levels between 17 to 34 μmol/l. Affected patients usually do not require splenectomy, but if they do, it usually is not needed until adulthood. In the moderate form, hemoglobin ranges from 8 to 12 g/dl with reticulocytosis greater than 6% and bilirubin levels greater than 34 μmol/l. Affected patients usually require splenectomy prior to puberty. In the severe form, hemoglobin levels range from 6 to 8 g/dl with reticulocytosis greater than 10% and bilirubin levels greater than 51%. Affected patients will typically need splenectomy due to the severity of hemolysis. In the most severe cases, inadequately treated patients can present similarly to those with severe thalassemia, with growth retardation and extramedullary erythropoiesis. Patients require chronic transfusions and can experience subsequent iron overload requiring chelation therapy. These most severe forms are usually inherited in an autosomal recessive fashion [171, 172, 174].

HS may be suspected with the previously described symptoms and lab findings as well as a characteristically elevated MCHC. In the case of a positive family history with spherocytes on the smear, reticulocytosis, and elevated MCHC on labs, confirmatory diagnosis is not needed [175]. Confirmatory diagnosis is pursued when the diagnosis is equivocal. Two recommended confirmatory methods exist

[175]. The first method, the eosin-5'-maleimide-binding test (EMA-binding test), employs flow cytometry to detect interactions with band 3, which are decreased in HS, resulting in decreased fluorescence. This method has been shown to have 90% sensitivity and 95% specificity [172, 175, 176]. The second method, the cryohemolysis test, exposes erythrocytes to hypertonic saline and assesses the degree of hemolysis under different cold temperature stresses. This method has been shown to have 95% sensitivity and 96% specificity [177–179]. The osmotic fragility test, which exposes both fresh and incubated blood to different concentrations of hypertonic saline, is no longer recommended, as it demonstrates lower sensitivity and specificity than the recommended testing, can be normal in mild and in compensated presentations, and can yield a false positive in the setting of autoimmune hemolytic anemia [171, 176]. If these tests are inconclusive, then sodium dodecyl sulfate polyacrylamide gel electrophoresis, or SDS-PAGE testing, can be pursued to assess for specific allelic mutations [171, 175]. Diagnosis of hereditary spherocytosis in neonates can be difficult because spherocytes might only be sporadically present or appear atypical on a smear; consequently, confirmatory diagnosis is usually delayed until infants reach 6 months of age [171, 175].

Treatment of HS depends on the severity of the disease. Red cell transfusions are provided as needed to support optimum hemoglobin levels. Patients receiving chronic transfusions will require iron chelation. Folate supplementation supports increased erythropoiesis in patients with moderate and severe cases. Children with HS should be seen annually with monitoring of anemia during viral illnesses that may cause aplastic crisis, especially if their disease is severe. Splenectomy is recommended in children with severe disease and in patients suffering from moderate to severe disease experiencing symptomatic hemolysis, such as cholelithiasis. Splenectomy is shown to decrease hemolysis and gallstone incidence, but it comes with the risk of increased infection. When cholelithiasis becomes symptomatic and burdensome, cholecystectomy can also be performed [171, 172, 175].

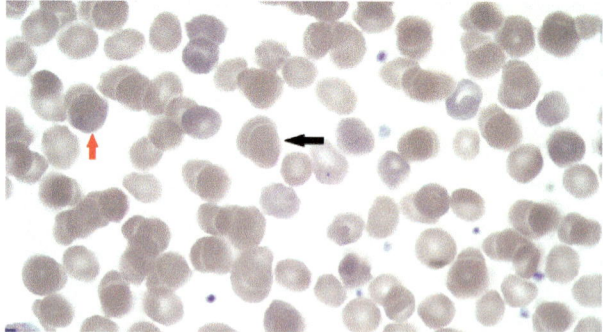

Fig. 6.4 Red blood cell morphology in hereditary spherocytosis. The smear shows numerous spherocytes (black arrow) which have no central pallor and are dense and hyperchromic. Reticulocytes (red arrow) are increased as well

Red Blood Cell Enzyme Defects

Glucose-6-Phosphate Dehydrogenase Deficiency

Glucose-6-phosphate dehydrogenase (G6PD) is a ubiquitous enzyme. It is the catalyst of the first reaction in the pentose phosphate pathway, allowing the cell to produce nicotinamide adenine dinucleotide phosphate hydrogen (NADPH). NADPH provides a reducing agent for reductive biosynthesis as well as maintains glutathione in its reduced form (Fig. 6.5). Reduced glutathione allows for reduction of free radicals and thus protection against oxidative stress. Red blood cells lack mitochondria and therefore depend on the pentose phosphate pathway to create NADPH and defend both the cell and its hemoglobin from oxidation [180, 181]. Typically, levels of G6PD decrease in the red blood cell as it ages. When not under oxidative stress, G6PD operates at about 2% of its potential. However, when exposed to oxidative stress, the activity level increases. Consequently, patients with deficient G6PD cannot mount the proper enzyme response, resulting in hemolysis and the physiologic features of G6PD deficiency. The older, more G6PD-deficient red blood cells hemolyze first, with younger red blood cells and reticulocytes less likely to hemolyze since they express higher levels of G6PD [180, 182]. Oxidative stressors of note that affect patients with G6PD deficiency include but are not limited to fava beans, the antimalarial drug primaquine, and the commonly used antibiotic sulfamethoxazole

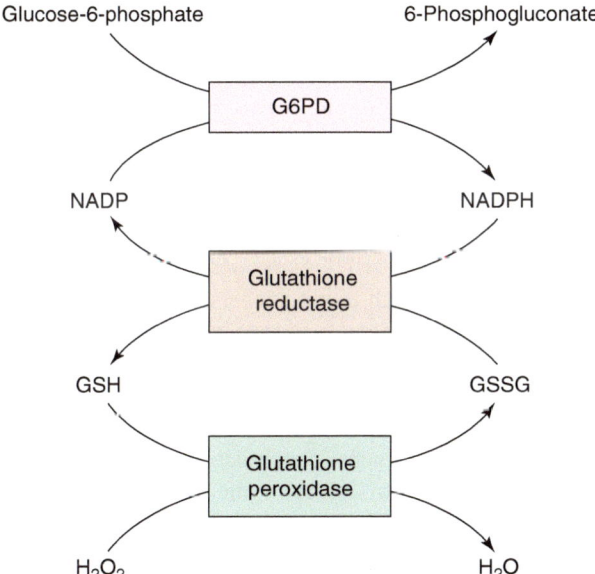

Fig. 6.5 Role of glucose-6-phospate dehydrogenase in prevention of oxidant injury. (Reprinted from McAdam et al. [249]. Copyright 2015, with permission from Elsevier)

[182, 183]. Infection can also trigger hemolysis, possibly via the release of free radicals during leukocyte-induced phagocytosis [183, 184]. Commonly implicated infections include viruses such as influenza A, *Salmonella*, beta-hemolytic strepto-cocci, and *Escherichia coli* [182].

G6PD is encoded for by the G6PD gene, which resides on the long arm of the X chromosome. Mutations in the G6PD gene result in G6PD deficiency [180]. G6PD deficiency is inherited in an X-linked fashion, with a higher incidence in males than females. Homozygous females with G6PD deficiency carry two copies of a mutated G6PD gene. Heterozygous females inherit one mutated copy and one functioning copy. Subsequent X chromosome inactivation (i.e., lyonization) causes two red blood cell lines to proliferate, one with functioning G6PD and one with deficient G6PD, leading to decreased G6PD expression relative to normal individuals [182, 185, 186]. Most mutations causing G6PD deficiency are missense mutations [183].

G6PD deficiency is the most prevalent enzyme deficiency across the globe, with over 400 million individuals affected [182, 187]. One recent meta-analysis estimated a global prevalence of 4.9% [188]. G6PD deficiency is more common in malaria-ridden nations, particularly sub-Saharan African countries. This geographic correla-tion is theorized to be secondary to a protective effect incurred by the deficiency, in that the *Plasmodium falciparum* parasites do not grow as well in G6PD-deficient red blood cells [187]. Affected individuals in the United States tend to be of Mediterranean and African descent [188]. The different biochemical variants causing G6PD defi-ciency, of which over 400 have been identified, are categorized into five classes based on clinical severity [180, 182]. Class I patients exhibit the most severe disease, with chronic non-spherocytic hemolytic anemia and severely deficient G6PD activ-ity. Classes II and III are characterized by severely deficient and moderately deficient G6PD activity, respectively, with acute episodes of hemolysis; these are the most commonly encountered variants. Classes IV and V tend to be clinically insignificant, with normal and increased levels of G6PD activity, respectively [180–182].

In the neonatal period, G6PD deficiency is a known risk factor for hyperbilirubine-mia, which sometimes progresses into irreversible bilirubin-induced neurologic dam-age (BIND). Such severe hyperbilirubinemia is thought to be related to acute hemolysis, even though the typical markers of hemolysis might remain within normal ranges [189, 190]. More common than BIND is moderate hyperbilirubinemia that usually responds to phototherapy although might need exchange transfusion, with hemolysis likely contributing. In both BIND and moderate hyperbilirubinemia in the patient with G6PD deficiency, a clear environmental trigger for the hemolysis might not be appar-ent. Other mediating factors contributing to hyperbilirubinemia are thought to be pres-ent, including concomitant genetic defects in bilirubin conjugation or other red blood cell abnormalities [180, 189]. Other research suggests that G6PD itself might play a role in bilirubin conjugation, with defects in the enzyme causing impaired bilirubin clearance and subsequent hyperbilirubinemia in the neonatal period [191].

Outside of the neonatal period, G6PD deficiency manifests clinically with acute episodes of hemolysis. Acute hemolytic episodes may be characterized by back and abdominal pain, jaundice, dark-colored urine secondary to hemoglobinuria, and transient splenomegaly. Labs will show anemia, reticulocytosis 4–7 days after the onset of hemolysis, decreased haptoglobin, and indirect hyperbilirubinemia [182, 192]. Examination of a peripheral blood smear during an episode might show red blood cell inclusions called Heinz bodies representing denatured hemoglobin. Heinz bodies tend to appear earlier during the episode or are rarely seen at all [182, 183]. Drug-induced hemolysis usually occurs within 1–3 days of drug exposure and can last from 4 days up to a week [182, 183, 192]. Fava bean-induced hemolysis, or favism, usually occurs within 24 h of fava bean ingestion. Of note, not all patients with G6PD deficiency will experience hemolysis after fava bean ingestion [180, 182, 183]. Oxidative drugs given to breastfeeding mothers can be transferred into breast milk, causing hemolytic crisis in G6PD-deficient neonates; hemolytic crises have been observed in exposed infants of breastfeeding mothers who have recently consumed fava beans [182, 193, 194]. Infection remains a more common cause of hemolysis in G6PD-deficient patients than drugs and fava beans [182]. Careful attention should be given to viral hepatitis in G6PD-deficient patients, which can lead to fulminant hepatic failure [195]. Diabetic ketoacidosis, myocardial infarction, and high-level physical activity have also been associated with hemolysis, but these links have not been proven [180, 196–198]. In class I G6PD deficiency, patients experience acute on chronic hemolysis, but the clinical manifestations range from mild disease to transfusion-dependent hemolytic anemia [182].

G6PD deficiency should be considered in patients with severe neonatal hyperbilirubinemia as well as patients who experience hemolysis after the previously described triggers, especially if they are of African or Mediterranean descent [180, 182]. Typically, screening and diagnosis for G6PD deficiency are performed with biochemical methods that assess G6PD activity by measuring the conversion of NADP to NADPH. The gold standard method is the spectrophotometric quantitative assay, but it takes longer to result and is less readily available than other methods. In countries with high prevalence of G6PD and malaria, semiqualitative methods that are inexpensive and result quickly tend to be used, such as the fluorescent spot test. Access to rapid results is especially important if the use of primaquine to treat malaria is being considered [180, 181, 199]. Unfortunately, these biochemical methods are not always accurate during an acute hemolytic episode, since reticulocytes and RBCs increase in number, thus falsely elevating the level of G6PD activity [200]. G6PD activity should ideally be measured after the patient has recovered from the hemolytic episode [183]. As an alternative to biochemical assays, molecular methods of diagnosis exist, such as gradient gel electrophoresis and gene microarray, which detect mutations in the G6PD gene. The molecular methods remain the definitive way to diagnose heterozygous females with G6PD deficiency, as these patients are often not detected by the biochemical methods [180, 201]. An alternative biochemical assay has been recommended for heterozygous females, which measures the ratio of G6PD to 6-phosphogluconate dehydrogenase, another enzyme in the pentose phosphate pathway; this method has been shown to be more sensitive than the previously described biochemical assays [201]. Neonatal screening is not performed universally, but the World Health Organization recommends that it be done in all populations where the disease prevalence in males is greater than 3–5% [182, 202].

Treatment of G6PD deficiency generally involves counseling patients to avoid the hemolytic triggers. Patients generally remain well between episodes without significant clinical changes. Blood transfusions may be necessary if the degree of anemia may impact hemodynamic stability during acute episodes. When infection triggers hemolysis, such as with hepatitis, renal failure can occur that necessitates dialysis. In the setting of neonatal hyperbilirubinemia, close monitoring of serum bilirubin levels is required, with possible phototherapy and exchange transfusion if the levels become too high. In chronic non-spherocytic hemolytic anemia, patients who become transfusion dependent might require chelation therapy [180, 182].

Pyruvate Kinase Deficiency

The pyruvate kinase (PK) enzyme acts in the glycolysis pathway, converting phosphoenolpyruvate to pyruvate such that ATP is produced. This conversion is responsible for half of the erythrocyte's adenosine triphosphate (ATP), which is critical for the various protein and membrane interactions that maintain the function and shape [203, 204]. Four different PK isoenzymes exist, with R-PK expressed in red blood cells; the other isoenzymes are L-PK, M_1-PK, and M_2-PK. The PK-LR gene encodes for R-PK as well as L-PK, which is notably expressed in the liver [204–206]. The decreased ATP production in PK-deficient red blood cells leads to impaired metabolism and decreased lifespan. Reticulocytes and younger RBCs, which have been shown to be more dependent on PK for functioning than older RBCs, are destroyed first. Hemolysis generally occurs as these cells pass through the splenic reticuloendothelial system and incur metabolic and mechanical stress with subsequent macrophage phagocytosis, although in some cases, secondary clearance occurs via the reticuloendothelial system in the liver [207–211].

The PK-LR gene is located on the long arm of chromosome 1 [212]. Defects in this gene result in PK deficiency. Even though the gene also encodes for the L-PK isoenzyme, hepatic manifestations are usually not seen, possibly because the persistent PK synthesis that occurs in hepatocytes compensates for the deficiency [213]. Over 200 known pathogenic mutations exist, and most are missense mutations [214]. The disease is inherited in an autosomal recessive fashion, with homozygosity for a given mutation or compound heterozygosity for two different mutations resulting in clinical disease [204, 206]. Research has been able to link genotype to disease phenotype based on amino acid substitutions affecting the structure of the aberrant enzyme [204, 215, 216]. Particularly severe disease has been associated with disruptive mutations, including those causing large deletions or affecting the stop codon, as well as with homozygous missense mutations [204, 217].

PK deficiency occurs worldwide and across ethnicities, with the majority of known variants located in Europe, followed by Asia and then the United States and Canada [214]. In the general Caucasian population, the estimated prevalence is approximately one per 20,000 individuals [218]. A high frequency is observed in the Pennsylvania Amish and other specific patient populations, likely due to the autosomal recessive nature of the disease and founder effect [206, 219, 220]. Limited evidence suggests that a co-distribution between endemic malaria and PK deficiency exists, particularly in sub-Saharan countries, but this link has not been as strongly studied as that between endemic malaria and the other congenital hemolytic anemias described in this chapter [221, 222]. Nonetheless, research has demonstrated impaired parasite survival in PK-deficient red blood cells, suggesting that the disease may confer a protective effect [223, 224].

PK deficiency is categorized as mild, moderate, and severe based on the phenotype. Severe disease is diagnosed at birth and early infancy, while mild and moderate diseases are not diagnosed until later childhood or adulthood [203, 204]. In the prenatal and neonatal period, PK deficiency demonstrates clinical variability [203, 225]. In the most severe of cases, PK deficiency can present with fetal anemia, causing hydrops fetalis and intrauterine death [226, 227]. In at least one case, death has been reported shortly after birth [225]. In the neonatal period, about 30–50% of patients with mild to moderate disease will have hyperbilirubinemia secondary to hemolysis, more likely requiring phototherapy with a few patients needing exchange transfusion. In severe disease, most patients will have hyperbilirubinemia, and they will most likely need exchange transfusion [225]. Neonates with severe disease may also develop cholestasis and liver failure [228].

Beyond the newborn period, PK deficiency ranges from mild, compensated hemolysis to transfusion-dependent hemolytic anemia [203]. Anemia that is present in infancy generally, although not always, seems to improve throughout childhood and sometimes self-resolves [229]. In adulthood, the level of anemia remains stable, although it can worsen in the setting of pregnancy and infection [206]. Patients with mild to moderate disease rarely need blood transfusions outside of acute hemolytic exacerbations, whereas those with severe disease are transfusion dependent [203].

PK deficiency can be associated with iron overload independent of transfusion history. The development of iron overload is multifactorial, likely related to a combination of chronic hemolysis and ineffective erythropoiesis, with further increased risk after splenectomy and possible co-inheritance of hemochromatosis [206, 230–232]. During pregnancy, maternal PK deficiency might manifest in increased hemolysis requiring multiple red blood cell transfusions, but the reported maternal and fetal outcomes have generally been positive [206, 233–236]. One case in the literature reported impaired fetal growth, in the setting of maternal iron overload and poor medication adherence [237]. Other disease complications related to chronic hemolysis include splenomegaly and cholelithiasis. Less commonly reported manifestations include aplastic crisis due to parvovirus, extramedullary hematopoiesis, leg ulcers, and thromboembolic events [206, 238, 239]. As seen in other hemolytic anemias, the incidence of thromboembolic events seems to increase after splenectomy [240].

Laboratory evaluation in PK deficiency is notable for a variable degree of anemia, with median pre-splenectomy hemoglobin values of 11 g/dl in mild disease, 9 g/dl in moderate disease, and 6.8 g/dl in severe disease. After splenectomy, which is rarely done for mild disease, median hemoglobin values increase by one or two points [203]. On peripheral blood smear, red blood cells commonly appear normal, but there may be a range of unequally sized cells, poikilocytes, and shrunken echinocytes [204, 206]. Labs will also show reticulocytosis, but that number does not reflect the degree of hemolysis that is occurring due to the splenic sequestration of reticulocytes. For that same reason, after splenectomy, the level of reticulocytosis might paradoxically increase [206]. Unconjugated hyperbilirubinemia is also seen, but levels above 6 mg/dl raise suspicion for concurrent Gilbert's syndrome [203, 204, 206].

A diagnosis of PK deficiency should be considered in several scenarios, including a positive family history and severe hyperbilirubinemia in the newborn period without a clear cause. Furthermore, it should be on the differential for DAT-negative, congenital, chronic non-spherocytic hemolytic anemia in which hemoglobinopathies, red blood cell membrane defects, and G6PD deficiency have been ruled out [203]. It should also be considered if a patient has worsening reticulocytosis or increased presence of shrunken echinocytes following a splenectomy [203, 206]. Diagnosis is usually done biochemically via an assay to measure red blood cell PK enzyme activity. However, several limitations exist with this method. The presence of donor red blood cells or incompletely removed leukocytes can falsely elevate PK activity. In some patients, older red blood cells express M_2-PK, which may errantly be measured. Furthermore, some patients may have increased but abnormally functioning PK activity, thus inflating the actual level of functional enzyme activity [206]. Thus, when the level of suspicion for disease is high and when confirmatory testing is needed, molecular diagnosis with possible genetic testing should be pursued [203].

Since a cure does not yet exist for PK deficiency, the mainstay of treatment includes supportive care and management of complications that arise. Blood transfusions may be needed either intermittently or chronically depending on the clinical circumstances. In the neonatal period, hyperbilirubinemia must be treated according to published guidelines, either with phototherapy or exchange transfusion, in order to avoid bilirubin-induced neurologic dysfunction. The ideal hemoglobin level and transfusion frequency for pediatric patients with PK deficiency have not been formally determined, but maintaining a level between 7 and 9 g/dl is likely optimal for growth and development [203]. Of note, patients may tolerate a lower hemoglobin concentration than expected because of a rightward shift in the hemoglobin-oxygen dissociation curve, due to the accumulation of 2,3-diphosphoglycerate [241].

During pregnancy, maternal hemoglobin levels should be maintained at 8 g/dl or above, with a hematologist closely involved. Patients will also likely need folic acid supplementation beyond the traditional requirements during pregnancy, in order to accommodate the increased hemolysis [203, 237]. Both pediatric and adult patients with reticulocytosis should be supplemented with folic acid in order to support their increased RBC production. Some patients may require cholecystectomy if gallstones become symptomatic [203].

There are no guidelines governing screening for iron overload in these patients. In affected children receiving multiple transfusions, screening should likely start once the patient has been transfused at least 10–20 times [203]. Even in intermittently transfused, asymptomatic patients, screening should occur by adulthood, since the degree of iron overload may not be clinically apparent [232]. Ferritin and transferrin saturation can be used for screening, but they may not accurately reflect tissue iron deposition. If available, T2* MRI should be performed once ferritin exceeds 500 ng/ml. Chelation therapy is indicated when ferritin exceeds 1000 ng/ml or typical findings are seen on MRI [203]. Successful use of desferroxamine, deferiprone, and deferasirox has been demonstrated, with one report in the literature of using concomitant erythropoietin [203, 206, 242, 243].

Patients with mild disease rarely need splenectomy. Splenectomy helps to mitigate transfusion dependence and frequency in patients with moderate to severe disease, with some patients no longer needing transfusions postoperatively [203, 204]. As with other patients with congenital hemolytic anemia, splenectomy in early childhood increases the risk of fulminant sepsis with encapsulated bacteria, so the timing must be carefully considered. Even with proper vaccination against encapsulated bacteria and penicillin prophylaxis following splenectomy, the risk for sepsis remains. A fatal case of *Klebsiella pneumoniae* sepsis has been reported; a vaccine directed toward this microbe does not exist [203, 244]. Splenectomy also increases the risk for thromboembolic events and iron overload.

Beyond transfusions and supportive care, nontraditional and experimental methods at treating PK deficiency have been attempted. Successful bone marrow transplantation has been performed in both mice and a pediatric patient [245, 246]. Furthermore, a successful murine gene therapy model has been studied [247].

References

1. Noronha SA. Acquired and congenital hemolytic anemia. Pediatr Rev. 2016;37(6):235–46.
2. Dhaliwal GC, Cornett PA, Tierney LM. Hemolytic anemia. Am Fam Physician. 2004;69(11):2599–606.
3. Robertson JJ, Brem E, Koyfman A. The acute hemolytic anemias: the importance of emergency diagnosis and management. J Emerg Med. 2017;53(2):202–11.
4. Forde DG, Cope A, Stone B. Acute parvovirus B19 infection in identical twins unmasking previously unidentified hereditary spherocytosis. BMJ Case Rep. 2014;2014:pii: bcr2013202957.
5. Musallam KM, et al. Clinical experience with fetal hemoglobin induction therapy in patients with beta-thalassemia. Blood. 2013;121(12):2199–212; quiz 2372
6. Origa R, Moi P. Alpha-thalassemia. In: Adam MP, et al., editors. GeneReviews(R). Seattle, WA: University of Washington, Seattle University of Washington; 1993. GeneReviews is a registered trademark of the University of Washington, Seattle. All rights reserved.: Seattle, WA.
7. Hatton CS, et al. Alpha-thalassemia caused by a large (62 kb) deletion upstream of the human alpha globin gene cluster. Blood. 1990;76(1):221–7.
8. Farashi S, Harteveld CL. Molecular basis of alpha-thalassemia. Blood Cells Mol Dis. 2018;70:43–53.

9. Thein SL. Molecular basis of beta thalassemia and potential therapeutic targets. Blood Cells Mol Dis. 2018;70:54–65.
10. Daikeler T, et al. New autoimmune diseases after cord blood transplantation: a retrospective study of EUROCORD and the Autoimmune Disease Working Party of the European Group for Blood and Marrow Transplantation. Blood. 2013;121(6):1059–64.
11. Karakas Z, et al. Evaluation of alpha-thalassemia mutations in cases with hypochromic microcytic anemia: the Istanbul perspective. Turk J Haematol. 2015;32(4):344–50.
12. Harteveld CL, Higgs DR. Alpha-thalassaemia. Orphanet J Rare Dis. 2010;5:13.
13. Flint J, et al. High frequencies of alpha-thalassaemia are the result of natural selection by malaria. Nature. 1986;321(6072):744–50.
14. Modiano G, et al. Protection against malaria morbidity: near-fixation of the alpha-thalassemia gene in a Nepalese population. Am J Hum Genet. 1991;48(2):390–7.
15. Vichinsky EP. Clinical manifestations of alpha-thalassemia. Cold Spring Harb Perspect Med. 2013;3(5):a011742.
16. Vichinsky EP, et al. Changes in the epidemiology of thalassemia in North America: a new minority disease. Pediatrics. 2005;116(6):e818–25.
17. Chui DH, Fucharoen S, Chan V. Hemoglobin H disease: not necessarily a benign disorder. Blood. 2003;101(3):791–800.
18. Farashi S, Najmabadi H. Diagnostic pitfalls of less well recognized HbH disease. Blood Cells Mol Dis. 2015;55(4):387–95.
19. Fucharoen S, Viprakasit V. Hb H disease: clinical course and disease modifiers. Hematology Am Soc Hematol Educ Program. 2009:26–34.
20. Galanello R, et al. HbH disease in Sardinia: molecular, hematological and clinical aspects. Acta Haematol. 1992;88(1):1–6.
21. Chui DH. Alpha-thalassemia: Hb H disease and Hb Barts hydrops fetalis. Ann N Y Acad Sci. 2005;1054:25–32.
22. Blouin P, et al. Evans' syndrome: a retrospective study from the ship (French Society of Pediatric Hematology and Immunology) (36 cases). Arch Pediatr. 2005;12(11):1600–7.
23. Yaegashi N, et al. Parvovirus B19 infection induces apoptosis of erythroid cells in vitro and in vivo. J Infect. 1999;39(1):68–76.
24. Songdej D, Babbs C, Higgs DR. An international registry of survivors with Hb Bart's hydrops fetalis syndrome. Blood. 2017;129(10):1251–9.
25. Caocci G, et al. Long-term survival of beta thalassemia major patients treated with hematopoietic stem cell transplantation compared with survival with conventional treatment. Am J Hematol. 2017;92(12):1303–10.
26. Taher AT, et al. Optimal management of beta thalassaemia intermedia. Br J Haematol. 2011;152(5):512–23.
27. Galanello R, Cao A. Relationship between genotype and phenotype. Thalassemia intermedia. Ann N Y Acad Sci. 1998;850:325–33.
28. Vehapoglu A, et al. Hematological indices for differential diagnosis of Beta thalassemia trait and iron deficiency anemia. Anemia. 2014;2014:576738.
29. Cappellini MD, et al. Coagulopathy in beta-thalassemia: current understanding and future perspectives. Mediterr J Hematol Infect Dis. 2009;1(1):e2009029.
30. Ben Salah N, et al. Revisiting beta thalassemia intermedia: past, present, and future prospects. Hematology. 2017;22(10):607–16.
31. Haddad A, et al. Beta-thalassemia intermedia: a bird's-eye view. Turk J Haematol. 2014;31(1):5–16.
32. Manfre L, et al. MR imaging of the brain: findings in asymptomatic patients with thalassemia intermedia and sickle cell-thalassemia disease. AJR Am J Roentgenol. 1999;173(6):1477–80.
33. Badens C, et al. Variants in genetic modifiers of beta-thalassemia can help to predict the major or intermedia type of the disease. Haematologica. 2011;96(11):1712–4.
34. Danjou F, et al. A genetic score for the prediction of beta-thalassemia severity. Haematologica. 2015;100(4):452–7.

35. Galanello R, et al. Amelioration of Sardinian beta0 thalassemia by genetic modifiers. Blood. 2009;114(18):3935–7.
36. Spanos T, et al. Red cell alloantibodies in patients with thalassemia. Vox Sang. 1990;58(1):50–5.
37. Taher A, et al. Prevalence of thromboembolic events among 8,860 patients with thalassaemia major and intermedia in the Mediterranean area and Iran. Thromb Haemost. 2006;96(4):488–91.
38. Taher AT, et al. Splenectomy and thrombosis: the case of thalassemia intermedia. J Thromb Haemost. 2010;8(10):2152–8.
39. Cappellini MD, et al. Venous thromboembolism and hypercoagulability in splenectomized patients with thalassaemia intermedia. Br J Haematol. 2000;111(2):467–73.
40. Karimi M, et al. Adverse effects of hydroxyurea in beta-thalassemia intermedia patients: 10 years' experience. Pediatr Hematol Oncol. 2010;27(3):205–11.
41. Bradai M, et al. Decreased transfusion needs associated with hydroxyurea therapy in Algerian patients with thalassemia major or intermedia. Transfusion. 2007;47(10):1830–6.
42. El-Beshlawy A, et al. Response to hydroxycarbamide in pediatric beta-thalassemia intermedia: 8 years' follow-up in Egypt. Ann Hematol. 2014;93(12):2045–50.
43. Foong WC, et al. Hydroxyurea for reducing blood transfusion in non-transfusion dependent beta thalassaemias. Cochrane Database Syst Rev. 2016;10:Cd011579.
44. Rutjanaprom W, et al. Heart rate variability in beta-thalassemia patients. Eur J Haematol. 2009;83(5):483–9.
45. Cazzola M, et al. A moderate transfusion regimen may reduce iron loading in beta-thalassemia major without producing excessive expansion of erythropoiesis. Transfusion. 1997;37(2):135–40.
46. Angelucci E, et al. Italian Society of Hematology practice guidelines for the management of iron overload in thalassemia major and related disorders. Haematologica. 2008;93(5):741–52.
47. Borgna-Pignatti C, Marsella M. Iron chelation in thalassemia major. Clin Ther. 2015;37(12):2866–77.
48. Borgna-Pignatti C, et al. Myocardial iron overload in thalassaemia major. How early to check? Br J Haematol. 2014;164(4):579–85.
49. Bayanzay K, Khan R. Meta-analysis on effectiveness of hydroxyurea to treat transfusion-dependent beta-thalassemia. Hematology. 2015;20:469–76.
50. Baronciani D, et al. Hemopoietic stem cell transplantation in thalassemia: a report from the European Society for Blood and Bone Marrow Transplantation Hemoglobinopathy Registry, 2000–2010. Bone Marrow Transplant. 2016;51(4):536–41.
51. Makis A, et al. 2017 Clinical trials update in new treatments of beta-thalassemia. Am J Hematol. 2016;91(11):1135–45.
52. Herrick JB. Peculiar elongated and sickle-shaped red blood corpuscles in a case of severe anemia. 1910. Reprint from Arch Int Med. 1910;5:517. Yale J Biol Med. 2001;74(3):179–84.
53. Beet EA. The genetics of the sickle-cell trait in a Bantu tribe. Ann Eugenics. 1949;14(4):279–84.
54. Neel JV. The inheritance of sickle cell anemia. Science. 1949;110(2846):64–6.
55. Pauling L, Itano HA, et al. Sickle cell anemia a molecular disease. Science. 2865;1949(110):543–8.
56. Piel FB, et al. Global epidemiology of sickle haemoglobin in neonates: a contemporary geostatistical model-based map and population estimates. Lancet. 2013;381(9861):142–51.
57. Gill FM, et al. Clinical events in the first decade in a cohort of infants with sickle cell disease. Cooperative study of sickle cell disease. Blood. 1995;86(2):776–83.
58. Noguchi CT, Schechter AN. Sickle hemoglobin polymerization in solution and in cells. Annu Rev Biophys Biophys Chem. 1985;14:239–63.
59. Ballas SK, Gupta K, Adams-Graves P. Sickle cell pain: a critical reappraisal. Blood. 2012;120(18):3647–56.
60. Manwani D, Frenette PS. Vaso-occlusion in sickle cell disease: pathophysiology and novel targeted therapies. Blood. 2013;122(24):3892–8.

61. Sheehan VA, et al. Genetic modifiers of sickle cell anemia in the BABY HUG cohort: influence on laboratory and clinical phenotypes. Am J Hematol. 2013;88(7):571–6.
62. Aleluia MM, et al. Comparative study of sickle cell anemia and hemoglobin SC disease: clinical characterization, laboratory biomarkers and genetic profiles. BMC Hematol. 2017;17:15.
63. Meier ER, Wright EC, Miller JL. Reticulocytosis and anemia are associated with an increased risk of death and stroke in the newborn cohort of the Cooperative Study of Sickle Cell Disease. Am J Hematol. 2014;89(9):904–6.
64. Miller ST, et al. Prediction of adverse outcomes in children with sickle cell disease. N Engl J Med. 2000;342(2):83–9.
65. Quinn CT, et al. Prediction of adverse outcomes in children with sickle cell anemia: a study of the Dallas Newborn Cohort. Blood. 2008;111(2):544–8.
66. Quinn CT, et al. Prognostic significance of early vaso-occlusive complications in children with sickle cell anemia. Blood. 2007;109(1):40–5.
67. Serjeant GR, et al. The painful crisis of homozygous sickle cell disease: clinical features. Br J Haematol. 1994;87(3):586–91.
68. Gonzalez ER, et al. Intermittent injection vs patient-controlled analgesia for sickle cell crisis pain. Comparison in patients in the emergency department. Arch Intern Med. 1991;151(7):1373–8.
69. van Beers EJ, et al. Patient-controlled analgesia versus continuous infusion of morphine during vaso-occlusive crisis in sickle cell disease, a randomized controlled trial. Am J Hematol. 2007;82(11):955–60.
70. Campbell CM, et al. An evaluation of central sensitization in patients with sickle cell disease. J Pain. 2016;17(5):617–27.
71. Dowell D, Haegerich TM, Chou R. CDC guideline for prescribing opioids for chronic pain – United States, 2016. MMWR Recomm Rep. 2016;65(1):1–49.
72. Haywood C Jr, et al. Perceived discrimination in health care is associated with a greater burden of pain in sickle cell disease. J Pain Symptom Manag. 2014;48(5):934–43.
73. Haywood C Jr, et al. Perceived discrimination, patient trust, and adherence to medical recommendations among persons with sickle cell disease. J Gen Intern Med. 2014;29(12):1657–62.
74. Wakefield EO, et al. Perceived racial bias and health-related stigma among youth with sickle cell disease. J Dev Behav Pediatr. 2017;38(2):129–34.
75. Schwartz LA, Radcliffe J, Barakat LP. Associates of school absenteeism in adolescents with sickle cell disease. Pediatr Blood Cancer. 2009;52(1):92–6.
76. Epping AS, et al. Academic attainment findings in children with sickle cell disease. J Sch Health. 2013;83(8):548–53.
77. Ladd RJ, Valrie CR, Walcott CM. Risk and resilience factors for grade retention in youth with sickle cell disease. Pediatr Blood Cancer. 2014;61(7):1252–6.
78. Pearson HA, et al. Developmental aspects of splenic function in sickle cell diseases. Blood. 1979;53(3):358–65.
79. Gaston MH, et al. Prophylaxis with oral penicillin in children with sickle cell anemia. A randomized trial. N Engl J Med. 1986;314(25):1593–9.
80. Quinn CT, et al. Improved survival of children and adolescents with sickle cell disease. Blood. 2010;115(17):3447–52.
81. Ellison AM, et al. Pneumococcal bacteremia in a vaccinated pediatric sickle cell disease population. Pediatr Infect Dis J. 2012;31(5):534–6.
82. Santoro JD, et al. A case of invasive Streptococcus pneumoniae in an afebrile adolescent with sickle cell disease. Clin Pediatr (Phila). 2013;52(12):1173–5.
83. Ellison AM, et al. Variation in pediatric emergency department care of sickle cell disease and fever. Acad Emerg Med. 2015;22(4):423–30.
84. Brousse V, et al. Acute splenic sequestration crisis in sickle cell disease: cohort study of 190 paediatric patients. Br J Haematol. 2012;156(5):643–8.
85. Switzer JA, et al. Pathophysiology and treatment of stroke in sickle-cell disease: present and future. Lancet Neurol. 2006;5(6):501–12.

86. Ohene-Frempong K, et al. Cerebrovascular accidents in sickle cell disease: rates and risk factors. Blood. 1998;91(1):288–94.
87. Balkaran B, et al. Stroke in a cohort of patients with homozygous sickle cell disease. J Pediatr. 1992;120(3):360–6.
88. Powars D, et al. The natural history of stroke in sickle cell disease. Am J Med. 1978;65(3):461–71.
89. Russell MO, et al. Effect of transfusion therapy on arteriographic abnormalities and on recurrence of stroke in sickle cell disease. Blood. 1984;63(1):162–9.
90. Wang WC, et al. High risk of recurrent stroke after discontinuance of five to twelve years of transfusion therapy in patients with sickle cell disease. J Pediatr. 1991;118(3):377–82.
91. Fasano RM, Meier ER, Hulbert ML. Cerebral vasculopathy in children with sickle cell anemia. Blood Cells Mol Dis. 2015;54(1):17–25.
92. Griessenauer CJ, et al. Encephaloduroarteriosynangiosis and encephalomyoarteriosynangiosis for treatment of moyamoya syndrome in pediatric patients with sickle cell disease. J Neurosurg Pediatr. 2015;16(1):64–73.
93. Hankinson TC, et al. Surgical treatment of moyamoya syndrome in patients with sickle cell anemia: outcome following encephaloduroarteriosynangiosis. J Neurosurg Pediatr. 2008;1(3):211–6.
94. Adams R, et al. The use of transcranial ultrasonography to predict stroke in sickle cell disease. N Engl J Med. 1992;326(9):605–10.
95. Adams RJ, et al. Long-term stroke risk in children with sickle cell disease screened with transcranial Doppler. Ann Neurol. 1997;42(5):699–704.
96. Adams RJ, et al. Prevention of a first stroke by transfusions in children with sickle cell anemia and abnormal results on transcranial Doppler ultrasonography. N Engl J Med. 1998;339(1):5–11.
97. Adams RJ, Brambilla D, Optimizing Primary Stroke Prevention in Sickle Cell Anemia Trial Investigators. Discontinuing prophylactic transfusions used to prevent stroke in sickle cell disease. N Engl J Med. 2005;353(26):2769–78.
98. Ware RE, et al. Hydroxycarbamide versus chronic transfusion for maintenance of transcranial doppler flow velocities in children with sickle cell anaemia-TCD With Transfusions Changing to Hydroxyurea (TWiTCH): a multicentre, open-label, phase 3, non-inferiority trial. Lancet. 2016;387(10019):661–70.
99. Kwiatkowski JL, et al. Silent infarcts in young children with sickle cell disease. Br J Haematol. 2009;146(3):300–5.
100. Wang WC, et al. Abnormalities of the central nervous system in very young children with sickle cell anemia. J Pediatr. 1998;132(6):994–8.
101. Armstrong FD, et al. Cognitive functioning and brain magnetic resonance imaging in children with sickle cell disease. Neuropsychology Committee of the Cooperative Study of Sickle Cell Disease. Pediatrics. 1996;97(6 Pt 1):864–70.
102. Bernaudin F, et al. Multicenter prospective study of children with sickle cell disease: radiographic and psychometric correlation. J Child Neurol. 2000;15(5):333–43.
103. DeBaun MR, et al. Controlled trial of transfusions for silent cerebral infarcts in sickle cell anemia. N Engl J Med. 2014;371(8):699–710.
104. Clarkson JG. The ocular manifestations of sickle-cell disease: a prevalence and natural history study. Trans Am Ophthalmol Soc. 1992;90:481–504.
105. Platt OS, et al. Mortality in sickle cell disease. Life expectancy and risk factors for early death. N Engl J Med. 1994;330(23):1639–44.
106. Vichinsky EP, et al. Causes and outcomes of the acute chest syndrome in sickle cell disease. National Acute Chest Syndrome Study Group. N Engl J Med. 2000;342(25):1855–65.
107. Strouse JJ, et al. Primary hemorrhagic stroke in children with sickle cell disease is associated with recent transfusion and use of corticosteroids. Pediatrics. 2006;118(5):1916–24.
108. Strouse JJ, et al. Corticosteroids and increased risk of readmission after acute chest syndrome in children with sickle cell disease. Pediatr Blood Cancer. 2008;50(5):1006–12.

130

A. L. Reinish and S. A. Noronha

109. Quinn CT, et al. Tapered oral dexamethasone for the acute chest syndrome of sickle cell disease. Br J Haematol. 2011;155(2):263–7.
110. Sylvester KP, et al. Pulmonary function abnormalities in children with sickle cell disease. Thorax. 2004;59(1):67–70.
111. MacLean JE, et al. Longitudinal decline in lung volume in a population of children with sickle cell disease. Am J Respir Crit Care Med. 2008;178(10):1055–9.
112. Rosen CL, et al. Obstructive sleep apnea and sickle cell anemia. Pediatrics. 2014;134(2):273–81.
113. Fonseca GH, et al. Pulmonary hypertension diagnosed by right heart catheterisation in sickle cell disease. Eur Respir J. 2012;39(1):112–8.
114. Mehari A, et al. Mortality in adults with sickle cell disease and pulmonary hypertension. JAMA. 2012;307(12):1254–6.
115. Parent F, et al. A hemodynamic study of pulmonary hypertension in sickle cell disease. N Engl J Med. 2011;365(1):44–53.
116. Gordeuk VR, Castro OL, Machado RF. Pathophysiology and treatment of pulmonary hypertension in sickle cell disease. Blood. 2016;127(7):820–8.
117. Gladwin MT, et al. Pulmonary hypertension as a risk factor for death in patients with sickle cell disease. N Engl J Med. 2004;350(9):886–95.
118. Karayalcin G, et al. Cholelithiasis in children with sickle cell disease. Am J Dis Child. 1979;133(3):306–7.
119. Lachman BS, et al. The prevalence of cholelithiasis in sickle cell disease as diagnosed by ultrasound and cholecystography. Pediatrics. 1979;64(5):601–3.
120. Mintz AA, Church G, Adams ED. Cholelithiasis in sickle cell anemia. J Pediatr. 1955;47(2):171–7.
121. Walker TM, Hambleton IR, Serjeant GR. Gallstones in sickle cell disease: observations from The Jamaican Cohort study. J Pediatr. 2000;136(1):80–5.
122. Shah R, Taborda C, Chawla S. Acute and chronic hepatobiliary manifestations of sickle cell disease: a review. World J Gastrointest Pathophysiol. 2017;8(3):108–16.
123. Ahn H, Li CS, Wang W. Sickle cell hepatopathy: clinical presentation, treatment, and outcome in pediatric and adult patients. Pediatr Blood Cancer. 2005;45(2):184–90.
124. Buchanan GR, Glader BE. Benign course of extreme hyperbilirubinemia in sickle cell anemia: analysis of six cases. J Pediatr. 1977;91(1):21–4.
125. Aygun B, et al. Hydroxyurea treatment decreases glomerular hyperfiltration in children with sickle cell anemia. Am J Hematol. 2013;88(2):116–9.
126. Falk RJ, et al. Prevalence and pathologic features of sickle cell nephropathy and response to inhibition of angiotensin-converting enzyme. N Engl J Med. 1992;326(14):910–5.
127. Yawn BP, et al. Management of sickle cell disease: summary of the 2014 evidence-based report by expert panel members. JAMA. 2014;312(10):1033–48.
128. Falletta JM, et al. Discontinuing penicillin prophylaxis in children with sickle cell anemia. Prophylactic Penicillin Study II. J Pediatr. 1995;127(5):685–90.
129. Zhang D, et al. Neutrophils, platelets, and inflammatory pathways at the nexus of sickle cell disease pathophysiology. Blood. 2016;127(7):801–9.
130. Platt OS, et al. Hydroxyurea enhances fetal hemoglobin production in sickle cell anemia. J Clin Invest. 1984;74(2):652–6.
131. Charache S, et al. Hydroxyurea and sickle cell anemia. Clinical utility of a myelosuppressive "switching" agent. The Multicenter Study of Hydroxyurea in Sickle Cell Anemia. Medicine (Baltimore). 1996;75(6):300–26.
132. Steinberg MH, et al. Effect of hydroxyurea on mortality and morbidity in adult sickle cell anemia: risks and benefits up to 9 years of treatment. JAMA. 2003;289(13):1645–51.
133. Voskaridou E, et al. The effect of prolonged administration of hydroxyurea on morbidity and mortality in adult patients with sickle cell syndromes: results of a 17-year, single-center trial (LaSHS). Blood. 2010;115(12):2354–63.

134. Steinberg MH, et al. The risks and benefits of long-term use of hydroxyurea in sickle cell anemia: a 17.5 year follow-up. Am J Hematol. 2010;85(6):403–8.
135. Kinney TR, et al. Safety of hydroxyurea in children with sickle cell anemia: results of the HUG-KIDS study, a phase I/II trial. Pediatric Hydroxyurea Group. Blood. 1999;94(5):1550–4.
136. Thornburg CD, et al. Impact of hydroxyurea on clinical events in the BABY HUG trial. Blood. 2012;120(22):4304–10; quiz 4448
137. Wang WC, et al. Hydroxyurea is associated with lower costs of care of young children with sickle cell anemia. Pediatrics. 2013;132(4):677–83.
138. Badawy SM, et al. Adherence to hydroxyurea, health-related quality of life domains, and patients' perceptions of sickle cell disease and hydroxyurea: a cross-sectional study in adolescents and young adults. Health Qual Life Outcomes. 2017;15(1):136.
139. Badawy SM, et al. Health-related quality of life and adherence to hydroxyurea in adolescents and young adults with sickle cell disease. Pediatr Blood Cancer. 2017;64(6):e26369.
140. Badawy SM, Thompson AA, Liem RI. Beliefs about hydroxyurea in youth with sickle cell disease. Hematol Oncol Stem Cell Ther. 2018; https://doi.org/10.1016/j.hemonc.2018.01.001.
141. Badawy SM, et al. Barriers to hydroxyurea adherence and health-related quality of life in adolescents and young adults with sickle cell disease. Eur J Haematol. 2017;98(6):608–14.
142. Haywood C Jr, et al. Examining the characteristics and beliefs of hydroxyurea users and nonusers among adults with sickle cell disease. Am J Hematol. 2011;86(1):85–7.
143. Oyeku SO, et al. Parental and other factors associated with hydroxyurea use for pediatric sickle cell disease. Pediatr Blood Cancer. 2013;60(4):653–8.
144. Morris CR, et al. Erythrocyte glutamine depletion, altered redox environment, and pulmonary hypertension in sickle cell disease. Blood. 2008;111(1):402–10.
145. Niihara Y, et al. Oral L-glutamine therapy for sickle cell anemia: I. Subjective clinical improvement and favorable change in red cell NAD redox potential. Am J Hematol. 1998;58(2):117–21.
146. Embury SH, et al. The contribution of endothelial cell P-selectin to the microvascular flow of mouse sickle erythrocytes in vivo. Blood. 2004;104(10):3378–85.
147. Luo W, et al. P-selectin glycoprotein ligand-1 inhibition blocks increased leukocyte-endothelial interactions associated with sickle cell disease in mice. Blood. 2012;120(18):3862–4.
148. Ataga KI, et al. Crizanlizumab for the prevention of pain crises in sickle cell disease. N Engl J Med. 2017;376(5):429–39.
149. Gluckman E. Allogeneic transplantation strategies including haploidentical transplantation in sickle cell disease. Hematology Am Soc Hematol Educ Program. 2013;2013:370–6.
150. Shenoy S, et al. A trial of unrelated donor marrow transplantation for children with severe sickle cell disease. Blood. 2016;128(21):2561–7.
151. Fitzhugh CD, et al. Cyclophosphamide improves engraftment in patients with SCD and severe organ damage who undergo haploidentical PBSCT. Blood Adv. 2017;1(11):652–61.
152. Brodsky RA, et al. Reduced intensity HLA-haploidentical BMT with post transplantation cyclophosphamide in nonmalignant hematologic diseases. Bone Marrow Transplant. 2008;42(8):523–7.
153. Frangoul H, et al. Haploidentical hematopoietic stem cell transplant for patients with sickle cell disease using thiotepa, fludarabine, thymoglobulin, low dose cyclophosphamide, 200 cGy tbi and post transplant cyclophosphamide. Bone Marrow Transplant. 2018;53(5):647–50.
154. Pawlowska AB, et al. HLA haploidentical stem cell transplant with pretransplant immunosuppression for patients with sickle cell disease. Biol Blood Marrow Transplant. 2018;24(1):185–9.
155. Lidonnici MR, Ferrari G. Gene therapy and gene editing strategies for hemoglobinopathies. Blood Cells Mol Dis. 2018;70:87–101.
156. Andolfo I, et al. New insights on hereditary erythrocyte membrane defects. Haematologica. 2016;101(11):1284–94.
157. Tse WT, Lux SE. Red blood cell membrane disorders. Br J Haematol. 1999;104(1):2–13.

158. Narla J, Mohandas N. Red cell membrane disorders. Int J Lab Hematol. 2017;39 Suppl 1:47–52.
159. Da Costa L, et al. Hereditary spherocytosis, elliptocytosis, and other red cell membrane disorders. Blood Rev. 2013;27(4):167–78.
160. Dhermy D, Schrevel J, Lecomte MC. Spectrin-based skeleton in red blood cells and malaria. Curr Opin Hematol. 2007;14(3):198–202.
161. Gallagher PG. Hereditary elliptocytosis: spectrin and protein 4.1R. Semin Hematol. 2004;41(2):142–64.
162. Gallagher PG, Forget BG. Hematologically important mutations: spectrin variants in hereditary elliptocytosis and hereditary pyropoikilocytosis. Blood Cells Mol Dis. 1996;22(3):254–8.
163. Figueiredo S, et al. Transient pure red blood cell aplasia as clinical presentation of congenital hemolytic anemia: a case report. Cases J. 2009;2:6814.
164. Debray FG, et al. A particular hereditary anemia in a two-month-old infant: elliptocytosis. Arch Pediatr. 2005;12(2):163–7.
165. Barcellini W, et al. Hereditary red cell membrane defects: diagnostic and clinical aspects. Blood Transfus. 2011;9(3):274–7.
166. Gallagher PG, et al. Mutation of a highly conserved residue of betaI spectrin associated with fatal and near-fatal neonatal hemolytic anemia. J Clin Invest. 1997;99(2):267–77.
167. Gallagher PG, et al. Recurrent fatal hydrops fetalis associated with a nucleotide substitution in the erythrocyte beta-spectrin gene. J Clin Invest. 1995;95(3):1174–82.
168. Bayhan T, Unal S, Gumruk F. Hereditary Elliptocytosis with Pyropoikilocytosis. Turk J Haematol. 2016;33(1):86–7.
169. Bogardus HH, et al. A de novo band 3 mutation in hereditary spherocytosis. Pediatr Blood Cancer. 2012;58(6):1004.
170. Konca C, et al. Hereditary spherocytosis: evaluation of 68 children. Indian J Hematol Blood Transfus. 2015;31(1):127–32.
171. Perrotta S, Gallagher PG, Mohandas N. Hereditary spherocytosis. Lancet. 2008;372(9647):1411–26.
172. Rencic J, et al. Circling back for the diagnosis. N Engl J Med. 2017;377(18):1778–84.
173. Mariani M, et al. Clinical and hematologic features of 300 patients affected by hereditary spherocytosis grouped according to the type of the membrane protein defect. Haematologica. 2008;93(9):1310–7.
174. Eber SW, Armbrust R, Schroter W. Variable clinical severity of hereditary spherocytosis: relation to erythrocytic spectrin concentration, osmotic fragility, and autohemolysis. J Pediatr. 1990;117(3):409–16.
175. Bolton-Maggs PH, et al. Guidelines for the diagnosis and management of hereditary spherocytosis--2011 update. Br J Haematol. 2012;156(1):37–49.
176. Bianchi P, et al. Diagnostic power of laboratory tests for hereditary spherocytosis: a comparison study in 150 patients grouped according to molecular and clinical characteristics. Haematologica. 2012;97(4):516–23.
177. Iglauer A, et al. Cryohemolysis test as a diagnostic tool for hereditary spherocytosis. Ann Hematol. 1999;78(12):555–7.
178. Streichman S, Gesheidt Y, Tatarsky I. Hypertonic cryohemolysis: a diagnostic test for hereditary spherocytosis. Am J Hematol. 1990;35(2):104–9.
179. Streichman S, Gescheidt Y. Cryohemolysis for the detection of hereditary spherocytosis: correlation studies with osmotic fragility and autohemolysis. Am J Hematol. 1998;58(3):206–12.
180. Cappellini MD, Fiorelli G. Glucose-6-phosphate dehydrogenase deficiency. Lancet. 2008;371(9606):64–74.
181. Glucose-6-phosphate dehydrogenase deficiency. WHO Working Group. Bull World Health Organ. 1989;67(6):601–11.
182. Frank JE. Diagnosis and management of G6PD deficiency. Am Fam Physician. 2005;72(7):1277–82.
183. Beutler E. G6PD deficiency. Blood. 1994;84(11):3613–36.

184. Baehner RL, Nathan DG, Castle WB. Oxidant injury of caucasian glucose-6-phosphate dehydrogenase-deficient red blood cells by phagocytosing leukocytes during infection. J Clin Invest. 1971;50(12):2466–73.
185. Beutler E, Yeh M, Fairbanks VF. The normal human female as a mosaic of X-chromosome activity: studies using the gene for C-6-PD-deficiency as a marker. Proc Natl Acad Sci U S A. 1962;48:9–16.
186. Kaplan M, et al. Acute hemolysis and severe neonatal hyperbilirubinemia in glucose-6-phosphate dehydrogenase-deficient heterozygotes. J Pediatr. 2001;139(1):137–40.
187. Ruwende C, Hill A. Glucose-6-phosphate dehydrogenase deficiency and malaria. J Mol Med (Berl). 1998;76(8):581–8.
188. Nkhoma ET, et al. The global prevalence of glucose-6-phosphate dehydrogenase deficiency: a systematic review and meta-analysis. Blood Cells Mol Dis. 2009;42(3):267–78.
189. Kaplan M, Hammerman C. Glucose-6-phosphate dehydrogenase deficiency and severe neonatal hyperbilirubinemia: a complexity of interactions between genes and environment. Semin Fetal Neonatal Med. 2010;15(3):148–56.
190. Kaplan M, et al. Severe hemolysis with normal blood count in a glucose-6-phosphate dehydrogenase deficient neonate. J Perinatol. 2008;28(4):306–9.
191. Kaplan M, et al. Conjugated bilirubin in neonates with glucose-6-phosphate dehydrogenase deficiency. J Pediatr. 1996;128(5 Pt 1):695–7.
192. Edwards CQ. Anemia and the liver. Hepatobiliary manifestations of anemia. Clin Liver Dis. 2002;6(4):891–907, viii.
193. Corchia C, et al. Favism in a female newborn infant whose mother ingested fava beans before delivery. J Pediatr. 1995;127(5):807–8.
194. American Academy of Pediatrics Committee on Drugs. Transfer of drugs and other chemicals into human milk. Pediatrics. 2001;108(3):776–89.
195. Moiz B, Ali SA. Fulminant hemolysis in glucose-6-phosphate dehydrogenase deficiency. Clin Case Rep. 2018;6(1):224–5.
196. Gellady AM, Greenwood RD. G-6-PD hemolytic anemia complicating diabetic ketoacidosis. J Pediatr. 1972;80(6):1037–8.
197. Lee DH, et al. Acute hemolytic anemia precipitated by myocardial infarction and pericardial tamponade in G6PD deficiency. Am J Hematol. 1996;51(2):174–5.
198. Ninfali P, Bresolin N. Muscle glucose 6-phosphate dehydrogenase (G6PD) deficiency and oxidant stress during physical exercise. Cell Biochem Funct. 1995;13(4):297–8.
199. Luzzatto L, Nannelli C, Notaro R. Glucose-6-phosphate dehydrogenase deficiency. Hematol Oncol Clin North Am. 2016;30(2):373–93.
200. Ringelhahn B. A simple laboratory procedure for the recognition of A – (African type) G-6-PD deficiency in acute haemolytic crisis. Clin Chim Acta. 1972;36(1):272–4.
201. Minucci A, et al. Glucose-6-phosphate dehydrogenase laboratory assay: how, when, and why? IUBMB Life. 2009;61(1):27–34.
202. Lam R, Li H, Nock ML, Assessment of G6PD screening program in premature infants in a NICU. J Perinatol. 2015;35(12):1027–9.
203. Grace RF, et al. Erythrocyte pyruvate kinase deficiency: 2015 status report. Am J Hematol. 2015;90(9):825–30.
204. Zanella A, et al. Pyruvate kinase deficiency: the genotype-phenotype association. Blood Rev. 2007;21(4):217–31.
205. Fothergill-Gilmore LA, Michels PA. Evolution of glycolysis. Prog Biophys Mol Biol. 1993;59(2):105–235.
206. Zanella A, et al. Red cell pyruvate kinase deficiency: molecular and clinical aspects. Br J Haematol. 2005;130(1):11–25.
207. Bowman HS, Oski FA. Laboratory studies of erythrocytic pyruvate kinase deficiency. Pathogenesis of the hemolysis. Am J Clin Pathol. 1978;70(2):259–70.
208. Bowman HS, Procopio F. Hereditary non-spherocytic hemolytic anemia of the pyruvate-kinase deficient type. Ann Intern Med. 1963;58:567–91.

209. Matsumoto N, et al. Sequestration and destruction of reticulocyte in the spleen in pyruvate kinase deficiency hereditary nonspherocytic hemolytic anemia. Nihon Ketsueki Gakkai Zasshi. 1972;35(4):525–37.
210. Mentzer WC Jr, et al. Selective reticulocyte destruction in erythrocyte pyruvate kinase deficiency. J Clin Invest. 1971;50(3):688–99.
211. Nathan DG, et al. Life-span and organ sequestration of the red cells in pyruvate kinase deficiency. N Engl J Med. 1968;278(2):73–81.
212. Satoh H, et al. The human liver-type pyruvate kinase (PKL) gene is on chromosome 1 at band q21. Cytogenet Cell Genet. 1988;47(3):132–3.
213. Nakashima K, et al. Characterization of pyruvate kinase from the liver of a patient with aberrant erythrocyte pyruvate kinase, PK Nagasaki. J Lab Clin Med. 1977;90(6):1012–20.
214. Canu G, et al. Red blood cell PK deficiency: an update of PK-LR gene mutation database. Blood Cells Mol Dis. 2016;57:100–9.
215. van Wijk R, et al. Fifteen novel mutations in PKLR associated with pyruvate kinase (PK) deficiency: structural implications of amino acid substitutions in PK. Hum Mutat. 2009;30(3):446–53.
216. Warang P, et al. Molecular and clinical heterogeneity in pyruvate kinase deficiency in India. Blood Cells Mol Dis. 2013;51(3):133–7.
217. Zanella A, Bianchi P. Red cell pyruvate kinase deficiency: from genetics to clinical manifestations. Baillieres Best Pract Res Clin Haematol. 2000;13(1):57–81.
218. Beutler E, Gelbart T. Estimating the prevalence of pyruvate kinase deficiency from the gene frequency in the general white population. Blood. 2000;95(11):3585–8.
219. Baronciani L, Beutler E. Molecular study of pyruvate kinase deficient patients with hereditary nonspherocytic hemolytic anemia. J Clin Invest. 1995;95(4):1702–9.
220. Christensen RD, et al. Six children with pyruvate kinase deficiency from one small town: molecular characterization of the PK-LR gene. J Pediatr. 2011;159(4):695–7.
221. Machado P, et al. Pyruvate kinase deficiency in sub-Saharan Africa: identification of a highly frequent missense mutation (G829A;Glu277Lys) and association with malaria. PLoS One. 2012;7(10):e47071.
222. Min-Oo G, Gros P. Erythrocyte variants and the nature of their malaria protective effect. Cell Microbiol. 2005;7(6):753–63.
223. Ayi K, et al. Pyruvate kinase deficiency and malaria. N Engl J Med. 2008;358(17):1805–10.
224. Min-Oo G, et al. Pyruvate kinase deficiency: correlation between enzyme activity, extent of hemolytic anemia and protection against malaria in independent mouse mutants. Blood Cells Mol Dis. 2007;39(1):63–9.
225. Pissard S, et al. Pyruvate kinase (PK) deficiency in newborns: the pitfalls of diagnosis. J Pediatr. 2007;150(4):443–5.
226. Ferreira P, et al. Hydrops fetalis associated with erythrocyte pyruvate kinase deficiency. Eur J Pediatr. 2000;159(7):481–2.
227. Hennekam RC, et al. Hydrops fetalis associated with red cell pyruvate kinase deficiency. Genet Couns. 1990;1(1):75–9.
228. Olivier F, et al. Cholestasis and hepatic failure in a neonate: a case report of severe pyruvate kinase deficiency. Pediatrics. 2015;136(5):e1366–8.
229. Boivin P, Ottenwaelter T. Hereditary haemolytic anaemia due to pyruvate kinase deficiency. Prognosis of neonatal forms (author's transl). Nouv Press Med. 1982;11(12):917–9.
230. Zanella A, et al. Iron status and HFE genotype in erythrocyte pyruvate kinase deficiency: study of Italian cases. Blood Cells Mol Dis. 2001;27(3):653–61.
231. Marshall SR, et al. The dangers of iron overload in pyruvate kinase deficiency. Br J Haematol. 2003;120(6):1090–1.
232. Andersen FD, et al. Unexpectedly high but still asymptomatic iron overload in a patient with pyruvate kinase deficiency. Hematol J. 2004;5(6):543–5.
233. Amankwah KS, Dick BW, Dodge S. Hemolytic anemia and pyruvate kinase deficiency in pregnancy. Obstet Gynecol. 1980;55(3 Suppl):42s–4s.

234. Esen UI, Olajide F. Pyruvate kinase deficiency: an unusual cause of puerperal jaundice. Int J Clin Pract. 1998;52(5):349–50.
235. Fanning J, Hinkle RS. Pyruvate kinase deficiency hemolytic anemia: two successful pregnancy outcomes. Am J Obstet Gynecol. 1985;153(3):313–4.
236. Wax JR, et al. Pyruvate kinase deficiency complicating pregnancy. Obstet Gynecol. 2007;109(2 Pt2):553–5.
237. Dolan LM, Ryan M, Moohan J. Pyruvate kinase deficiency in pregnancy complicated by iron overload. BJOG. 2002;109(7):844–6.
238. Pincus M, Stark RA, O'Neill JH. Ischaemic stroke complicating pyruvate kinase deficiency. Intern Med J. 2003;33(9–10):473–4.
239. Muller-Soyano A, et al. Pyruvate kinase deficiency and leg ulcers. Blood. 1976;47(5):807–13.
240. Chou R, DeLoughery TG. Recurrent thromboembolic disease following splenectomy for pyruvate kinase deficiency. Am J Hematol. 2001;67(3):197–9.
241. Oski FA, et al. The role of the left-shifted or right-shifted oxygen-hemoglobin equilibrium curve. Ann Intern Med. 1971;74(1):44–6.
242. Deeren D. Deferasirox in pyruvate kinase deficiency. Ann Hematol. 2009;88(4):397.
243. Vukelja SJ. Erythropoietin in the treatment of iron overload in a patient with hemolytic anemia and pyruvate kinase deficiency. Acta Haematol. 1994;91(4):199–200.
244. Zahid MF, Bains APS. Rapidly fatal Klebsiella pneumoniae sepsis in a patient with pyruvate kinase deficiency and asplenia. Blood. 2017;130(26):2906.
245. Morimoto M, et al. Pyruvate kinase deficiency of mice associated with nonspherocytic hemolytic anemia and cure of the anemia by marrow transplantation without host irradiation. Blood. 1995;86(11):4323–30.
246. Tanphaichitr VS, et al. Successful bone marrow transplantation in a child with red blood cell pyruvate kinase deficiency. Bone Marrow Transplant. 2000;26(6):689–90.
247. Garcia-Gomez M, et al. Safe and efficient gene therapy for pyruvate kinase deficiency. Mol Ther. 2016;24(7):1187–98.
248. Steinberg MH. Sickle cell disease and other hemoglobinopathies. In: Goldman L, Shafer A, editors. Goldman-cecil medicine. 25th ed. Philadelphia, PA: Elsevier Saunders; 2016. p. 1095–104.
249. McAdam AJ, Milner DA, Sharpe AH. Red blood cell and bleeding disorders. In: Kumar V, Abbas AK, Aster JC, editors. Robbins and Cotran pathologic basis of disease. 9th ed. Philadelphia, PA: Elsevier Saunders; 2015. p. 629–67.

Chapter 7
Immune-Mediated Hemolytic Anemia

Ilene Weitz

Autoimmune hemolytic anemia (AIHA) is an acquired autoimmune disorder characterized by the development of antibodies directed against antigens on autologous erythrocytes [1]. It is a rare disorder with an incidence of 1–3 cases in 100,000 persons per year [2]. Antibodies may be IgG, IgM or on rare occasions IgA. The thermal amplitude of the antibody determines whether or not the antibody binds at cold (4–22 °C) versus warm (37 °C) temperature. The focus of this paper will be on warm mediated autoimmune hemolytic anemias (AIHA) most often characterized by IgG autoantibodies.

Warm, autoimmune hemolytic anemia accounts for 65–70% of the autoimmune hemolytic anemias. The antibodies are most often IgG which bind to the RBC at 37 °C. Hemolysis occurs mostly in the spleen, in which the macrophage has a receptor for the Fc domain of IgG [3–5]. Depending on the IgG subtype, the antibodies may fix complement (IgG1, IgG3). These may result in a component of intravascular hemolysis as well as extracellular clearance by macrophage complement C3b receptors in the spleen and liver. Eight percent of AIHA involve both IgG and IgM autoantibodies [6]. On rare occasions, IgM antibodies will have a higher thermal amplitude resulting in a "warm" antibody phenotype, but with prominent intravascular hemolysis. In addition to the thermal amplitude of the antibody, the degree of hemolysis may also depend on the concentration of the antibody, the presence of complement binding, and the affinity of the autoantibody to the RBC antigens. Hemolysis can occur with low-affinity autoantibodies, low concentration of RBC-bound autoantibodies (<200 IgG), or rare IgA autoantibodies which may be associated with a negative antiglobulin (Coombs) test and require specialized laboratory studies for detection [7, 8]. Warm autoantibodies can be classified into two distinct categories, depending on their reactivity with reticulocyte-enriched (younger) or

I. Weitz, MD
Jane Anne Nohl Division of Hematology, USC Keck School of Medicine,
Los Angeles, CA, USA
e-mail: iweitz@med.usc.edu

© Springer Nature Switzerland AG 2019
R. T. Means Jr. (ed.), *Anemia in the Young and Old*,
https://doi.org/10.1007/978-3-319-96487-4_7

reticulocyte-poor (older) red cell fractions. Type I autoantibodies demonstrate preferential reactivity with older red cells; type II autoantibodies reacted with both older and younger (reticulocyte rich) red cells. Type II antibodies are associated with more severe anemia most likely due to antibody binding to and suppression of the reticulocytes response which can be observed in up to 30% of patients [9–11].

Autoimmune hemolytic anemia can occur as a primary (idiopathic) disorder or occur in association with other immune or nonimmune disorders (secondary AIHA). Secondary forms of AIHA may account for 40–50% of all patients with AIHA [1, 12, 13]. Secondary AIHA may occur in other autoimmune disorders such as systemic lupus erythematosus (SLE), rheumatoid arthritis (RA), scleroderma, mixed connective tissue disease, and autoimmune thyroid disease. It can occur with lymphoproliferative disorders such as chronic lymphocytic leukemia, Hodgkin's and non-Hodgkin's lymphomas, or large granular lymphocytic leukemia [14–16]. Autoimmune hemolytic anemia can also be seen in association with immune dysregulatory disorders such as common variable immunodeficiency (CVID) and autoimmune lymphoproliferative syndrome (ALPS) [17]. ALPS in pediatric cases and some adults has also been associated with concomitant immune thrombocytopenia (Evan's syndrome) [18]. Unlike mycoplasma pneumonia which is associated with cold agglutinins, viral syndromes such as Epstein-Barr virus (EBV) and human immunodeficiency virus (HIV) have been associated with warm AIHA [19].

Paroxysmal cold hemoglobinuria is a rare form of IgG + C3b-mediated hemolysis causing cold hemolytic anemia due to the Donath-Landsteiner antibody which binds to the "P" RBC antigen [20]. The antibody has a low thermal amplitude, so it will bind at low temperature but stay bound to the cell, fixing and activating complement as the core temperature increases. The disease is often secondary to chronic syphilis infection and after an acute viral often infection in children [20].

Medication-related AIHA is well recognized. Several mechanisms have been described to explain how medications can induce autoimmune hemolytic anemia [21]. Haptene protein complex formation, such as has been described with penicillin results in the creation of a new immunogenic small protein complex on the red cell membrane leading to antibody formation. Some drugs such as quinine, quinidine, or second- or third-generation cephalosporins can form antibodies wherein the antibody-drug immune complex can bind to the red blood cell membrane after which the RBC undergoes hemolysis as an innocent bystander. Autoantibodies have been also described in association with oxaliplatin and fludarabine. A medication that can induce autoantibodies directed to specific RBC antigens, such as in the case of alpha methyldopa, can also cause hemolysis [21–24].

Drug-induced antibodies can be classified as either drug-independent antibodies, which do not require drug to be added into in vitro test systems, or drug-dependent antibodies which require the drug to be present in the test system. Drug-independent antibodies (DI-AIHA) are true RBC autoantibodies, not antibodies to a drug, and can be the cause of a true autoimmune hemolytic anemia. The laboratory and clinical findings can be indistinguishable from those associated with idiopathic AIHA. It is thought that drugs evoking these antibodies do it by having a direct effect on the immune system possibly due to molecular mimicry that can induce AIHA. The more common forms of antibodies are drug-dependent antibodies causing drug-dependent immune hemolytic anemia (DD-IHA). These antibodies react only when drug is present. They can be classified into two major subtypes, defined by in vitro activity. Type I antibodies that react with RBCs that are coated with the dru. Some drugs bind covalently to the RBC membrane will remain on the RBCs after several washes in vitro. Type II antibodies can be detected by incubating the patient's serum (containing drug antibody), drug, and ABO-compatible RBCs [24].

Lymphoproliferative disorders, such as chronic lymphocytic leukemia (CLL) and lymphomas, are also associated with the development of AIHA. The presentation of AIHA may be a harbinger of or may occur concurrently with the diagnosis of leukemia/lymphoma. Waldenstrom's macroglobulinemia is most often associated with cold hemolytic anemia. All patients with AIHA should be screened for possible lymphoproliferative disorders [14–16, 25].

AIHA is associated with a high incidence of venous thrombosis [26, 27]. In a retrospective analysis of patients at a large urban hospital, 25% of patient with AIHA presented with concurrent venous thromboembolic complication (VTE) [26]. Thrombosis as a cause of death is common [1]. The antiphospholipid syndrome (APLS) occurs in 1/3 of patients [27]. However, even without laboratory evidence of APLS, 15% of patient will have a potentially life-threatening VTE [27]. In view of this, it is strongly recommended that patients be tested for D-dimer, lupus anticoagulant, anticardiolipin, and B2 glycoprotein 1 antibodies. Duplex scans of the legs and, if the patients have pulmonary symptoms, a high-resolution computerized tomography pulmonary angiography (CTPA) should be performed. If there is no evidence of thrombosis, prophylactic anticoagulation is recommended as long as there is evidence of hemolysis. Full dose anticoagulation is recommended if there is evidence of active thrombosis.

Clinical Presentation

Patients with AIHA may have sudden onset of weakness, dyspnea, and jaundice. Or the presentation may be somewhat more insidious, with fatigue and generalized malaise, joint pain [28]. The degree of anemia will depend on the concentration of antibody, the presence of complement binding, as well as the reticulocyte response. Anemia, reticulocytosis, increased lactic dehydrogenase, and indirect hyperbilirubinemia will be found on laboratory testing. Rare patients (5–10%) may present with reticulocytopenia due to antibodies binding to the reticulocytes [9–11]. The blood smear characteristically demonstrated anisopoikilocytosis, microspherocytes, and shift cells. Nucleated RBCs may also be seen. Mild leukocytosis and an increase in RBC mean corpuscular volume (MCV) due to reticulocytosis may also be noted. Direct antiglobulin (DAT) will identify the presence of an IgG antibody bound to the RBC with or without C3b. Specific identification of the RBC antigen to which the antibody is bound versus a pan antibody should be done. The DAT will detect

≥200 IgG antibodies on the RBCs. However, if the DAT is negative but the smear and clinical presentation are suggestive, then specialized testing for low-level antibody or IgA should be considered [7].

Treatment

AIHA can be difficult to treat. Multiple therapies have been used with varying success (Table 7.1). Corticosteroids and immune modulation remains the mainstay of therapy. Corticosteroids are associated with a high response rate (82%) in acutely decreasing the hemolysis. Prednisone 1–1.5 mg/kg orally daily or dexamethasone can be used [29–31, 49, 50]. Unfortunately, 80–85% of patients will relapse as the steroids are lowered or discontinued. Because of the toxicities of long-term corticosteroid treatment, the use of other immune modulation may be indicated.

Azathioprine remains among the most effective second-line treatments for steroid-refractory and steroid-dependent patients with warm antibody AIHA. Overall responses are 40–60%, with 10–20% of patients obtaining a complete response

Table 7.1 Treatment recommendations in warm antibody autoimmune hemolytic anemia

Intervention	Outcomes	Reference
Corticosteroids	85% acute response Relapse 80–85%	[28–31]
Immune modulators		
B cell		
Rituximab 375 mg/week ×4 1000 mg q 2 weeks	79% (95% CI, 60%–90%). Complete response 42% (95% CI, 27%–58%). 79%	[32–34] [35]
T cell		
Mycophenolate mofetil Cyclosporine 5 mg/kg bid × 5 days then tapered to 3 mg/kg bid	90% (children) 75% CR, 25% PR	[36, 37] [38]
B & T cell		
Azathioprine 2–3 mg/kg/day	40%–60% complete response = 10–20%	[39]
Cyclophosphamide (CTX) 50 mg/kg × 4 days + GCSF	5/8 patients (62.5%)	[40]
CTX (750–1000 mg) + rituximab + dexamethasone	100% response duration of response 22 months[a] 96% response rate[b]	[41] [42]
Splenectomy	40–80% 20% long-term responses	[43, 44] [45–47]
Sirolimus	3/3 with AIHA = CR	[48]

[a]CLL
[b]Non-leukemia-associated AIHA

[29–31, 49, 50]. The usual treatment dose azathioprine is 2–3 mg/kg/d (100–250 mg). The long-term use of azathioprine appears to be well tolerated by most patients. Toxicities include pancytopenia and transaminitis.

Evidence suggest that although AIHA is an antibody-mediated disorder, there is significant T-cell dysregulation with the loss of regulatory T cells (Tregs) [39, 51]. T-cell modulators such as cyclosporine, mycophenolate mofetil, and cyclophosphamide have been used to treat refractory patients [36–38, 40, 52, 53].

Antibody-producing B cells can be depleted using rituximab, a monoclonal antibody to circulating and tissue CD 20 + B cells. In addition, rituximab has been demonstrated to restore Tregs to normal levels [54]. The ORR for warm AIHA in 154 patients was 79% (95% CI, 60–90%). The complete response rate for warm AIHA was 42% (95% CI, 27–58%). There does not appear to be a significant difference in response between patients with primary versus secondary AIHA [32–34, 54]. Michel et al., conducted a phase III trial using rituximab versus placebo in newly diagnosed AIHA. Rituximab was given at a dose of 1000 mg every 2 weeks for two doses. Corticosteroids were used concurrently but tapered rapidly over 2 weeks. The overall response rate at 1 year was 75% (95% CI, 47.6–92.7) with 11 CR and 1 PR with rituximab versus 31% (11.0–58.7) (5 CR) with placebo ($P = 0.032$). At 2 years, 10/16 patients receiving rituximab versus 3/16 with placebo remained in CR ($P = 0.011$). The rate of infection was lower in the rituximab-treated group compared to the placebo group [35]. Combination treatment with cyclophosphamide, rituximab, and corticosteroids appears to be very effective in treating warm AIHA associated with lymphoproliferative malignancies (100% response) [41]. The application of this combination to non-leukemia-associated AIHA appears to yield similar response rates (96%) [42]. Cyclophosphamide (50 mg/kg), as a single agent, has also been used [49]. Toxicities of cyclophosphamide treatment include nausea, bone marrow suppression with cytopenias, male and female sterility, hemorrhagic cystitis, myelodysplasia, and leukemia.

Splenectomy

Before corticosteroids became available, splenectomy was the only treatment for patients with AIHA. In an early retrospective study of splenectomy in AIHA, 57 patients with AIHA were analyzed for response and survival. Thirty-four patients were deemed have to be primary or idiopathic AIHA. Of these 34 primary AIHA patients, splenectomy was performed in 27 patients (79%) [2, 43]. Of these 27 patients, 9 died due to persistent AIHA, sepsis post splenectomy, or cardiac failure [43]. Of the surviving 18 patients, 10 patients had "good" response, hemoglobin >10 g/dl, with survivals ranging from 26 to 99 months. Seven patients had a "fair" response, hemoglobin of 10 g/dl or less, although their survivals were comparable (22–120 months) [43]. One patient had a poor response. Most contemporary reports on the use of splenectomy for the treatment of AIHA report a 40–80% initial response, with up to a 20% long-term remission [31, 44, 45].

The advent of laparoscopic splenectomy combined with postsurgical antibiotic and thrombotic prophylaxis has significantly reduced surgery-related morbidity and mortality [46]. However, a long-term increased risk of overwhelming sepsis remains even with appropriate immunizations [45–47, 50, 55, 56]. The risk of severe infection is approximately 3–7%, with a nearly 50% mortality [47, 55]. The subsequent use of immune modulatory therapy in patients who do not respond to the procedure may increase the risk of severe infection. In addition, an increased risk of venous thromboembolism and pulmonary hypertension has been observed in patients treated for immune thrombocytopenia and thalassemia with splenectomy [47, 57].

Future Directions for AIHA

Immune modulation with agents other than those discussed above is in or pending clinical trials. MTOR inhibitors such as rapamycin, which increase regulatory T cells and induce apoptosis of abnormal lymphocytes, have been used with some efficacy in ALPS and a small pediatric series of AIHA [48].

FcgR activation induces the activation of Syk, which leads to increased phagocytosis. The Syk pathway inhibitor has shown some activity in immune thrombocytopenic purpura (ITP). There are ongoing clinical trials in AIHA (ClinicalTrials.gov NCT02612558). FcRn is a receptor that internalizes IgG antibody decreasing its degradation. Inhibitors to FCR enhance the catabolism of these abnormal antibodies. A phase I clinical trial underway in AIHA (ClinicalTrials.gov NCT03075878).

Complement activation due to IgG or IgM binding to the RBC can result in both intravascular hemolysis and increased clearance of C3b-coated RBC via the spleen and liver. Blockade of the complement system at various points is being evaluated in clinical trials. The binding of complement 1q following antibody binding can propel further complement activation and C3b deposition on the RBC. Inhibition by C1q esterase inhibitor has demonstrated some preliminary efficacy in warm IgM-mediated hemolytic anemia [58].

In summary, AIHA is a responsive but chronically relapsing immune disorder. It can be primary or secondary due to medications, underlying autoimmune diseases, or lymphoma/leukemia. Immune suppression with corticosteroids as well as B- and T-cell modulators remains the mainstay of therapy. However, no advances in our understanding of the pathologic immune mechanisms causing AIHA have resulted in new and innovative therapies.

References

1. Dacie JV, Worlledge SM. Autoimmune hemolytic anemia. In: Brown EB, Morre CV, editors. Progress in hematology VI. New York: Grune & Stratton; 1969.
2. Bottiger LE, Westerholm B. Acquired haemolytic anaemia. Acta Med Scand. 1973;193:223–6.

3. Engelfriet CC, Overbeeke MAM, von dem Borne AEG. Autoimmune hemolytic anemia. Semin Hematol. 1992;29:3–12.
4. Quist E, Koepsell S. Autoimmune hemolytic anemia and red blood cell auto-antibodies. Arch Pathol Lab Med. 2015;139:1455–68.
5. Nailk R. Warm autoimmune hemolytic anemia. Hematol Oncol Clin North Am. 2015;29:445–53.
6. Shulman IA, Branch DR, Nelson JM, et al. Autoimmune hemolytic anemia with both cold and warm autoantibodies. JAMA. 1985;253:1746–58.
7. Segel GB, Lichtman MA. Direct antiglobulin ("Coombs") test-negative autoimmune hemolytic anemia. Blood Cells Mol Dis. 2014;52:152–60.
8. Lai M, Visconti E, D'Onofrio G, Tamburrini E, Cauda R, Leone G. Lower hemoglobin levels in human immunodeficiency virus-infected patients with a positive direct antiglobulin test (DAT): relationship with DAT strength and clinical stages. Transfusion. 2006;46:1237–43.
9. Branch DR, Shulman IA, Sy Siok Hian AL, Petz LD. Two distinct categories of warm autoantibody reactivity with age fractionated red cells. Blood. 2004;63(1):177–80.
10. Conely CL, Lippman SM, Ness PM, Petz LD, Branch DR, Gallagher MT. Autoimmune hemolytic anemia with reticulocytopenia and erythroid marrow. N Engl J Med. 1982;306:281–6.
11. Liesveld JL, Rowe JM, Lichtman MA. Variability of the erythropoietic response in autoimmune hemolytic anemia: analysis of 109 cases. Blood. 1987;69:820–8.
12. Sokol RJ, Booker DJ, Stamps R. The pathology of autoimmune haemolytic anaemia. J Clin Pathol. 1992;45:1047–52.
13. Pirofsky B. Clinical aspects of autoimmune hemolytic anemia. Semin Hematol. 1976;13:251–65.
14. Mauro F, Foa R, Cerretti R, Giannarelli D, Coluzzi S, Mandelli F, Girelli G. Autoimmune hemolytic anemia in chronic lymphocytic leukemia. Clinical, therapeutic and prognostic features. Blood. 2000;95:2786–92.
15. Feng Q, Zak D, Daya R. Autoimmune hemolytic anemia and classical Hodgkin lymphoma: a case report and literature review. Clin Adv Hematol Oncol. 2012;10:270–6.
16. Qin X, Yu Y, Yan S, Wang R, Liu X, Chen C. Pure red cell aplasia and autoimmune hemolytic anemia sequentially occurring in a patient with large granular T-lymphocytic leukemia. Intern Med. 2016;55:1491–6.
17. Seve P, Bourdillon L, Sarrot-Reynauld F, Ruivard M, Jaussaud R, Bouhour D, Bonotte B, Gardembas M, Poindron V, Thiercelin MF, Broussolle C, Oksenhendler E, DEF-I Study Group. Autoimmune hemolytic anemia and common variable immunodeficiency: a case-control study of 18 patients. Medicine. 2008;87:177–84.
18. Seif AE, Manno CS, Sheen C, Grupp SA, Teachey DT. Identifying autoimmune lymphoproliferative syndrome in children with Evans syndrome: a multi-institutional study. Blood. 2010;115:2142–5.
19. Koduri PR, Singa P, Nikolinakos P. Autoimmune hemolytic anemia in patients infected with human immunodeficiency virus-1. Am J Hematol. 2012;70:174–6.
20. Shanbhag S, Spivak J. Paroxysmal cold hemoglobinuria. Hematol Oncol Clin North Am. 2015;29:473–8.
21. Arndt PA, Garrety G. The changing spectrum of drug-induced immune hemolytic anemia. Semin Hematol. 2005;42:137–44.
22. Salama A. Drug-induced immune hemolytic anemia. Expert Opin Drug Saf. 2009;8:73–9.
23. Garbe E, Andersohn F, Bronder E, et al. Drug induced immune haemolytic anaemia in the Berlin case-control surveillance study. Br J Haematol. 2011;154:644–53.
24. Garrety G. Immune hemolytic anemia caused by drugs. J Expert Opin Drug Saf. 2012;11:635–42.
25. Sallah S, Wan JY, Hanrahan LR. Future development of lymphoproliferative disorders in patients with autoimmune hemolytic anemia. Clin Cancer Res. 2001;7(4):791–4.
26. Roumier M, Loustau V, Guillaud C, et al. Characteristics and outcome of warm autoimmune hemolytic anemia in adults: new insights based on a single-center experience with 60 patients. Am J Hematol. 2014;89:E150–1555.

27. Pullarkat V, Ngo M, Iqbal S, et al. Detection of lupus anticoagulant identifies patients with autoimmune hemolytic anemia at increased risk for venous thrombosis. Br J Haematol. 2002;118:1166–9.
28. Petz LD, Garratty G. Immune hemolytic anemias. 2nd ed. Philadelphia: Churchill Livingstone; 2004.
29. Ozsoylu F. Megadose methylprednisolone for treatment of patients with Evan's syndrome. Pediatr Hematol Oncol. 2004;21:739–40.
30. Meyer O, Stahl D, Beckhove P, et al. Pulse high-dose dexamethasone in chronic autoimmune hemolytic anaemia of warm type. Br J Haematol. 1997;98:860–2.
31. Zupanska B, Sylwestrowicz T, Pawelski S. The results of prolonged treatment of autoimmune haemolytic anaemia. Haematologica. 1981;14:425–33.
32. Barcellini W, Zaja F, Zaninoni A, et al. Low-dose rituximab in adult patients with idiopathic autoimmune hemolytic anemia: clinical efficacy and biologic studies. Blood. 2012;119:3691–7.
33. Reynaud Q, Durieu I, Dutertre M, et al. Efficacy and safety of rituximab in autoimmune hemolytic anemia: a meta-analysis of 21 studies. Autoimmun Rev. 2015;14:304–13.
34. Birgens H, Frederiksen H, Hasselbalch HC, et al. A phase III randomized trial comparing glucocorticoid monotherapy versus glucocorticoid and rituximab in patients with autoimmune haemolytic anaemia. Br J Haematol. 2013;163:393–9.
35. Michel M, Terriou L, Roudot-Thoraval F, Hamidou M, Ebbo M, Le Guenno G, Audia S, Royer B, Morin AS, Michot JM, Jaccard A, Frenzel L, Khellaf M, Godeau B. Randomized and double blind trial evaluating safety and efficacy of rituximab for warm auto-immune hemolytic anemia in adults (RIAHA). Am J Hematol. 2017;92:23–7.
36. Howard J, Hoffbrand AV, Prentice HG, et al. Mycophenolate mofetil for treatment of refractory auto-immune haemolytic anaemia and auto-immune thrombocytopenia. Br J Haematol. 2002;117:712–5.
37. Miano M, Ramenghi U, Russo G, Rubert L, Barone A, Tucci F, Farruggia P, Petrone A, Mondino A, Lo Valvo L, Crescenzio N, Bellia F, Olivieri I, Palmisani E, Caviglia I, Dufour C, Fioredda F. Mycophenolate mofetil for the treatment of children with immune thrombocytopenia and Evans syndrome. A retrospective data review from the Italian association of paediatric haematology/oncology. Br J Haematol. 2016;175:490–5.
38. Emilia G, Messora C, Longo G, et al. Long-term salvage treatment by cyclosporine in refractory haematologic disorders. Br J Haematol. 1996;93:341–4.
39. Barcellini W. Current treatment strategies in autoimmune hemolytic disorders. Expert Rev Hematol. 2015;8:681–91.
40. Moyo VM, Smith D, Brodsky I, et al. High-dose cyclophosphamide for refractory autoimmune hemolytic anemia. Blood. 2002;100:704–6.
41. Kaufman M, Limaye SA, Driscoll N, Johnson C, Caramanica A, Lebowicz Y, Patel D, Kohn N, Rai K. A combination of rituximab, cyclophosphamide and dexamethasone effectively treats immune cytopenias of chronic lymphocytic leukemia. Leuk Lymphoma. 2009;50:892–9.
42. Piatek C, Bocian H, O'Connell C, Weitz IC, Liebman H. Combination treatment of rituximab, cyclophoaphamide and dexamethasone hemotalogica. Hematologica. 2018; abstract 3963.
43. Crosby WH, Rappaport H. Autoimmune hemolytic anemia. Analysis of hematologic observations with particular reference to their prognostic value. A survey of 57 cases. Blood. 1957;12:42–55.
44. Bowdler AS. The role of the spleen and splenectomy in autoimmune hemolytic anemia. Semin Hematol. 1976;13:335–85.
45. Crowther M, Chan YL, Garbett IK, et al. Evidence-based focused review of treatment of idiopathic warm immune hemolytic anemia in adults. Blood. 2011;118:4036–40.
46. Casaccia M, Torelli IP, Squarcia S, et al. Laparoscopic splenectomy for hematologic diseases: a preliminary analysis performed on the Italian registry of laparoscopic surgery of the spleen. Surg Endosc. 2006;20:1214–20.
47. Boyle S, White R, Brunson A, et al. Splenectomy and the incidence of venous thromboembolism and sepsis in patients with immune thrombocytopenia. Blood. 2013;121:4782–90.

48. Miano M, Calvillo M, Palmisani E, et al. Sirolimus for the treatment of multi-resistant autoimmune haemolytic in children. Br J Haematol. 2014;167:571–4.
49. Murphy S, LoBuglio AF. Drug therapy of autoimmune hemolytic anemia. Semin Hematol. 1976;13:323–48.
50. Zanella A, Barcellini W. Treatment of autoimmune hemolytic anemias. Haematologica. 2014;99:1547–54.
51. Ahmad E, Elgohary T, Ibrahim H. Regulatory T cells essential to prevent the loss of self-tolerance in murine models of erythrocyte-specific autoantibody responses. J Investig Allergol Clin Immunol. 2011;21:297–304.
52. Hershko C, Sonneblick M, Ashkenazi J. Control of steroid-resistant autoimmune hemolytic anaemia by cyclosporine. Br J Haematol. 1990;76:436–7.
53. Rao VK, Dugan F, Dale JK, et al. Use of mycophenolate mofetil for chronic, refractory immune cytopenias in children with autoimmune lymphoproliferative syndrome. Br J Haematol. 2005;129:534–8.
54. Stasi R, Cooper N, Del Poeta G, Stipa E, Laura Evangelista M, Abruzzese E, Amadori S. Analysis of regulatory T-cell changes in patients with idiopathic thrombocytopenic purpura receiving B cell-depleting therapy with rituximab. Blood. 2008;112:1147–50.
55. Bisharat N, Omari H, Lavi I, et al. Risk of infection and death among post- splenectomy patients. J Infect. 2001;43:182–6.
56. Kyaw MH, Holmes EM, Toolis F, et al. Evaluation of severe infection and survival after splenectomy. Am J Med. 2006;119:276.e1–7.
57. Fayed MA, Abdel-Hady HE, Hafez MM, Salama OS, Al-Tonbary YA. Study of platelet activation, hypercoagulable state, and the association with pulmonary hypertension in children with beta-thalassemia. Hematol Oncol Stem Cell Ther. 2018;11(2):65–74.
58. Wouters D, Stephan F, Strengers P, de Haas M, Brouwer C, Hagenbeek A, et al. C1 esterase inhibitor concentrate rescues erythrocytes from complement-mediated destruction in autoimmune hemolytic anemia. Blood. 2013;128(22):4817.

Chapter 8
Anemia of Renal Failure/Chronic Kidney Disease

Robert T. Means Jr.

The anemia seen with chronic kidney disease (CKD), also called the anemia of renal failure or (in the older literature) anemia of uremia, affects patients of all ages. However, it represents a significant proportion of the anemia observed in the elderly. The development of recombinant human erythropoietin (rhEpo) as a therapeutic modality changed the management of anemia in CKD and enhanced our understanding of the weight of different mechanisms in its development. In this chapter, the pathogenetic processes producing this syndrome will be reviewed. Following that discussion, frequency of anemia of CKD in the elderly will be discussed. The chapter will conclude with discussion of treatment of anemia due to CKD.

Anemia is extremely common in patients with significant CKD [1]. Prior to the availability of rhEpo for treatment, nearly all hemodialysis patients were anemic [2], and even with rhEpo therapy readily available, approximately a quarter of dialysis patient and almost half of pre-dialysis severe CKD patients have significant anemia (hemoglobin ≤ 10 g/dL)d [3, 4]. As Fig. 8.1 demonstrates, anemia begins to increase in prevalence at an estimated glomerular filtration rate (eGFR) of 45 mL/min/1.73 m^2 [5], defined as CKD stage 3 [6], and becomes more prevalent as renal function declines. With the exception of polycystic kidney disease, where the cysts can produce Epo and hemoglobin concentration is frequently preserved [7], the nature of the disease causing chronic renal insufficiency does not change the degree or frequency of anemia. Precise hemoglobin concentrations vary due to alterations in plasma volume, but hemoglobin concentrations less than 7–8 g/dL are uncommon.

R. T. Means Jr., MD
James H. Quillen College of Medicine, East Tennessee State University,
Johnson City, TN, USA
e-mail: MEANSR@mail.etsu.edu

© Springer Nature Switzerland AG 2019
R. T. Means Jr. (ed.), *Anemia in the Young and Old*,
https://doi.org/10.1007/978-3-319-96487-4_8

Fig. 8.1 Predicted
prevalence of hemoglobin
level less than 11, less than
12, and less than 13 g/dL
among men (**a**) and women
(**b**) 20 years and older who
participated in the Third
National Health and
Nutrition Examination
Survey (1988–1994).
(Reprinted from Astor
et al. [5] with permission
from the American
Medical Association)

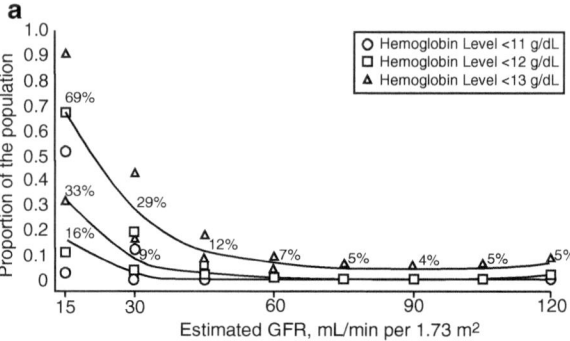

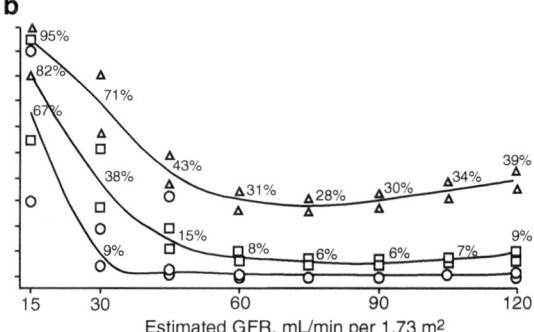

Laboratory Features/Approach

Red cell morphology is usually normocytic and normochromic. With severe uremia, echinocytes or "burr" cells may be seen. It is the author's impression that this is an uncommon event at the present time, as renal failure is typically detected prior to development of severe uremia. The reticulocyte percentage may be in the normal range or even slightly increased [8], but absolute reticulocyte count is always decreased. In the absence of a concurrent inflammatory process or of splenomegaly, white count and platelet count are typically normal, although the percentage of neutrophils on the differential count may be increased.

Assessment of anemia in CKD patients largely resembles that in any other anemic patient. Estimated GFR less than 45 mL/min/1.73 m^2 is permissive but not diagnostic. Screening for multiple myeloma using serum free light chains [9, 10] should be performed, since renal insufficiency and anemia are a common dyad at presentation for that disease. Particular attention should be paid to iron status. Iron deficiency has been reported in 17–44% of CKD patients [11, 12] and frequently coexists with anemia induced by Epo deficiency. Serum ferritin may be low in CKD patients with iron deficiency but usually is normal or somewhat increased and elevated out of proportion to iron stores due to inflammation [11]. Measurement of serum soluble transferrin receptor concentration may be helpful in identifying iron deficiency in CKD patients [13]. Iron absorption is impaired in CKD: this process is under the physiologic regulation of hepcidin, which tends to be elevated in renal patients [14, 15].

Bone marrow examination is rarely required but when performed shows a moderately hypercellular marrow with normal erythroid maturation. Iron may be absent [12, 16]. While Epo deficiency is the main cause of anemia in CKD, measurement of serum or plasma Epo concentration is not helpful or recommended for the assessment of anemia in CKD. The usual feedback relationship between hemoglobin concentrations and Epo is lost [17]. While Epo concentrations are always detectable, they are very low for the degree of anemia [18]. Some portion of Epo production in CKD derives from extrarenal sites like the liver, which retain some capacity for Epo production from earlier in embryonic development [18, 19]. However, extrarenal Epo secretion does not increase sufficiently to compensate for deficiencies in the kidney, the primary physiologic site of production [20].

Pathogenesis

Somewhat analogous to the anemia of inflammation\chronic disease (AICD; Chap. 9), three processes contribute to anemia in CKD. These are Epo deficiency, suppression of the marrow response to anemia, and shortened red cell survival. The first and most dominant is an absolute deficiency of Epo. As renal function deteriorates, renal Epo secretion decreases [21, 22]. Since Epo is the primary driver of erythropoiesis, anemia results. Classic animal studies [23] provided proof of principle for the dominant role of Epo deficiency in anemia due to CKD, confirmed by subsequent clinical trials of rhEpo in renal failure patients [24, 25].

There is no single mechanism by which the second pathophysiologic process exerts its effects. The most common and best studied is probably cytokine-mediated suppression of erythropoiesis in the context of inflammation, by mechanisms previously described for AICD and discussed in detail in that chapter [26, 27]. Like AICD, the iron regulatory peptide hepcidin plays a significant role in this effect [28, 29]. Polyamines such as spermine accumulate in renal failure and have been demonstrated to suppress erythroid colony formation in vitro. Some of these polyamines are more effectively removed by peritoneal dialysis than by hemodialysis, possibly contributing to a lower severity of anemia in peritoneal dialysis [30, 31]. Secondary hyperparathyroidism or pseudohypoparathyroidism may contribute to anemia, either by direct inhibition of erythroid progenitors [32] or by contributing to marrow fibrosis (osteitis fibrosa cystica) [33, 34].

There is a modest shortening of red cell survival also [35]. As in AICD, this shortened red cell survival, while small in itself, creates demand for red cell production that cannot be met due to Epo deficiency and marrow suppression. In addition to neocytolysis, the process contributing to shortened red cell survival in AICD [36], erythrocyte oxidative stress [37], abnormal cation flux [38], and red cell membrane lipid peroxidation [39] play a role in shortened red cell survival in CKD.

Apart from the anemia of CKD per se, patients with CKD, particularly those on hemodialysis, are susceptible to other causes of anemia, including iron deficiency (discussed above) and dialysis-exacerbated folate deficiency [40].

Anemia of CKD in the Elderly

Renal function tends to decline with age. It is debated whether this decrease in GFR is an intrinsic consequence of aging or rather reflects comorbid conditions, particularly hypertension [41]. It has been suggested that progressive vascular insufficiency leads to this decline [42]. The decline in GFR with aging is not strictly linear – in the oldest old, it appears that the GFR decline levels off [43].

In four surveys of etiology of anemia in the elderly cited in Chap. 3 [44–47], the frequency of CKD as an etiology of anemia ranged between 1.2% and 15%. One study from Brazil identified CKD as a contributor to anemia in 62% of elderly patients [48].

Treatment

This section only addresses treatment of the anemia of CKD as defined above. Iron deficiency, folate deficiency, or other specific diagnoses would be managed as appropriate for those conditions.

Renal replacement therapy. The most common approach to renal replacement therapy when CKD is at an advanced stage is *functional* replacement by dialysis. In general, this does not correct anemia significantly, since it does not restore Epo production. If uremic toxins that are removable by dialysis are contributing to anemia by suppressing marrow or increasing hemolysis, dialysis may mitigate anemia to some degree. This is the proposed explanation for the observation that peritoneal dialysis is associated with less severe anemia than is hemodialysis [49, 50], since some of the polyamines implicated in suppression of erythropoiesis are removed less effectively by hemodialysis. While hemodialysis itself does not mitigate anemia, inadequate hemodialysis intensity can be a significant contributor to rhEpo resistance and consequent worsened anemia in dialysis patients [51].

Renal transplantation corrects anemia in CKD patients through native Epo produced from the transplanted kidney. Approximately 80% of patients will correct their anemia to some degree over an 8–10-week period following a successful renal allograft [52, 53]. A sustained peak in renal allograft Epo production begins around day 8 and continues until hemoglobin concentration is approximately 10 g/dL. In patients with delayed allograft function, an early peak in Epo production occurs and then returns to baseline by day 7. This early peak is not associated with correction of anemia [53, 54].

rhEpo and rhEpo analogs. rhEpo or an rhEpo analog such as darbepoetin is the treatment of choice for anemia in CKD requiring therapy in patients on either hemodialysis or peritoneal dialysis or in predialysis patients with measured or estimated GFR less than 45 mL/min/1.73 m^2 [55]. The introduction of rhEpo in the 1980s markedly changed management, relegating modalities such as androgens to the category of "historical treatments" [25, 56]. Due to complications observed with complete normalization of hemoglobin concentration [57, 58], rhEpo treatment is initiated when hemoglobin concentration is persistently less than 10 g/dL and rhEpo should be discontinued at a target hemoglobin concentration between 11 and 12 g/dL [57, 59]. The desired hemoglobin concentration is typically attained within 6–8 weeks [60]. It is widely believed that rhEpo therapy improves quality of life in treated CKD patients [61, 62]; but meta-analysis has generally not supported this belief, primarily because of methodology issues making individual studies difficult to compare [59]. Specific dosing and administration instructions for rhEpo administration should be obtained from current guidelines [63, 64]. There is no high-quality evidence indicating that any Epo analog is more effective or safer than any other [65].

Iron supplementation (as distinct from iron *replacement*, the management of actual iron deficiency) is nearly always required, particularly in patients on hemodialysis [66]. As noted earlier, ferritin is elevated out of proportion to iron stores in CKD patients. Iron should be administered with caution at ferritin concentrations in the 500–800 μg/L and should not be given at all when the ferritin is >800 μg/L [55]. Intravenous iron should be used for dialysis patients and may allow comparable hemoglobin concentrations to be obtained with less rhEpo [67–70].

Despite the effectiveness of rhEpo and its analogs in correcting anemia in CKD, roughly a quarter of dialysis patients remain significantly anemic. This is referred to as *Epo resistance*. The main cause of Epo resistance is concurrent iron deficiency. This was noted in the earliest studies of rhEpo therapy in CKD [71]. Another major cause of Epo resistance is inflammation and consequent cytokine suppression of erythropoiesis [72]. The role of inadequate dialysis intensity has already been noted. Other causes of rhEpo resistance are listed in Table 8.1 and have been reviewed in detail elsewhere [72].

The safety profile of rhEpo and its analogs is excellent, but adverse effects occur and seem to occur primarily in dialysis/CKD patients. Hypertension is the most common of such effects [73] and may be severe and complicated by encephalopathy on rare occasions [74]. It tends to be a transient phenomenon occurring in the first few months of treatment, and attention to patient blood pressure allows preemptive management. The mechanism is not entirely clear. The observation that occurrence of hypertension is more closely related to the rate of increase in the blood hemoglobin level than to the dose of rhEpo [75] led to the reasonable hypothesis that it resulted from changes in the relative balance between red cell mass and plasma volume for which CKD or dialysis patients could not compensate rapidly. However, it is likely more complicated, involving nitric oxide-mediated vascular effects which are apparently unique to CKD [76]. Beginning in the late 1990s and continuing for several years thereafter, there were a number of reports of rhEpo-induced anti-Epo neutralizing antibodies causing Epo resistance and even pure red cell aplasia. These

Table 8.1 Causes of resistance/unresponsiveness to recombinant erythropoietin [72]

Systemic causes
Iron deficiency
Concurrent inflammation
Folate deficiency
Secondary hypoparathyroidism
Primary renal causes
Insufficient dialysis intensity
Renal allograft failure
Aluminum toxicity (from dialysate; now rare)
Pharmacologic causes
Angiotensin converting enzyme inhibitors
Angiotensin receptor blocking agents
Recombinant erythropoietin-induced antierythropoietin antibodies (now uncommon; discussed in text)
Myelosuppressive drugs
Primary hematologic causes
Marrow failure disorders (primary or induced)
Hemolysis
Hematologic malignancies
Hemoglobinopathy
Splenomegaly

cases were almost exclusively in CKD/dialysis patients and largely confined to Western Europe and Canada. Epidemiologic investigation ultimately attributed this phenomenon to unanticipated adjuvant effects of the stoppers in prefilled syringes distributed in those regions. The problem was largely eliminated by packaging changes, and new cases are rare [77, 78]. Allergic reactions to rhEpo, including anaphylaxis, have been reported but are extremely rare [79]. The author has been treating patients with rhEpo for more than 30 years, beginning with pre-approval clinical trials in the 1980s. To the best of my recollection, I have encountered only one definite allergic reaction in a patient treated with rhEpo, and it is possible that it was a reaction to a protein used as a stabilizer in the formulation in those days.

New agents. Orally administered hypoxia-inducible factor (HIF) stabilizing compounds are in development for treatment of anemia in CKD and may eventually become an alternative to, or replace, rhEpo if studies show them to be to be safe, effective, and available at an appropriate cost [80].

References

1. Desforges JF. Anemia in uremia. Arch Intern Med. 1970;126(5):808–11.
2. Charles G, Lundin AP 3rd, Delano BG, Brown C, Friedman EA. Absence of anemia in maintenance hemodialysis. Int J Artif Organs. 1981;4(6):277–9.

3. End Stage Renal Disease Core Indicators Project. 1997 annual report. Baltimore, MD: US Department of Health and Human Services/Health Care Financing Administration; 1997.
4. Voormolen N, Grootendorst DC, Urlings TA, et al. Prevalence of anemia and its impact on mortality and hospitalization rate in predialysis patients. Nephron Clin Pract. 2010;115(2):c133–41.
5. Astor BC, Muntner P, Levin A, Eustace JA, Coresh J. Association of kidney function with anemia: the Third National Health and Nutrition Examination Survey (1988-1994). Arch Intern Med. 2002;162(12):1401–8.
6. Delanaye P, Cavalier E. Staging chronic kidney disease and estimating glomerular filtration rate: an opinion paper about the new international recommendations. Clin Chem Lab Med. 2013;51(10):1911–7.
7. Eckardt KU, Mollmann M, Neumann R, et al. Erythropoietin in polycystic kidneys. J Clin Invest. 1989;84(4):1160–6.
8. Talwar VK, Gupta HL, Shashinarayan. Clinicohaematological profile in chronic renal failure. J Assoc Physicians India. 2002;50:228–33.
9. Dejoie T, Corre J, Caillon H, et al. Serum free light chains, not urine specimens, should be used to evaluate response in light-chain multiple myeloma. Blood. 2016;128(25):2941–8.
10. Vermeersch P, Van HL, Delforge M, Marien G, Bossuyt X. Diagnostic performance of serum free light chain measurement in patients suspected of a monoclonal B-cell disorder. Br J Haematol. 2008;143(4):496–502.
11. Lukaszyk E, Lukaszyk M, Koc-Zorawska E, Tobolczyk J, Bodzenta-Lukaszyk A, Malyszko J. Iron status and inflammation in early stages of chronic kidney disease. Kidney Blood Press Res. 2015;40(4):366–73.
12. Stancu S, Stanciu A, Zugravu A, et al. Bone marrow iron, iron indices, and the response to intravenous iron in patients with non-dialysis-dependent CKD. Am J Kidney Dis. 2010;55(4):639–47.
13. de Paoli Vitali E, Ricci G, Perini L, et al. The determination of plasma transferrin receptor as good index of erythropoietic activity in renal anemia and after renal transplantation. Nephron. 1996;72(4):552–6.
14. Valenti L, Messa P, Pelusi S, Campostrini N, Girelli D. Hepcidin levels in chronic hemodialysis patients: a critical evaluation. Clin Chem Lab Med. 2014;52(5):613–9.
15. Jelic M, Cvetkovic T, Djordjevic V, et al. Hepcidin and iron metabolism disorders in patients with chronic kidney disease. Vojnosanit Pregl. 2013;70(4):368–73.
16. Weng CH, Lu KY, Hu CC, Huang WH, Wang IK, Yen TH. Bone marrow pathology predicts mortality in chronic hemodialysis patients. Biomed Res Int. 2015;2015:160382.
17. Pavlovic-Kentera V, Clemons GK, Djukanovic L, Biljanovic-Paunovic L. Erythropoietin and anemia in chronic renal failure. Exp Hematol. 1987;15(7):785–9.
18. Caro J, Brown S, Miller O, Murray T, Erslev AJ. Erythropoietin levels in uremic nephric and anephric patients. J Lab Clin Med. 1979;93(3):449–58.
19. Naets JP, Wittek M. Erythropoiesis in anephric man. Lancet. 1968;1(7549).941–3.
20. Zucker S, Lysik RM, Mohammad G. Erythropoiesis in chronic renal disease. J Lab Clin Med. 1976;88(4):528–35.
21. Radtke HW, Claussner A, Erbes PM, Scheuermann EH, Schoeppe W, Koch KM. Serum erythropoietin concentration in chronic renal failure: relationship to degree of anemia and excretory renal function. Blood. 1979;54(4):877–84.
22. McGonigle RJ, Wallin JD, Shadduck RK, Fisher JW. Erythropoietin deficiency and inhibition of erythropoiesis in renal insufficiency. Kidney Int. 1984;25(2):437–44.
23. Eschbach JW, Mladenovic J, Garcia JF, Wahl PW, Adamson JW. The anemia of chronic renal failure in sheep. Response to erythropoietin-rich plasma in vivo. J Clin Invest. 1984;74(2):434–41.
24. Eschbach JW, Kelly MR, Haley NR, Abels RI, Adamson JW. Treatment of the anemia of progressive renal failure with recombinant human erythropoietin. N Engl J Med. 1989;321(3):158–63.
25. Winearls CG, Oliver DO, Pippard MJ, Reid C, Downing MR, Cotes PM. Effect of human erythropoietin derived from recombinant DNA on the anaemia of patients maintained by chronic haemodialysis. Lancet. 1986;2:1175–8.

26. Allen DA, Breen C, Yaqoob MM, Macdougall IC. Inhibition of CFU-E colony formation in uremic patients with inflammatory disease: role of IFN-gamma and TNF-alpha. J Investig Med. 1999;47:204–11.
27. Rafiean-Kopaie M, Nasri H. Impact of inflammation on anemia of hemodialysis patients who were under treatment of recombinant human erythropoietin. J Renal Inj Prev. 2013;2(3):93–5.
28. Goyal H, Mohanty S, Sharma M, Rani A. Study of anemia in nondialysis dependent chronic kidney disease with special reference to serum hepcidin. Indian J Nephrol. 2017;27(1):44–50.
29. Ganz T, Nemeth E. Iron balance and the role of hepcidin in chronic kidney disease. Semin Nephrol. 2016;36(2):87–93.
30. Hotta T, Maeda H, Suzuki I, Chung TG, Saito A. Selective inhibition of erythropoiesis by sera from patients with chronic renal failure. Proc Soc Exp Biol Med. 1987;186(1):47–51.
31. Radtke HW, Rege AB, LaMarche MB, et al. Identification of spermine as an inhibitor of erythropoiesis in patients with chronic renal failure. J Clin Invest. 1981;67(6):1623–9.
32. Potasman I, Better OS. The role of secondary hyperparathyroidism in the anemia of chronic renal failure. Nephron. 1983;33(4):229–31.
33. Touam M, Martinez F, Lacour B, et al. Aluminum induced reversible microcytic anemia in chronic renal failure: clinical and experimental studies. Clin Nephrol. 1983;19:295–8.
34. Zingraff J, Drueke T, Marie P, Man NK, Jungers P, Bordier P. Anemia and secondary hyperparathyroidism. Arch Intern Med. 1978;138(11):1650–2.
35. Korell J, Vos FE, Coulter CV, Schollum JB, Walker RJ, Duffull SB. Modeling red blood cell survival data. J Pharmacokinet Pharmacodyn. 2011;38(6):787–801.
36. Alfrey CP, Fishbane S. Implications of neocytolysis for optimal management of anaemia in chronic kidney disease. Nephron Clin Pract. 2007;106(4):c149–56.
37. Rosenmund A, Binswanger U, Straub PW. Oxidative injury to erythrocytes, cell rigidity, and splenic hemolysis in hemodialyzed uremic patients. Ann Intern Med. 1975;82(4):460–5.
38. Cheng JT, Kahn T, Kaji DM. Mechanism of alteration of sodium potassium pump of erythrocytes from patients with chronic renal failure. J Clin Invest. 1984;74(5):1811–20.
39. Gallucci MT, Lubrano R, Meloni C, et al. Red blood cell membrane lipid peroxidation and resistance to erythropoietin therapy in hemodialysis patients. Clin Nephrol. 1999;52(4):239–45.
40. Teschner M, Kosch M, Schaefer RM. Folate metabolism in renal failure. Nephrol Dial Transplant. 2002;17(Suppl 5):24–7.
41. Krol E, Rutkowski B, Czarniak P, Kraszewska E. Aging or comorbid conditions – what is the main cause of kidney damage? J Nephrol. 2010;23(4):444–52.
42. Buckalew VM Jr. Ischemic nephropathy: an important cause of renal disease in the elderly. Geriatr Nephrol Urol. 1998;8(3):155–9.
43. Feinfeld DA, Keller S, Somer B, et al. Serum creatinine and blood urea nitrogen over a six-year period in the very old. Creatinine and BUN in the very old. Geriatr Nephrol Urol. 1998;8(3):131–5.
44. Artz AS, Thirman MJ. Unexplained anemia predominates despite an intensive evaluation in a racially diverse cohort of older adults from a referral anemia clinic. J Gerontol A Biol Sci Med Sci. 2011;66(8):925–32.
45. Guralnik JM, Eisenstaedt RS, Ferrucci L, Klein HG, Woodman RC. Prevalence of anemia in persons 65 years and older in the United States: evidence for a high rate of unexplained anemia. Blood. 2004;104(8):2263–8.
46. Tettamanti M, Lucca U, Gandini F, et al. Prevalence, incidence and types of mild anemia in the elderly: the "Health and Anemia" population-based study. Haematologica. 2010;95(11):1849–56.
47. Michalak SS, Rupa-Matysek J, Gil L. Comorbidities, repeated hospitalizations, and age ≥80 years as indicators of anemia development in the older population. Ann Hematol. 2018;97:1337.
48. Santos IS, Scazufca M, Lotufo PA, Menezes PR, Bensenor IM. Causes of recurrent or persistent anemia in older people from the results of the Sao Paulo Ageing & Health Study. Geriatr Gerontol Int. 2013;13(1):204–8.
49. House AA, Pham B, Page DE. Transfusion and recombinant human erythropoietin requirements differ between dialysis modalities. Nephrol Dial Transplant. 1998;13:1763–9.

50. De Paepe MB, Schelstraete KH, Ringoir SM, Lameire NH. Influence of continuous ambulatory peritoneal dialysis on the anemia of endstage renal disease. Kidney Int. 1983;23(5): 744–8.
51. Ifudu O, Feldman J, Friedman EA. The intensity of hemodialysis and the response to erythropoietin in patients with end-stage renal disease. N Engl J Med. 1996;334(7):420–5.
52. Hoffman GC. Human erythropoiesis following kidney transplantation. Ann N Y Acad Sci. 1968;149(1):504–8.
53. Kessler M. Erythropoietin and erythropoiesis in renal transplantation. Nephrol Dial Transplant. 1995;10(Suppl 6):114–6.
54. Abbrecht PH, Greene JA Jr. Serum erythropoietin after renal homotransplantation. Ann Intern Med. 1966;65(5):908–21.
55. Conditions NCCfC. Anaemia Management in Chronic Kidney Disease: National Clinical Guideline for Management in Adults and Children. Anaemia management in chronic kidney disease: national clinical guideline for management in adults and children. London: Royal College of Physicians (UK) Royal College of Physicians of London; 2006.
56. Eschbach JW, Egrie JC, Downing MR, Browne JK, Adamson JW. Correction of the anemia of end-stage renal disease with recombinant human erythropoietin. Results of a combined phase I and II clinical trial. N Engl J Med. 1987;316(2):73–8.
57. Besarab A, Bolton WK, Browne JK. The effects of normal as compared with low hematocrit values in patients with cardiac disease who are receiving hemodialysis and epoetin. N Engl J Med. 1998;339:584–90.
58. Besarab A, Goodkin D, Nissenson AR. The normal hematocrit study—follow-up. N Engl J Med. 2008;358:433–4.
59. Collister D, Komenda P, Hiebert B, et al. The effect of erythropoietin-stimulating agents on health-related quality of life in Anemia of chronic kidney disease: a systematic review and meta-analysis. Ann Intern Med. 2016;164(7):472–8.
60. Locatelli F, Aljama P, Barany P. Revised European best practice guidelines for the management of anaemia in patients with chronic renal failure. Nephrol Dial Transplant. 2004;19:ii1–ii47.
61. Temple RM, Deary IJ, Winney RJ. Recombinant erythropoietin improves cognitive function in patients maintained on chronic ambulatory peritoneal dialysis. Nephrol Dial Transplant. 1995;10(9):1733–8.
62. Mayer G, Thum J, Cada EM, Stumvoll HK, Graf H. Working capacity is increased following recombinant human erythropoietin treatment. Kidney Int. 1988;34:525–8.
63. Mikhail A, Brown C, Williams JA, et al. Renal association clinical practice guideline on Anaemia of Chronic Kidney Disease. BMC Nephrol. 2017;18(1):345.
64. National Clinical Guideline Centre. National Institute for Health and Care Excellence: Clinical Guidelines. Anaemia management in chronic kidney disease: partial update 2015. London: Royal College of Physicians (UK) National Clinical Guideline Centre; 2015.
65. Palmer SC, Saglimbene V, Mavridis D, et al. Erythropoiesis-stimulating agents for anaemia in adults with chronic kidney disease: a network meta-analysis. Cochrane Database Syst Rev. 2014;12:Cd010590.
66. Tanaka S, Tanaka T. How to supplement iron in patients with renal anemia. Nephron. 2015;131(2):138–44.
67. Pollak VE, Lorch JA, Means RT Jr. Unanticipated favorable effects of correcting iron deficiency in chronic hemodialysis patients. J Investig Med. 2001;49(2):173–83.
68. Fishbane S, Frei GL, Maesaka J. Reduction in recombinant human erythropoietin doses by the use of chronic intravenous iron supplementation. Am J Kidney Dis. 1995;26(1):41–6.
69. Sepandj F, Jindal K, West M, Hirsch D. Economic appraisal of maintenance parenteral iron administration in treatment of anaemia in chronic haemodialysis patients. Nephrol Dial Transplant. 1996;11(2):319–22.
70. KDOQI. Clinical practice guidelines and clinical practice recommendations for anemia in chronic kidney disease. Am J Kidney Dis. 2006;47:S11–S145.
71. Eschbach JW, Adamson JW. Guidelines for recombinant human erythropoietin therapy. Am J Kidney Dis. 1989;14(2 Suppl 1):2–8.

72. Johnson DW, Pollock CA, Macdougall IC. Erythropoiesis-stimulating agent hyporesponsiveness. Nephrology (Carlton). 2007;12(4):321–30.
73. Jones MA, Kingswood JC, Dallyn PE, et al. Changes in diurnal blood pressure variation and red cell and plasma volumes in patients with renal failure who develop erythropoietin-induced hypertension. Clin Nephrol. 1995;44(3):193–200.
74. Beccari M. Seizures in dialysis patients treated with recombinant erythropoietin. Review of the literature and guidelines for prevention. Int J Artif Organs. 1994;17(1):5–13.
75. Kokot F, Wiecek A. Arterial hypertension in uraemic patients treated with erythropoietin. Nephron. 1995;71(2):127–32.
76. Vaziri ND, Zhou XJ, Naqvi F, et al. Role of nitric oxide resistance in erythropoietin-induced hypertension in rats with chronic renal failure. Am J Physiol Endocrinol Metab. 1996;271(1):E113–22.
77. Bennett CL, Starko KM, Thomsen HS, et al. Linking drugs to obscure illnesses: lessons from pure red cell aplasia, nephrogenic systemic fibrosis, and Reye's syndrome. A report from the Southern Network on Adverse Reactions (SONAR). J Gen Intern Med. 2012;27(12):1697–703.
78. McKoy JM, Stonecash RE, Cournoyer D, et al. Epoetin-associated pure red cell aplasia: past, present, and future considerations. Transfusion. 2008;48(8):1754–62.
79. Garcia JE, Senent C, Pascual C, et al. Anaphylactic reaction to recombinant human erythropoietin. Nephron. 1993;65:636–7.
80. Malyszko J, Malyszko JS. Emerging drugs for the treatment of kidney disease-induced anemia. Expert Opin Emerg Drugs. 2016;21(3):315–30.

Chapter 9
The Anemia of Inflammation/Chronic Disease and the Unexplained Anemia of the Elderly

Robert T. Means Jr.

Anemia of Inflammation/Chronic Disease

Introduction

The clinical syndrome formerly known as the "anemia of chronic disease" is likely the most common anemia syndrome encountered in medical practice after anemia due to blood loss and subsequent iron deficiency. Initially characterized in the mid-twentieth century by Wintrobe and Cartwright, this disorder was traditionally associated with infectious, inflammatory, or neoplastic diseases persisting for greater than 2 months [1]. Subsequent studies showed that the original categories of associated diseases were too narrow [2], and that in fact, the "anemia of chronic disease" could be encountered in acute situations. Although an association between the pathogenetic mechanisms underlying the development of anemia in this syndrome and the cytokine mediators of the immune and inflammatory response has been known for many years [3], the demonstration of the central pathogenetic role of hepcidin, a mediator of innate immunity with iron regulatory properties, led to wider use of the term "anemia of inflammation" [4]. In this chapter and related chapters therefore, the syndrome will be referred to as "anemia of inflammation/chronic disease" (AICD).

R. T. Means Jr., MD
James H. Quillen College of Medicine, East Tennessee State University, Johnson City, TN, USA
e-mail: MEANSR@mail.etsu.edu

© Springer Nature Switzerland AG 2019
R. T. Means Jr. (ed.), *Anemia in the Young and Old*,
https://doi.org/10.1007/978-3-319-96487-4_9

Pathogenesis of AICD

As depicted in Fig. 9.1, the pathogenesis of AICD reflects a balance of various processes. A modest (<10%) shortening of red cell survival, probably as result of selective hemolysis of the youngest red cells (neocytolysis) [5], creates an increased demand for red cell production. Under normal conditions, such a small increase in red cell demand could be compensated easily by the marrow. However, in the situations associated with AICD, the marrow is not able to respond adequately due to a combination of three processes. The first process is a blunted erythropoietin response to anemia: for any given decrease in hemoglobin concentration, the increment in erythropoietin is less than would be seen in a comparable degree of anemia due to uncomplicated iron deficiency [6]. While the erythropoietin response is relatively decreased, the actual erythropoietin concentrations observed in patients are as high or higher than are seen in patients without anemia. This implies an impaired response of erythroid progenitors to erythropoietin. Such an impaired response has been demonstrated in in vitro models of AICD [7–11]. Finally, there is impairment of iron mobilization from reticuloendothelial stores and of iron utilization for erythropoiesis, contributing to the pathogenesis of the disease and providing the characteristic iron parameter findings (hypoferremia with adequate or increased iron stores) which make the laboratory diagnosis [12]. These processes are not present in equal proportions in all circumstances – in juvenile rheumatoid arthritis, for example, the iron abnormalities are predominant [13].

The mathematics of the balance between the small reduction in red cell survival and the degree accounts for the slow onset of anemia observed by Wintrobe and Cartwright in chronic infections [1] (hence the name "anemia of chronic disease"). When "acute" anemia of chronic disease arises, as with critically ill hospital patients

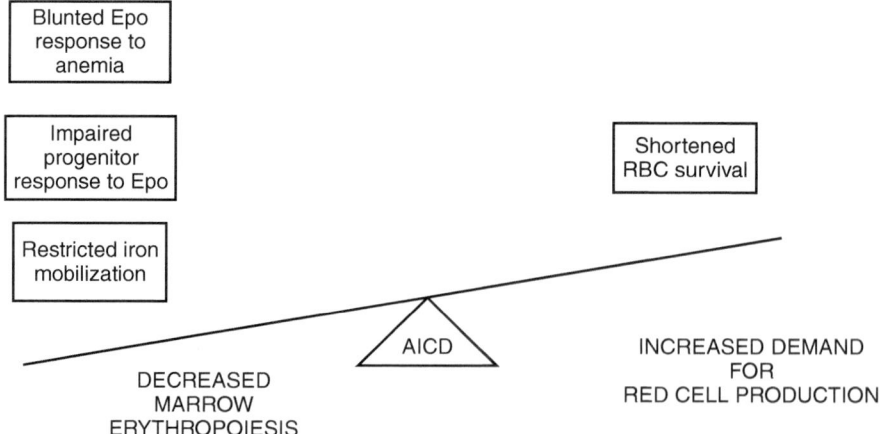

Fig. 9.1 Pathogenetic processes involved in anemia of inflammation/chronic disease. AICD – anemia of inflammation/chronic disease, Epo – erythropoietin, RBC – red blood cell

[14–16], it is likely that a combination of disease-related and iatrogenic blood loss adds to the small decrease in red cell survival and allows a more rapid establishment of a pathophysiologically identical anemia.

All the pathogenetic mechanisms of AICD have been linked to effects of various cytokine mediators of inflammation, such as tumor necrosis factor (TNF), interleukin (IL)-1 and IL-6, and the interferons (IFNs), particularly IFNγ. These clinical and in vitro associations have been reviewed elsewhere [12, 17]. Neocytolysis appears to be a consequence of relative or absolute erythropoietin deficiency [18, 19], which can itself be attributed to cytokine effects.

However, the mediator of these cytokine effects appears to be hepcidin in most cases [4, 20, 21]. Hepcidin is a type II acute-phase-reacting peptide produced in the liver and largely but not exclusively regulated by IL-6 [4, 22, 23]. Hepcidin production in patients who have anemia with an elevated serum ferritin concentration compared to iron-deficient patients [4]. Hepcidin promotes macrophage iron retention by causing internalization of the iron export protein ferroportin [24].

Considering involvement of hepcidin in the pathogenetic processes shown in Fig. 9.1, hepcidin clearly drives the abnormalities in iron metabolism. Transgenic mice overexpressing hepcidin show an impaired erythropoietic response to erythropoietin as well as the characteristic iron abnormalities [25], and dialysis patients with increased circulating hepcidin have a higher degree of resistance to recombinant erythropoietin therapy [26]. Under conditions of limited erythropoietin availability mimicking those seen in AICD, hepcidin is associated with impaired erythroid colony formation in vitro [27]. Hepcidin and erythropoietin expression both appear to be regulated by hypoxia-inducible factor (HIF) [28] and other interrelated processes [29], potentially linking hepcidin with the relative erythropoietin deficiency of AICD and, by extension, with neocytolysis. While hepcidin is clearly the most significant mediator of AICD pathogenesis, AICD can develop independently of its effects in response to other mediators of inflammation [30].

Diagnosis

AICD is typically normocytic or slightly microcytic. A mean corpuscular volume value less than 78 fL should prompt consideration of other diagnoses. The absolute reticulocyte count is low for the degree of anemia, although the value of reticulocyte percentage may be in the normal range. The hallmark of the diagnosis is a low serum iron with normal or increased iron stores. If the serum ferritin (usually the best chemical estimate of iron stores) is equivocal, serum-soluble transferrin receptor, typically as a ratio with the logarithm of serum ferritin concentration [31], will rule out iron deficiency. The Thomas plot, whether using the transferrin/ferritin index or serum hepcidin concentration, can also be a useful diagnostic tool [32, 33]. Some investigators advocate using a specific marker of inflammation or cytokine activation, such as IL-6 or C-reactive protein (CRP), to confirm the presence of inflammation [34].

In principle, measuring serum or plasma hepcidin should confirm the diagnosis [35]. However, availability for purposes other than research is limited.

Unexplained Anemia of the Elderly (UAE)

Table 9.1 lists the percentage of patients diagnosed with either AICD or UAE in five reports of anemia in the elderly. In three of these series, UAE was the single most common diagnosis. If it represents a single entity (which it most likely does not), it is the most common etiology of anemia in the elderly.

Pathogenesis

There are several possible pathogenetic mechanisms for UAE.

Consequence of Normal Processes of Aging As discussed in Part I. Chap. 3, anemia should not be considered "normal" in aging, but it may be a consequence of processes that are part of the physiologic state of aging, analogous to the physiologic anemia of pregnancy. A decline in renal function (and hence in erythropoietin production) is a well-known consequence of normal aging and may contribute to anemia [41]. The age-related decline in serum testosterone in men and of insulin-like growth factor (IGF)-1 in patients of both sexes appears to correlate independently with a decline in hemoglobin [42, 43]. Plasma concentration of the cytokine IL-6 increases with age [44]. This may have particular consequences apart from its effects on hepcidin production, discussed earlier. IL-6 administration is associated with increased plasma volume, and it has been postulated that IL-6-induced anemia is primarily dilutional rather than the result of decreased red cell mass [45–47]. It has been proposed that age-related arterial stiffness, with consequent impaired renal perfusion, may lead to unexplained anemia [48].

Table 9.1 Prevalence of anemia of inflammation/chronic disease (AICD) and unexplained anemia of the elderly (UAE) in five reports from different countries

Country of origin, year of report	AICD (%)	UAE (%)
USA, 2004 [36]	19.7	33.6
USA, 2011 [37]	9.8	43.7
Italy, 2010 [38]	17.4	26.4
Poland, 2018 [39]	33.1	28.4
Brazil, 2013[a] [40]	35.1	12.3

[a]Participants in this study could be assigned more than one etiology of anemia

A Forme Fruste of AICD UAE may be an incomplete form of AICD that has not risen to meet the diagnostic criteria. There are many similarities between the disorders:

1. Both occur in clinical circumstance of cytokine activation. Evidence of cytokine activation and inflammation is frequent in the elderly, including elevated levels of cytokine mediators of inflammation and nonspecific mediators of inflammation such as CRP [49–53]. The inflammatory markers seen in aging are associated with a number of the comorbidities associated with anemia including frailty, mobility limitation, and cognitive impairment [54–56].
2. Individuals with UAE appear to have a relatively blunted erythropoietin response to anemia [57, 58]. This appears not to be due to normal aging. Elderly individuals with definable iron-deficiency anemia appear to have an intact erythropoietin response [57], as do the healthy elderly [59].
3. Abnormalities of iron stores, as manifested by changes in serum ferritin concentrations, are also associated with aging. Iron stores tend to be elevated in the elderly, whether anemic or not [60]. While the percentile distribution of ferritin concentrations in adults becomes relatively flat after age 32, the 97.5 percentile ferritin concentration rises steadily with age [61]. In some reports, this increase in ferritin concentration is associated with a reduction in serum iron concentration [62]. Serum sTfR reportedly does not vary with age in adults [63].
4. Studies of hematopoietic progenitors in the elderly have yielded differing results. Some investigators have reported that erythroid colony-forming units (CFU-E) are decreased in anemic elderly individuals [64], consistent with reports that CFU-E colony formation is decreased in some AICD patients [65]. Others argue that the hematopoietic stem cell, rather than progenitors, becomes intrinsically abnormal during aging [66–69]. However, even if this is the case, it manifests itself primarily under circumstances of stress, as supported by the predominantly normal hematologic profile of most elderly individuals [66]. Alterations in the bone marrow microenvironment may still play a significant role in hematopoietic progenitor regulation in the elderly [70]. In addition, the increased prevalence of anemia in the elderly with erythropoietin concentrations that, though relatively decreased, are still higher than are seen in individuals without anemia suggests an impaired progenitor response to EPO.
5. The role of hepcidin is less clear than in AICD, and it may be that a lower degree of hepcidin involvement may distinguish UAE and AICD. Some but not all investigators have reported elevated hepcidin levels in UAE [71, 72].

A Mixed Bag of Other Diagnoses UAE may, and to some degree certainly does, represent a collection of patients with different disorders not otherwise diagnosed. Approximately half of elderly men with unexplained anemia and low testosterone levels showed significant correction of anemia with testosterone treatment in a large trial [73]. The corollary of this finding is that half of the men with unexplained anemia and low testosterone did *not* correct their anemia with testosterone. Ferritin concentrations rise with age as a normal finding [74], and it can be (and has been

[75]) argued that UAE populations include patients with iron-deficiency missed due to age-inappropriate normal ferritin ranges. In a study similar to that described for testosterone above, a subgroup of UAE patients with serum ferritin concentrations 20–200 ng/mL responded to intravenous iron [76]. Unsuspected clonal disorders of hematopoiesis may be present also [77].

Diagnosis

UAE is a diagnosis of exclusion [78] – it represents the cases of anemia remaining after anemia due to vitamin or mineral deficiency, renal insufficiency/chronic kidney disease, and AICD are ruled out, usually by specific testing, and other possibilities, such as hemolysis, clonal hematopoietic disorders, or hemoglobinopathies, have been evaluated or felt to be unlikely. It is therefore reasonable to wonder if UAE is a specific entity or a "mixed bag" of diagnoses. The observation that patients with UAE have survival comparable to elderly individuals who are not anemic, and better than patients with a specific anemia diagnosis [79], suggests that UAE is a distinct prognostic category if perhaps not a pathophysiologic one.

Management of AICD and UAE

In most cases, neither of these syndromes require specific treatment. In general, management of AICD follows from management of the underlying disorder that has led to activation of the cytokine mediators of inflammation. The vast majority of these patients (more than 80%) have hemoglobin values greater than 9 g/dL [2] and are not symptomatic on the basis of their anemia. Although iron therapy in and of itself is typically not indicated, there have been some reports of effective results with intravenous iron [80, 81]. A significant portion (although a minority) of cases of AICD are associated with concurrent iron deficiency [80, 82]. Anemia in these patients will respond to iron replacement to the extent that the anemia is a consequence of iron deficiency. Intravenous iron is typically more effective than oral iron. In some cases, iron-restricted erythropoiesis may be correctable by intravenous iron in AICD. A subset of patients with serum ferritin levels greater than 200 ng/mL (where iron stores are almost certainly present) have elevated serum-soluble transferrin receptor concentrations (a finding typical of iron deficiency) [83]. This may be a marker for individuals with AICD in whom parenteral iron therapy may be beneficial.

Recombinant erythropoietin therapy has been demonstrated to correct anemia in AICD [84], although there is debate about how significant this is for individual patients [85]. Concurrent iron support (oral or parenteral) is a significant contributor to the response to erythropoietin treatment in AICD [86].

In UAE, therapy is generally not indicated. The anemia is of modest degree, and anemia sufficiently severe to require therapy or to be symptomatic should likely lead to a reconsideration of the diagnosis. Although there is one study showing an improvement in hemoglobin concentration and quality of life in elderly African-American women with unexplained chronic anemia treated with erythropoietin [87], there has not been systematic investigation of erythropoietin therapy in UAE. As discussed earlier, a significant proportion of men with UAE and low testosterone will have an increase in hemoglobin concentration with testosterone therapy [73]. Some individuals with UAE and ferritin values in the normal range but less than 200 ng/mL will respond to parenteral iron [76]. In these individuals, the assumption should be that this was previously undiagnosed iron deficiency, and they should undergo an investigation for sources of blood loss appropriate for their overall clinical status and wishes.

References

1. Wintrobe MM, Cartwright GE. Studies on the mechanism of the anemia of infection. Proc Am Fed Clin Res. 1945;2:112.
2. Cash JM, Sears DA. The anemia of chronic disease: spectrum of associated diseases in a series of unselected hospitalized patients. Am J Med. 1989;87(6):638–44.
3. Means RT. Pathogenesis of the anemia of chronic disease: a cytokine-mediated anemia. Stem Cells. 1995;13:32–7.
4. Nemeth E, Valore EV, Territo M, Schiller G, Lichtenstein A, Ganz T. Hepcidin, a putative mediator of anemia of inflammation, is a type II acute phase protein. Blood. 2003;101:2461–3.
5. Rice L, Alfrey CP. The negative regulation of red cell mass by neocytolysis: physiologic and pathophysiologic manifestations. Cell Physiol Biochem. 2005;15(6):245–50.
6. Baer AN, Dessypris EN, Goldwasser E, Krantz SB. Blunted erythropoietin response to anaemia in rheumatoid arthritis. Br J Haematol. 1987;66:559–64.
7. Means RT, Krantz SB. Inhibition of human erythroid colony-forming units by tumor necrosis factor requires beta interferon. J Clin Investig. 1993;91:416–9.
8. Means RT, Krantz SB. Inhibition of human erythroid colony forming units by gamma interferon can be corrected by recombinant human erythropoietin. Blood. 1991;78:2564–7.
9. Means RT, Dessypris EN, Krantz SB. Inhibition of human erythroid colony-forming units by interleukin-1 is mediated by gamma interferon. J Cell Physiol. 1992;150:59–64.
10. Means RT, Krantz SB, Luna J, Marsters SA, Ashkenazi A. Inhibition of murine erythroid colony formation in vitro by gamma interferon and correction by interferon inhibitor. Blood. 1994;83:911–5.
11. Dallalio G, Means RT. Effects of oxidative stress on human erythroid colony formation: modulation by gamma interferon. J Lab Clin Med. 2003;141:395–400.
12. Means RT. Recent developments in the anemia of chronic disease. Curr Hematol Rep. 2003;2:116–21.
13. Cazzola M, Ponchio L, de Benedetti F, et al. Defective iron supply for erythropoiesis and adequate endogenous erythropoietin production in the anemia associated with systemic-onset juvenile chronic arthritis. Blood. 1996;87(11):4824–30.
14. Rodriguez RM, Corwin HL, Gettinger A, Corwin MJ, Gubler D, Pearl RG. Nutritional deficiencies and blunted erythropoietin response as causes of the anemia of critical illness. J Crit Care. 2001;16:36–41.
15. Asare K. Anemia of critical illness. Pharmacotherapy. 2008;28(10):1267–82.
16. Lasocki S, Longrois D, Montravers P, Beaumont C. Hepcidin and anemia of the critically ill patient: bench to bedside. Anesthesiology. 2011;114(3):688–94.
17. Means RT. Advances in the anemia of chronic disease. Int J Hematol. 1999;70:7–12.

18. Trial J, Rice L, Alfrey CP. Erythropoietin withdrawal alters interactions between young red blood cells, splenic endothelial cells, and macrophages: an in vitro model of neocytolysis. J Investig Med. 2001;49:335–45.
19. Trial J, Rice L. Erythropoietin withdrawal leads to the destruction of young red cells at the endothelial-macrophage interface. Curr Pharm Des. 2004;10(2):183–90.
20. Weinstein DA, Roy CN, Fleming MD, Loda MF, Wolfsdorf JI, Andrews NC. Inappropriate expression of hepcidin is associated with iron refractory anemia: implications for the anemia of chronic disease. Blood. 2002;100(10):3776–81.
21. Fleming RE, Sly WS. Hepcidin: a putative iron-regulatory hormone relevant to hereditary hemochromatosis and the anemia of chronic disease. Proc Natl Acad Sci U S A. 2001;98:8160–2.
22. Rivera S, Gabayan V, Ganz T. In chronic inflammation, there exists an IL-6-independent pathway for the induction of hepcidin (abstract). Blood. 2004;104:875a.
23. Armitage AE, Eddowes LA, Gileadi U, et al. Hepcidin regulation by innate immune and infectious stimuli. Blood. 2011;118(15):4129–39.
24. Nemeth E, Tuttle MS, Powelson J, et al. Hepcidin regulates iron efflux by binding to ferroportin and inducing its internalization. Science. 2004;306:2090–3.
25. Roy CN, Mak HH, Akpan I, Losyev G, Zurakowski D, Andrews NC. Hepcidin antimicrobial peptide transgenic mice exhibit features of the anemia of inflammation. Blood. 2007;109(9):4038–44.
26. Kato A. Increased hepcidin-25 and erythropoietin responsiveness in patients with cardio-renal anemia syndrome. Futur Cardiol. 2010;6(6):769–71.
27. Dallalio G, Law E, Means RT Jr. Hepcidin inhibits in vitro erythroid colony formation at reduced erythropoietin concentrations. Blood. 2006;107:2702–4.
28. Liu Q, Davidoff O, Niss K, Haase VH. Hypoxia-inducible factor regulates hepcidin via erythropoietin-induced erythropoiesis. J Clin Invest. 2012;122(12):4635–44.
29. Camaschella C, Pagani A, Nai A, Silvestri L. The mutual control of iron and erythropoiesis. Int J Lab Hematol. 2016;38(Suppl 1):20–6.
30. Langdon JM, Yates SC, Femnou LK, et al. Hepcidin-dependent and hepcidin-independent regulation of erythropoiesis in a mouse model of anemia of chronic inflammation. Am J Hematol. 2014;89(5):470–9.
31. Punnonen K, Irjala K, Rajamaeki A. Serum transferrin receptor and its ratio to serum ferritin in the diagnosis of iron deficiency. Blood. 1997;89(3):1052–7.
32. Thomas C, Kirschbaum A, Boehm D, Thomas L. The diagnostic plot: a concept for identifying different states of iron deficiency and monitoring the response to epoetin therapy. Med Oncol. 2006;23(1):23–36.
33. Thomas C, Kobold U, Balan S, Roedddiger R, Thomas L. Serum hepcidin-25 may replace the ferritin index in the Thomas plot in assessing iron status in anemic patients. Int J Lab Hematol. 2011;33:187–93.
34. Weiss G, Goodnough LT. Anemia of chronic disease. N Engl J Med. 2005;352(10):1011–23.
35. Means RT Jr. Hepcidin in differential diagnosis: ready for the clinic? Eur J Haematol. 2015;94(1):2–3.
36. Guralnik JM, Eisenstaedt RS, Ferrucci L, Klein HG, Woodman RC. Prevalence of anemia in persons 65 years and older in the United States: evidence for a high rate of unexplained anemia. Blood. 2004;104(8):2263–8.
37. Artz AS, Thirman MJ. Unexplained anemia predominates despite an intensive evaluation in a racially diverse cohort of older adults from a referral anemia clinic. J Gerontol A Biol Sci Med Sci. 2011;66(8):925–32.
38. Tettamanti M, Lucca U, Gandini F, et al. Prevalence, incidence and types of mild anemia in the elderly: the "Health and Anemia" population-based study. Haematologica. 2010;95(11):1849–56.
39. Michalak SS, Rupa-Matysek J, Gil L. Comorbidities, repeated hospitalizations, and age ≥80 years as indicators of anemia development in the older population. Ann Hematol. 2018;97:1337–47.

40. Santos IS, Scazufca M, Lotufo PA, Menezes PR, Bensenor IM. Causes of recurrent or persistent anemia in older people from the results of the Sao Paulo Ageing & Health Study. Geriatr Gerontol Int. 2013;13(1):204–8.
41. Ble A, Fink JC, Woodman RC, et al. Renal function, erythropoietin, and anemia of older persons: the InCHIANTI study. Arch Intern Med. 2005;165(19):2222–7.
42. Yeap BB, Beilin J, Shi Z, et al. Serum testosterone levels correlate with haemoglobin in middle-aged and older men. Intern Med J. 2009;39(8):532–8.
43. Nilsson-Ehle H, Bengtsson BA, Lindstedt G, Mellstrom D. Insulin-like growth factor-1 is a predictor of blood haemoglobin concentration in 70-yr-old subjects. Eur J Haematol. 2005;74(2):111–6.
44. Forsey RJ, Thompson JM, Ernerudh J, et al. Plasma cytokine profiles in elderly humans. Mech Ageing Dev. 2003;124:487–93.
45. Goyal KK, Saha A, Sahi PK, et al. Hepcidin and proinflammatory markers in children with chronic kidney disease: a case-control study. Clin Nephrol. 2018;89:363–70.
46. Nieken J, Mulder NH, Buter J, et al. Recombinant human interleukin-6 induces a rapid and reversible anemia in cancer patients. Blood. 1995;86(3):900–5.
47. Atkins MB, Kappler K, Mier JW, Isaacs RE, Berkman EM. Interleukin-6-associated anemia: determination of the underlying mechanism. Blood. 1995;86(4):1288–91.
48. Montero D, Diaz-Canestro C, Flammer A, Lundby C. Unexplained anemia in the elderly: potential role of arterial stiffness. Front Physiol. 2016;7:485.
49. Bruunsgaard H, Pedersen M, Pedersen BK. Aging and proinflammatory cytokines. Curr Opin Hematol. 2001;8(3):131–6.
50. Leng S, Xue QL, Huang Y, et al. Total and differential white blood cell counts and their associations with circulating interleukin-6 levels in community-dwelling older women. J Gerontol A Biol Sci Med Sci. 2005;60(2):195–9.
51. Ferrucci L, Corsi A, Lauretani F, et al. The origins of age-related proinflammatory state. Blood. 2005;105(6):2294–9.
52. Roubenoff R. Catabolism of aging: is it an inflammatory process? Curr Opin Clin Nutr Metab Care. 2003;6(3):295–9.
53. Roubenoff R, Parise H, Payette HA, et al. Cytokines, insulin-like growth factor 1, sarcopenia, and mortality in very old community-dwelling men and women: the Framingham Heart Study. Am J Med. 2003;115(6):429–35.
54. Puts MT, Visser M, Twisk JW, Deeg DJ, Lips P. Endocrine and inflammatory markers as predictors of frailty. Clin Endocrinol (Oxf). 2005;63(4):403–11.
55. Bautmans I, Njemini R, Lambert M, Demanet C, Mets T. Circulating acute phase mediators and skeletal muscle performance in hospitalized geriatric patients. J Gerontol A Biol Sci Med Sci. 2005;60(3):361–7.
56. Dik MG, Jonker C, Hack CE, Smit JH, Comijs HC, Eikelenboom P. Serum inflammatory proteins and cognitive decline in older persons. Neurology. 2005;64(8):1371–7.
57. Kario K, Matsuo T, Kodama K, Nakao K, Asada R. Reduced erythropoietin secretion in senile anemia. Am J Hematol. 1992;41(4):252–7.
58. Joosten E, Van Hove L, Lesaffre E, et al. Serum erythropoietin levels in elderly inpatients with the anemia of chronic disorders and iron deficiency anemia. J Am Geriatr Soc. 1993;41:1301–4.
59. Mori M, Murai Y, Hirai M, et al. Serum erythropoietin titers in the aged. Mech Ageing Dev. 1988;46(1–3):105–9
60. Fleming DJ, Jacques PF, Tucker KL, et al. Iron status of the free-living, elderly Framingham Heart Study cohort: an iron-replete population with a high prevalence of elevated iron stores. Am J Clin Nutr. 2001;73(3):638–46.
61. Custer EM, Finch CA, Sobel RE, Zettner A. Population norms for serum ferritin. J Lab Clin Med. 1995;126(1):88–94.
62. Malaguarnera M, Di Fazio I, Vinci E, Bentivegna P, Mangione G, Romano M. Haematologic pattern in healthy elderly subjects. Panminerva Med. 1999;41(3):227–31.
63. Allen J, Backstrom KR, Cooper JA, et al. Measurement of soluble transferrin receptor in serum of healthy adults. Clin Chem. 1998;44:35–9.

64. Lipschitz DA, Udupa KB, Milton KY, Thompson CO. Effect of age on hematopoiesis in man. Blood. 1984;63(3):502–9.
65. Smith MA, Knight SM, Maddison PJ, Smith JG. Anaemia of chronic disease in rheumatoid arthritis: effect of the blunted response to erythropoietin and of interleukin 1 production by marrow macrophages. Ann Rheum Dis. 1992;51(6):753–7.
66. Fuller J. Hematopoietic stem cells and aging. Sci Aging Knowledge Environ. 2002;2002(25):e11.
67. Van Zant G, Holland BP, Eldridge PW, Chen JJ. Genotype-restricted growth and aging patterns in hematopoietic stem cell populations of allophenic mice. J Exp Med. 1990;171(5):1547–65.
68. Kamminga LM, van Os R, Ausema A, et al. Impaired hematopoietic stem cell functioning after serial transplantation and during normal aging. Stem Cells. 2005;23(1):82–92.
69. de Haan G, Lazare SS. Aging of hematopoietic stem cells. Blood. 2018;131(5):479–87.
70. Morra L, Moccia F, Mazzarello GP, Bessone G, Del NE, Ponassi GA. Defective burst-promoting activity of T lymphocytes from anemic and nonanemic elderly people. Ann Hematol. 1994;68(2):67–71.
71. Ferrucci L, Semba RD, Guralnik JM, et al. Proinflammatory state, hepcidin and anemia in older persons. Blood. 2010;115(18):3810–6.
72. Lee P, Gelbart T, Waalen J, Beutler E. The anemia of ageing is not associated with increased plasma hepcidin levels. Blood Cells Mol Dis. 2008;41(3):252–4.
73. Roy CN, Snyder PJ, Stephens-Shields AJ, et al. Association of testosterone levels with anemia in older men: a controlled clinical trial. JAMA Intern Med. 2017;177(4):480–90.
74. Woo J, Mak YT, Law LK, Swaminathan R. Plasma ferritin in an elderly population living in the community. J Med. 1989;20(2):123–34.
75. Eisenga MF, Stam SP, Bakker SJL. Redefining unexplained anemia in elderly. JAMA Intern Med. 2017;177(9):1394–5.
76. Price E, Artz AS, Barnhart H, et al. A prospective randomized wait list control trial of intravenous iron sucrose in older adults with unexplained anemia and serum ferritin 20-200 ng/mL. Blood Cells Mol Dis. 2014;53(4):221–30.
77. Steensma DP, Bejar R, Jaiswal S, et al. Clonal hematopoiesis of indeterminate potential and its distinction from myelodysplastic syndromes. Blood. 2015;126(1):9–16.
78. Goodnough LT, Schrier SL. Evaluation and management of anemia in the elderly. Am J Hematol. 2014;89(1):88–96.
79. Shavelle RM, MacKenzie R, Paculdo DR. Anemia and mortality in older persons: does the type of anemia affect survival? Int J Hematol. 2012;95(3):248–56.
80. Auerbach M, Witt D, Toler W, Fierstein M, Lerner RG, Ballard H. Clinical use of the total dose intravenous infusion of iron dextran. J Lab Clin Med. 1988;111:566–70.
81. Anthony L, Means R, Rigby PW. Defining the "acquired iron insufficiency syndrome" (abstract). Support Care Cancer. 2007;15:766.
82. Baer AN, Dessypris EN, Krantz SB. The pathogenesis of anemia in rheumatoid arthritis. A clinical and laboratory analysis. Semin Arthritis Rheum. 1990;14:209–23.
83. North M, Dallalio G, Donath AS, Melink R, Means RT. Serum transferrin receptor levels in patients undergoing evaluation of iron stores: correlation with other parameters, and observed versus predicted results. Clin Lab Haematol. 1997;19:93–7.
84. Pincus T, Olsen NJ, Russell IJ, et al. Multicenter study of recombinant human erythropoietin in correction of anemia in rheumatoid arthritis. Am J Med. 1990;89:161–8.
85. Marti-Carvajal AJ, Agreda-Perez LH, Sola I, Simancas-Racines D. Erythropoiesis-stimulating agents for anemia in rheumatoid arthritis. Cochrane Database Syst Rev. 2013;(2):Cd000332.
86. Eschbach JW. Iron requirements in erythropoietin therapy. Best Pract Res Clin Haematol. 2005;18(2):347–61.
87. Agnihotri P, Telfer M, Butt Z, et al. Chronic anemia and fatigue in elderly patients: results of a randomized, double-blind, placebo-controlled, crossover exploratory study with epoetin alfa. J Am Geriatr Soc. 2007;55(10):1557–65.

Chapter 10
Pure Red Cell Aplasia

Robert T. Means Jr.

Pure red cell aplasia (PRCA) is a syndrome defined by a normocytic normochromic anemia with severe reticulocytopenia and marked reduction or the absence of erythroid precursors from the bone marrow [1]. As discussed below, PRCA is not a single pathogenetic entity but rather reflects a collection of disorders that results in a common morphology and characteristic blood counts. There is no specific clinical presentation of PRCA: the signs and symptoms are only those associated with anemia. Since PRCA is a pure underproduction anemia, the decline in hemoglobin concentration is gradual and allows preservation of total blood volume with some opportunity for physiologic and symptomatic adaptation resulting. This may mean PRCA patients present with relatively severe anemia at the time of diagnosis. Patients with secondary PRCA may manifest the symptomatology of the associated syndrome. Abnormalities in PRCA are limited to the red cell lineage: abnormalities in other cell lines usually reflect another concurrent disorder.

Classification

A classification of PRCA is outlined in Table 10.1 [1]. Congenital PRCA largely consists of Diamond-Blackfan anemia and Pearson syndrome, discussed in the chapter on inherited bone marrow failure syndromes. Each arises from specific gene defects affecting ribosomes and mitochondria, respectively [2, 3]. Myelodysplastic primary acquired PRCA is an uncommon presentation of myelodysplastic syndrome morphologically characterized by erythroid hypoplasia but that behaves in

R. T. Means Jr., MD
James H. Quillen College of Medicine, East Tennessee State University,
Johnson City, TN, USA
e-mail: MEANSR@mail.etsu.edu

Table 10.1 Classification of pure red cell aplasia

Congenital PRCA
Diamond-Blackfan anemia
Acquired PRCA
Primary
Primary autoimmune PRCA (includes TEC)
Primary myelodysplastic PRCA
Secondary, associated with
Autoimmune/collagen vascular disorders
Systemic lupus erythematosus
Rheumatoid arthritis
Inflammatory bowel disease
Other immunologic mechanisms
ABO-incompatible stem cell transplantation
Pyoderma gangrenosum
Lymphoproliferative disorders
Chronic lymphocytic leukemia
LGL leukemia
Hodgkin disease
Non-Hodgkin lymphomas
Angioimmunoblastic lymphadenopathy
Multiple myeloma
Waldenstrom macroglobulinemia
Castleman disease
Other hematologic malignancies
Chronic myelogenous leukemia
Chronic myelomonocytic leukemia
Myelofibrosis with myeloid metaplasia
Essential thrombocythemia
Acute lymphocytic leukemia
Solid tumors
Thymoma
Gastric cancer
Breast cancer
Biliary cancer
Lung cancer
Thyroid cancer
Renal cell carcinoma
Carcinoma of unknown primary site
Infections
B19 parvovirus
Human immunodeficiency virus
T-cell leukemia-lymphoma virus
Infectious mononucleosis
Viral hepatitis (hepatitis A, B, C, and E)
Cytomegalovirus
Bacterial infections
Group C streptococcus
Tuberculosis
Bacterial sepsis

Table 10.1 continued

Drugs and toxins
Rh erythropoietin-induced erythropoietin antibody-associated PRCA
Other drugs – see Table 10.2
Other disorders
Pregnancy
Riboflavin deficiency

Reproduced with permission from Means [1]

Abbreviations: *LGL* large granular lymphocyte, *PRCA* pure red cell aplasia, *rh* recombinant human, *TEC* transient erythroblastopenia of childhood

Table 10.2 Selected drugs associated with PRCA reported in PubMed

Agent	Multiple reports	Mechanism investigated
Alemtuzumab		
Allopurinol	✓	
Ampicillin		
Azathioprine	✓	✓
Carbamazepine	✓	
Cephalothin		
Cladribine		
Chlorpropamide	✓	
Chloroquine		
Clopidogrel		
Dapsone/pyrimethamine	✓	
Diphenylhydantoin	✓	✓
Recombinant erythropoietin	✓	✓
Estrogens		
Fenoprofen	✓	
Fludarabine	✓	
Interferon-α	✓	
Isoniazid	✓	✓
Lamivudine	✓	
Leuprolide	✓	
Linezolid	✓	
Micafungin		
Mycophenolate mofetil	✓	
d-Penicillamine	✓	
Phenylbutazone		
Procainamide	✓	
Ribavirin	✓	
Rifampicin		✓
Sulfasalazine	✓	
Sulindac		
Tacrolimus	✓	
Trimethoprim/sulfamethoxazole	✓	
Valproic acid	✓	✓
Zidovudine	✓	

Reproduced with permission from Means [1]

other respects like the particular myelodysplastic syndrome it resembles at the molecular level [4]. These disorders will not be discussed in this chapter.

Diagnosis and Evaluation

Peripheral blood counts. The first step in diagnosis is a complete blood count with reticulocyte determination. Red cells in PRCA are normochromic and normocytic. The absolute reticulocyte count is always less than 10,000/μL (reticulocyte percent <1%) and in many cases much lower. The diagnosis of PRCA should be questioned with higher reticulocyte values or if the reticulocyte percentage is only less than 1% when corrected for the degree of anemia. In general, the white blood count, white blood cell differential, and platelet count are normal. In the setting of concurrent inflammation, there may be some modest reduction in the total white blood count or a mild abnormality (either slightly high or slightly low) in the platelet count. There may also be a mild relative lymphocytosis.

Bone marrow morphology. The diagnosis of PRCA requires a bone marrow examination. In primary acquired (autoimmune) PRCA, marrow cellularity and myeloid and megakaryocyte maturation are normal. The diagnosis of PRCA is based on the absence or near absence of erythroblasts from an otherwise normal marrow. Since the marrow is normocellular and there are no abnormal cells present, pathologists accustomed to looking for marrow infiltration or immature cell forms may occasionally fail to notice the reduction in erythroid lineage. A differential count on the bone marrow and the marked elevation of the myeloid/erythroid ratio will lead to the diagnosis in these cases (<1% erythroblasts on the marrow differential count). In some cases, a few proerythroblasts and/or basophilic erythroblasts are seen, not exceeding 5% of the differential count [5]. Large proerythroblasts with vacuolated cytoplasm and pseudopodia ("giant pronormoblasts") are suggestive of B19 parvovirus infection but are not diagnostic [6]. There may be some slight increase in lymphocytes, lymphoid aggregates, and/or plasma cells, reflecting a degree of immune/inflammatory activation. Iron stains will typically be normal. Due to the paucity of erythroid precursors, ring sideroblasts are difficult to see. If present, ring sideroblasts favor a myelodysplastic syndrome, as would marked hypercellularity.

Other diagnostic tests on bone marrow specimen. Material should be collected for cellular immunology and cytogenetics, as would be done for evaluation of any cytopenia. Clonal analysis of T-cell receptors should also be included in the evaluation of suspected PRCA [7]. Abnormal cytogenetics in the setting of a characteristic marrow for PRCA indicates the myelodysplastic variant of PRCA. If increased lymphocytes or plasma cells are present, they should be polyclonal in acquired immune PRCA but would be monoclonal in PRCA secondary to an associated lymphoproliferative disorder.

Parvovirus studies. As will be discussed below, the presence of B19 parvovirus has specific therapeutic implications in PRCA. In all patients with marrows diagnostic of PRCA, B19 parvovirus testing should be performed. It is particularly important to consider this in immunocompromised patients and in individuals who are pregnant. The test of choice is polymerase chain reaction (PCR) testing on peripheral blood. Parvovirus serology is frequently ineffective for diagnosis in the immunocompromised patients for whom this agent is a major cause of PRCA [8].

Other studies. In adults with PRCA and no evidence of parvovirus infection or of a disorder associated with secondary PRCA, a CT scan of the chest should be performed to rule out a thymoma, which would have potential implications for therapy.

Pathophysiology

Primary Acquired PRCA

Primary acquired PRCA is an autoimmune disorder in which an immune mechanism interrupts erythroid differentiation. This may be mediated by an autoantibody or by another immunologic process. When an autoantibody is involved, the specific target of the antibody on the erythroid precursor or progenitor is generally unknown, although in rare cases, antibodies directed against the erythropoietin receptor have been found in primary acquired PRCA [9, 10]. Transient erythroblastopenia of childhood (TEC) is an uncommon self-limited variant of primary acquired autoimmune PRCA occurring between the ages of 3 months and 4 years [11]. Other than being self-limited, it resembles acquired autoimmune PRCA in adults both pathophysiologically and clinically.

Secondary Acquired PRCA

Secondary acquired PRCA may be associated with autoimmune/collagen vascular disorders; lymphoproliferative disorders; infections especially B19 parvovirus; pregnancy; non-lymphoproliferative hematologic malignancies; non-hematologic neoplasms, of which the association with thymoma is the best known; and drugs and toxic agents. In a number of cases of the less common associations of disorders with PRCA, particularly non-lymphoproliferative hematologic malignancies like chronic myelogenous leukemia or non-thymoma solid tumors, the observation that the clinical course of PRCA typically runs independently of the course of the associated syndrome suggests that the association is coincidental rather than pathophysiologic [12].

Some specific syndromes of secondary PRCA and relevant pathophysiologic processes are outlined below:

PRCA associated with autoimmune/collagen vascular disorders. The collagen vascular disorder most strongly associated with PRCA is systemic lupus erythematosus [13], although it has been reported also with rheumatoid arthritis and related diseases [14, 15]. The mechanism in these cases is typically autoimmune but may or may not be antibody-mediated [16, 17].

Lymphoproliferative disorder-associated PRCA. The lymphoproliferative disorders most frequently associated with PRCA are CLL and large granular lymphocyte (LGL) leukemia [18, 19], although it has been reported with other disorders shown in Table 10.1. A number of small studies have suggested an increased frequency of otherwise unapparent clonal T-cell disorders in primary acquired PRCA [7]. As with collagen vascular disorders, PRCA is typically immune-mediated in these patients although not by antibody-dependent mechanisms [20].

B19 parvovirus-associated PRCA. Human B19 parvovirus can produce chronic PRCA in immunocompromised patients and self-limited aplastic crises in patients with sickle cell disease or other forms of congenital hemolytic anemia [21]. B19 parvovirus directly infects human erythroid progenitors through the red cell surface P antigen (globoside). Individuals whose erythroid progenitors do not express P antigen are resistant to parvovirus infection [22].

Thymoma-associated PRCA. Thymoma is the disorder with the strongest historical association with secondary PRCA. The finding of PRCA may precede the finding of a thymoma or may occur after its resection. Recent series suggest the frequency of thymoma is 7–10% in presenting PRCA patients [5, 23], with an overall frequency of PRCA in thymoma patients less than 5% [24].

Drugs and chemicals. A PubMed review (Table 10.2) easily identified more than 30 drugs associated with PRCA. A number of other agents (e.g., benzene [25], halothane [26], methazolamide [5], phenobarbital [27], sulfathiazole [5], thiamphenicol [28], tolbutamide [5]) have well-established reports of PRCA that are not locatable in PubMed possibly because they antedate the reporting range. Many of these are single case reports, and mechanisms are rarely defined. PRCA associated with diphenylhydantoin and rifampicin has been linked to IgG-mediated inhibition of erythropoiesis [29, 30].

The best-known association between PRCA and a drug is the association with recombinant human (rh) erythropoietin. Beginning in the 1990s, reports of PRCA associated with anti-erythropoietin neutralizing antibodies in patients treated with rh erythropoietin began to appear [31]. These cases were predominantly associated with subcutaneous erythropoietin administration, were all or nearly all in renal failure patients (in whom endogenous erythropoietin production is decreased), primarily occurred outside the United States, and more than 90% of cases involved a particular erythropoietin product. Epidemiologic studies eventually implicated potential adjuvant effects of leachates from rubber stoppers in pre-filled syringes and particular stabilizers in the specific erythropoietin formulation. With resolution of these issues, new cases have become rare [32].

ABO-incompatible stem cell transplantation. PRCA following ABO-incompatible bone marrow or stem cell transplant is observed most commonly with the combination of a blood group A donor and a blood group O recipient. PRCA complicated 7.5% of cases of ABO-incompatible transplant in one recent series [33].

Treatment

The goal of treatment in PRCA is to attain a normal hemoglobin concentration without any requirement for transfusion. This is the standard used to define a complete response in most reported studies. A partial response is defined as attainment of transfusion independence with a low but clinically acceptable hemoglobin concentration [34]. The general approach to treatment of PRCA is immunosuppression. Table 10.3 lists indications for use of immunosuppression as initial therapy. In some circumstances, other modalities should be used initially. If the patient is using a medication associated with PRCA and no other PRCA-associated syndrome is present, a trial of drug discontinuation should be considered. If an infectious disorder associated with PRCA is present, specific treatment for that disorder should be initiated. Similarly, if CLL, Hodgkin or non-Hodgkin lymphoma, or other lymphoproliferative disorders other than LGL leukemia are complicating PRCA and treatment of these disorders is otherwise indicated, specific chemotherapy for those disorders should be initiated. PRCA secondary to autoimmune/collagen vascular disorders may respond to therapy specific to the management of those disorders. However, the treatment of collagen vascular disorders is usually immunosuppression in any event, and such patients found to have PRCA are referred to hematologists at diagnosis.

Table 10.3 Indications for immunosuppressive/immunomodulatory therapy in pure red cell aplasia (PRCA)

As initial therapy
Primary PRCA
Primary autoimmune PRCA
Secondary PRCA
PRCA associated with large granular lymphocyte (LGL) leukemia
PRCA associated with solid tumors other than thymoma
As second-line therapy
Any cause of secondary PRCA where initial, disease-directed therapy is unsuccessful (parvovirus has a high recurrence rate after immunoglobulin therapy, and repeat immunoglobulin therapy is indicated rather than immunosuppression)

There are specific nuances in treatment of PRCA associated with thymoma, B19 parvovirus infection, ABO-incompatible stem cell transplantation, antibody-mediated inhibition induced by rh erythropoietin, or pregnancy, that will be discussed below.

Immunosuppression/Immunomodulation

A large number of immunosuppressive/immunomodulatory agents have been shown to be effective in PRCA. The agents that have been studied in the largest number of patients are corticosteroids (for many years the first-line therapy), cytotoxic agents such as azathioprine or cyclophosphamide typically with concurrent corticosteroids, antithymocyte globulin, and cyclosporine A. Overall, these agents used in succession can produce a response in 65–70% of PRCA patients [5, 34–36].

Cyclosporine A appears to be the most effective immunosuppressive agent in PRCA and should be considered the agent of choice for immunosuppression in PRCA [34]. Since it is more expensive than corticosteroids and has definite though manageable toxicity, some would reasonably contend that a trial of corticosteroids should be used first. The overall response rate to cyclosporine A is greater than 75% in pooled series [5, 34–36]. This is a particularly impressive number since many since many of the patients receiving cyclosporine in the reported series had failed a number of other agents. A reasonable starting dose is 6 mg/kg daily. It is sometimes used in association with prednisone 30 mg/d [9]. Cyclosporine trough levels should be monitored with target levels of 150–250 ng/mL [34]. Renal and hepatic function should also be monitored. After normalization of the hemoglobin concentration, cyclosporine can be tapered slowly. Maintenance therapy may be required [23].

The oral corticosteroid of choice in PRCA is prednisone. The usual dose for starting therapy is similar to that used for immune thrombocytopenia or autoimmune hemolytic anemia (1 mg/kg). The overall response rate to prednisone is 40%, but relapses are common [5, 34–36]. Prednisone is tapered, after a response is obtained, or decreased and either discontinued or utilized in association with another agent if remission is not obtained. Cytotoxic agents such as azathioprine or cyclophosphamide (usually in combination with oral corticosteroids) have been utilized in patients unresponsive to corticosteroids alone or in patients who do not respond to cyclosporine. Like prednisone, the response rate is approximately 40%, and like prednisone, relapses are frequent [5, 34–36]. Antithymocyte globulin, in the doses used for treatment of aplastic anemia, has a 50% historic response rate in primary autoimmune PRCA [5, 34–36]. It is the author's strong impression that the effectiveness of cyclosporine A has largely eliminated antithymocyte globulin as a therapeutic modality in PRCA.

A number of other agents have been reported to produce responses in PRCA but generally are described in small series or as isolated case reports. Tacrolimus and sirolimus each have been reported to be effective in PRCA and may provide alternatives to cyclosporine [37, 38]. The anti-CD20 monoclonal antibody rituximab appears to be effective against primary autoimmune PRCA [39] but is mainly used in PRCA secondary to lymphoproliferative disorders [40]. "Rescue treatments" with fairly low response rates include intravenous immunoglobulin [41], plasma exchange [42], splenectomy [43], and bone marrow transplantation [44].

Long-term follow-up data on PRCA patients following immunosuppressive therapy is available [23]. The median survival for patients with primary autoimmune PRCA followed by the Japanese PRCA Consortium was not reached at 250 months. For patients with LGL or thymoma-associated PRCA, median survivals were similar at 147.8 and 142.1 months, respectively. The principal causes of death were infection and organ failure. Factors predictive of death were refractoriness to therapy and relapse from response [23].

Treatment of B19 Parvovirus-Associated PRCA

As noted above, nearly every patient with diagnosis of PRCA should be tested for B19 parvovirus. Intravenous immunoglobulin G (IVIgG) is a specific and highly effective therapy for B19 parvovirus-associated PRCA. The usual therapeutic dose is 2 g/kg divided over 5 days (400 mg/kg/d) [21]. In a review of an institutional experience and the published literature, the vast majority of patients were significantly immunocompromised. PRCA is corrected after a first course of IVIgG in 93% of patients, but approximately one-third relapse, at mean time to relapse of 4.3 months [45].

Thymoma-Associated PRCA

If a thymoma is present in a patient with PRCA, it generally should be resected. Although earlier studies reported more optimistic results, no more than a third of patients will respond, and the responses are usually partial [46]. Relapses are frequent, and PRCA may develop after resection of a thymoma in patients who did not have PRCA previously [47]. Adjuvant immunosuppressive therapy is typically required [46, 47].

PRCA Following ABO-Incompatible Stem Cell Transplantation

As discussed earlier, ABO-incompatible stem cell transplantation can result in the generation of isohemagglutinins directed against donor red cell antigens that are also expressed on red cell precursors, leading to PRCA [33, 48]. There is a high frequency of spontaneous resolution but prolonged transfusion support may be required. If anti-donor isohemagglutinins persist longer than 2 months after transplant, then the likelihood of spontaneous remission is reported to be low [48]. Approaches taken to mitigate this problem include adjustment in the posttransplant immunosuppressive regimen, donor leukocyte infusion, plasma exchange, and rituximab treatment [48].

Rh Erythropoietin-Induced Antibody-Mediated PRCA

Immunosuppression should be initiated, with cyclosporine A (with or without corticosteroids) as the probable first choice. Since these nearly all these patients have erythropoietin deficiency from renal failure and the kidney is the site of erythropoietin production, renal transplantation should be considered, if that is an option [49]. Successful rechallenge with rh erythropoietin in patients who no longer have detectable antibodies has been described in various case reports, but this author believes it is high risk and does not recommend it [50].

Pregnancy-Associated PRCA

Due to the rarity of this syndrome, there has been little if any systematic investigation of management. Most patients will have resolution of PRCA at the end of pregnancy and can be supported with transfusion as needed; prednisone has also been used for immunosuppression [51, 52]. The majority of reported pregnancies result in a live delivery at term if anemia is controlled [51, 53]. Occurrence of PRCA with a pregnancy does not necessarily predict recurrence with a subsequent pregnancy. Cyclosporine and other immunosuppressive agents may have significant effects on fetal outcome and maternal morbidity and probably should be avoided.

References

1. Means RT. Pure red cell aplasia. Blood. 2016;128(21):2504–9.
2. Arbiv OA, Cuvelier G, Klaassen RJ, et al. Molecular analysis and genotype-phenotype correlation of Diamond-Blackfan anemia. Clin Genet. 2018;93(2):320–8.
3. Bergmann AK, Campagna DR, McLoughlin EM, et al. Systematic molecular genetic analysis of congenital sideroblastic anemia: evidence for genetic heterogeneity and identification of novel mutations. Pediatr Blood Cancer. 2010;54(2):273–8.
4. Cerchione C, Catalano L, Cerciello G, et al. Role of lenalidomide in the management of myelodysplastic syndromes with del(5q) associated with pure red cell aplasia (PRCA). Ann Hematol. 2015;94(3):531–4.
5. Dessypris EN. Pure red cell aplasia. Baltimore: Johns Hopkins University Press; 1988.
6. Au WY, Cheng VC, Wan TS, Ma SK. Myelodysplasia masquerading as parvovirus-related red cell aplasia with giant pronormoblasts. Ann Hematol. 2004;83(10):670–1.
7. Masuda M, Teramura M, Matsuda A, et al. Clonal T cells of pure red-cell aplasia. Am J Hematol. 2005;79(4):332–3.
8. Frickhofen N, Abkowitz JL, Safford M, et al. Persistent B19 parvovirus infection in patients infected with human immunodeficiency virus type 1 (HIV-1): a treatable cause of anemia in AIDS. Ann Intern Med. 1990;113(12):926–33.
9. Means RT, Dessypris EN, Krantz SB. Treatment of refractory pure red cell aplasia with cyclosporine A: in vitro correlation of clinical response. Br J Haematol. 1991;78:114–9.

10. Peschle C, Marmont AM, Marone G, Genovese A, Sasso GF, Condorelli M. Pure red cell aplasia: studies on an IgG serum inhibitor neutralizing erythropoietin. Br J Haematol. 1975;30(4):411–7.
11. van den Akker M, Dror Y, Odame I. Transient erythroblastopenia of childhood is an underdiagnosed and self-limiting disease. Acta Paediatr. 2014;103(7):e288–94.
12. Dessypris EN, McKee CL Jr, Metzantonakis C, Teliacos M, Krantz SB. Red cell aplasia and chronic granulocytic leukaemia. Br J Haematol. 1981;48(2):217–25.
13. Chalayer E, Costedoat-Chalumeau N, Beyne-Rauzy O, et al. Bone marrow involvement in systemic lupus erythematosus. QJM. 2017;110(11):701–11.
14. Parida PK, Shukla SN, Talati SS, Parikh SK. Acquired pure red cell aplasia in a patient of rheumatoid arthritis. Indian J Hematol Blood Transfus. 2014;30(Suppl 1):255–7.
15. Cavazzana I, Ceribelli A, Franceschini F, Cattaneo R. Unusual association between pure red cell aplasia and primary Sjogren's syndrome: a case report. Clin Exp Rheumatol. 2007;25(2):309–11.
16. Arcasoy MO, Chao NJ. T-cell-mediated pure red-cell aplasia in systemic lupus erythematosus: response to cyclosporin A and mycophenolate mofetil. Am J Hematol. 2005;78(2):161–3.
17. Kiely PD, McGuckin CP, Collins DA, Bevan DH, Marsh JC. Erythrocyte aplasia and systemic lupus erythematosus. Lupus. 1995;4(5):407–11.
18. Fujishima N, Sawada K, Hirokawa M, et al. Long-term responses and outcomes following immunosuppressive therapy in large granular lymphocyte leukemia-associated pure red cell aplasia: a Nationwide Cohort Study in Japan for the PRCA Collaborative Study Group. Haematologica. 2008;93(10):1555–9.
19. Visco C, Barcellini W, Maura F, Neri A, Cortelezzi A, Rodeghiero F. Autoimmune cytopenias in chronic lymphocytic leukemia. Am J Hematol. 2014;89(11):1055–62.
20. Hirokawa M, Sawada K, Fujishima N, et al. Acquired pure red cell aplasia associated with malignant lymphomas: a nationwide cohort study in Japan for the PRCA Collaborative Study Group. Am J Hematol. 2009;84(3):144–8.
21. Frickhofen N, Chen ZJ, Young NS, Cohen BJ, Heimpel H, Abkowitz JL. Parvovirus B19 as a cause of acquired chronic pure red cell aplasia. Br J Haematol. 1994;87(4):818–24.
22. Brown KE, Hibbs JR, Gallinella G, et al. Resistance to parvovirus B19 infection due to lack of virus receptor (erythrocyte P antigen). N Engl J Med. 1994;330(17):1192–6.
23. Hirokawa M, Sawada K, Fujishima N, et al. Long-term outcome of patients with acquired chronic pure red cell aplasia (PRCA) following immunosuppressive therapy: a final report of the nationwide cohort study in 2004/2006 by the Japan PRCA collaborative study group. Br J Haematol. 2015;169(6):879–86.
24. Bernard C, Frih H, Pasquet F, et al. Thymoma associated with autoimmune diseases: 85 cases and literature review. Autoimmun Rev. 2016;15(1):82–92.
25. Aksoy M, Dincol K, Agun T, Erdem S, Dincol G. Haematological effects of chronic benzene poisoning in 217 workers. Br J Ind Med. 1971;28:296–302.
26. Jurgensen JC, Abrahams JP, Hardy WW. Erythroid aplasia after halothane hepatitis: report of a case. Am J Dig Dis. 1970;15:577–81.
27. Gasser C. Akute Erythroblastopenie: 10 Falle aplasticher Erythroblastenkrisen mit Riesenproerythroblasten bei allergish toxischen Zustandsbildern. Helv Pediatr Acta. 1949;4:107.
28. Estavoyer JM, Singer P, Broda C, Bauflc GH. Toxicite hematologique du thiamphenicol: a propos de deux observations d'erythroblastopenie aigue. Sem Hop. 1981;57:1970–2.
29. Dessypris EN, Redline S, Harris JW, Krantz SB. Diphenylhydantoin-induced pure red cell aplasia. Blood. 1985;65:789–94.
30. Mariette X, Mitjavila MT, Moulinie JP, et al. Rifampicin-induced pure red cell aplasia. Am J Med. 1989;87(4):459–60.
31. Carson KR, Evens AM, Bennett CL, Luminari S. Clinical characteristics of erythropoietin-associated pure red cell aplasia. Best Pract Res Clin Haematol. 2005;18(3):467–72.
32. Bennett CL, Starko KM, Thomsen HS, et al. Linking drugs to obscure illnesses: lessons from pure red cell aplasia, nephrogenic systemic fibrosis, and Reye's syndrome. A report from the Southern Network on Adverse Reactions (SONAR). J Gen Intern Med. 2012;27(12):1697–703.

33. Aung FM, Lichtiger B, Bassett R, et al. Incidence and natural history of pure red cell aplasia in major ABO-mismatched haematopoietic cell transplantation. Br J Haematol. 2013;160(6):798–805.
34. Sawada K, Fujishima N, Hirokawa M. Acquired pure red cell aplasia: updated review of treatment. Br J Haematol. 2008;142(4):505–14.
35. Lacy MQ, Kurtin PJ, Tefferi A. Pure red cell aplasia: association with large granular lymphocyte leukemia and the prognostic value of cytogenetic abnormalities. Blood. 1996;87(7):3000–6.
36. Charles RJ, Sabo KM, Kidd PG, Abkowitz JL. The pathophysiology of pure red cell aplasia: implications for therapy. Blood. 1996;87(11):4831–8.
37. Yoshida S, Konishi T, Nishizawa T, Yoshida Y. Effect of tacrolimus in a patient with pure red-cell aplasia. Clin Lab Haematol. 2005;27(1):67–9.
38. Jiang H, Zhang H, Wang Y, et al. Sirolimus for the treatment of multi-resistant pure red cell aplasia. Br J Haematol. 2018; https://doi.org/10.1111/bjh.15245.
39. Auner HW, Wolfer A, Beham-Schmid C, Strunk D, Linkesch W, Still H. Restoration of erythropoiesis by rituximab in an adult patient with primary acquired pure red cell aplasia refractory to conventional treatment. Br J Haematol. 2002;116:727–8.
40. D'Arena G, Vigliotti ML, Dell'Olio M, et al. Rituximab to treat chronic lymphoproliferative disorder-associated pure red cell aplasia. Eur J Haematol. 2009;82(3):235–9.
41. Mouthon L, Guillevin L, Tellier Z. Intravenous immunoglobulins in autoimmune- or parvovirus B19-mediated pure red-cell aplasia. Autoimmun Rev. 2005;4(5):264–9.
42. Freund LG, Hippe E, Strandgaard S, Pelus LM, Erslev AJ. Complete remission in pure red cell aplasia after plasmapheresis. Scand J Haematol. 1985;35(3):315–8.
43. Zaentz DS, Krantz SB, Sears DA. Studies on pure red cell aplasia. VII. Presence of proerythroblasts and response to splenectomy: a case report. Blood. 1975;46(2):261–70.
44. Kochethu G, Baden HS, Jaworska E, Chang J, Chopra R. Reduced intensity conditioning bone marrow transplantation for pure red cell aplasia: successful outcome but difficult post transplant course. Bone Marrow Transplant. 2005;36(1):81–2.
45. Crabol Y, Terrier B, Rozenberg F, et al. Intravenous immunoglobulin therapy for pure red cell aplasia related to human parvovirus b19 infection: a retrospective study of 10 patients and review of the literature. Clin Infect Dis. 2013;56(7):968–77.
46. Thompson CA, Steensma DP. Pure red cell aplasia associated with thymoma: clinical insights from a 50-year single-institution experience. Br J Haematol. 2006;135(3):405–7.
47. Hirokawa M, Sawada K, Fujishima N, et al. Long-term response and outcome following immunosuppressive therapy in thymoma-associated pure red cell aplasia: a nationwide cohort study in Japan by the PRCA collaborative study group. Haematologica. 2008;93(1):27–33.
48. Worel N. ABO-mismatched allogeneic hematopoietic stem cell transplantation. Transfus Med Hemother. 2016;43(1):3–12.
49. Macdougall IC, Roger SD, de Francisco A, et al. Antibody-mediated pure red cell aplasia in chronic kidney disease patients receiving erythropoiesis-stimulating agents: new insights. Kidney Int. 2012;81(8):727–32.
50. Shimizu H, Saitoh T, Ota F, et al. Pure red cell aplasia induced only by intravenous administration of recombinant human erythropoietin. Acta Haematol. 2011;126(2):114–8.
51. Choudry MA, Moffett BK, Laber DA. Pure red-cell aplasia secondary to pregnancy, characterization of a syndrome. Ann Hematol. 2007;86(4):233–7.
52. Moussa M, Hassan MF. Newly diagnosed adult-onset Still's disease with pure red cell aplasia in pregnancy. Arch Gynecol Obstet. 2014;290(1):195–8.
53. Kashyap R, Pradhan M. Maternal and fetal outcome in pregnancy-associated pure red cell aplasia. J Obstet Gynaecol. 2010;30(7):733–4.

Chapter 11
Anemia in Elderly Patients: State of Art, with a Focus on Nutritional Anemia

Emmanuel Andrès, Thomas Vogel, and Abrar Zulfiqar

Introduction

Anemia is a common condition, especially in elderly patients ($\geq$65–70 years), and its prevalence increases with age in geriatric population [1, 2]. Apart from its own complications, anemia is a factor of aggravation or poor prognosis of chronic diseases, e.g., chronic heart failure (CHF), chronic obstructive pulmonary disease (COPD), and cerebrovascular disorders, especially in frailty elderly patients [2, 3]. Anemia affects cognitive and physical function [1]. It also affects quality of life in all elderly patients. Anemia is even associated with a risk of death. Thus, it should not be accepted as an unavoidable condition or a consequence of aging [1, 3]. Importantly, all the anemias deserve a consideration, a diagnostic procedure, and a treatment, even in very elderly patients ($\geq$75–80 years). In the elderly, many underlying conditions can lead to anemia such as chronic diseases, e.g., renal failure, chronic inflammation, myelodysplastic syndromes, cancer, and unexplained anemia [2, 3]. However, the most common anemias are related to nutrient deficiencies, especially iron, vitamin B9 (folic acid), and vitamin B12 (cobalamin) [4]. In clinical practice, recognition of these deficiencies is essential for optimal management and treatment.

E. Andrès, MD, PhD (✉)
Department of Internal Medicine, Diabetes and Metabolic Disorders,
University Hospital of Strasbourg, Strasbourg, France
e-mail: emmanuel.andres@chru-strasbourg.fr

T. Vogel, MD, PhD
Department of Internal Medicine and Geriatrics, University Hospital of Strasbourg,
Strasbourg, France

A. Zulfiqar, MD
Department of Geriatrics, University Hospital of Rouen, Rouen, France

© Springer Nature Switzerland AG 2019
R. T. Means Jr. (ed.), *Anemia in the Young and Old*,
https://doi.org/10.1007/978-3-319-96487-4_11

In this chapter, we report and discuss the current literatures of anemia in elderly patients, with a focus on nutrient-deficiency also called nutritional anemia.

Definition of Anemia

The *World Health Organization* (WHO) defines anemia in the adult as hemoglobin (Hb) concentration <12 g/dL (<120 g/L) for nonpregnant women and <13 g/dL (<130 g/L) for men [5, 6]. However, the validity of these reference values for older patients, which were developed 40 years ago by a WHO expert group, is controversial [2, 5]. In fact, several studies have shown that application of WHO criteria for anemia definition is not appropriate for aged patients. Not only was a reverse J-shaped association between Hb and risk for all-cause mortality shown but also an increasing mortality risk at elevated Hb levels [2, 5]. Thus, there is an ongoing quest for what can be considered a normal Hb reference value in older patients. Nevertheless in practice, an Hb concentration <12 g/dL (<120 g/L) is commonly considered as an "established" anemia (under strict sense of the academic definition), regardless of the sex of the patient [3, 6]. In clinical practice, an Hb level <10 g/dL is often considered to be a cutoff level where investigation in the elderly ("anemia to explore") and treatment should be performed [3, 7]. Indeed, at this Hb level, several recent studies have shown a benefit from investigating the anemia and for treating, in regard to the frequency of discovery of a curable etiology [7].

Nutrient-deficiency or nutritional anemia refers to types of anemia that can be directly attributed to "nutritional disorders" [4, 8]. Thus, the term nutrient-deficiency or nutritional anemia covers any anemia resulting from a deficiency of nutrients essential for red blood cell formation, for example, iron and vitamins, especially vitamin B9 (folate) but also vitamin B12 (cobalamin) and vitamin C (in scurvy). More rarely, other nutrient deficiencies may be responsible for nutritional anemia, as vitamin A, vitamin E, and vitamin B2 (riboflavin), vitamin B3 (in pellagra), and vitamin B6 (pyridoxine); selenium, zinc, and copper; and protein (in case of Kwashiorkor or anorexia nervosa) [8]. In geriatric population, anemia with nutrient deficiency is often associated with or related to malnutrition, which is an important health-affecting factor among older patients.

Hematopoiesis in the Elderly

Alterations host defenses as in lymphocyte immunophenotype and function with age have been clearly documented as has a decrease in neutrophil function [1, 5]. However, controversy continues to surround the significance of "unexplained anemia" in the elderly patient and the extent to which this could be a physiological occurrence. Thus although low hemoglobin levels (approximately 1 g/dL lower than the WHO standard) are often seen with advancing age, anemia should not be assumed to be a normal consequence of aging [4, 5]. The weight of evidence from animal and human studies would suggest that anemia is not a physiological occurrence but may have a multifactorial pathogenesis. Several age-related physiological changes such as renal insufficiency, stem cell aging, androgen insufficiency, and chronic inflammation may contribute either to a decline in red blood cell production or shortened red blood cell survival. Age may be associated with compromised hematopoietic reserve and consequently with an increased susceptibility to anemia in the presence of hematopoietic stress induced by an underlying disorder [5, 7]. Moreover, the loss of DNA telomeres from hematopoietic progenitor cells with aging implies that stem cell collections from an older patient may have compromised replicative capacity with a reduced response to hematopoietic growth factors [1, 5, 7].

Links Between Anemia and Frailty

Anemia and frailty are two common findings in geriatric patients. Recent studies have contributed to the growing evidence of a possible association. Several recent studies have shown a link between anemia and fragility marker [9]. Moreover, anemia has been shown to be associated with poor outcomes and mortality in frailty elderly patients [1, 9]. Thus, the link between frailty and anemia seems strong. Nevertheless to date, the precise meaning of this association remains to be determined. In this setting a prospective study was carried out in an acute geriatric unit, in the University Hospital of Rouen (Rouen France) [10]. This study has been conducted in 141 elderly patients (mean age of 86.7 years), including 67 anemic patients (57.5%). In bivariate analysis, the anemic patients have been reported as more fragile, as documented by the Fried score (3.88 IC95 [3.64; 4.12] versus non-anemic subjects: 2.01 IC95 [1.73; 2.30], $p < 0.0001$) and SEGA (*short emergency geriatric assessment*) (18.04 IC95 [17.22; 18.87] versus non-anemic subjects: 12.01 IC95 [10.90; 13.12], $p < 0.0001$). In multivariate analysis, the Fried score was increased by 1.89 (1.52; 2.27) in anemic patients compared to non-anemic patients. Adjusted to serum albumin level (albuminemia), age, sex, and heart failure, the result is virtually unchanged 1.84 (1.47; 2.21) and remains significant ($p < 0.0001$). Regarding SEGA, IADL (*instrumental activities of daily living*), and ADL (*activities of daily living*), the results are significant and independent to albuminemia, age, sex, and heart failure. Outside of fragility, anemia in older patients has been shown to be associated with increased physical impairment, falls, cognitive decline, depression, all knower factors of frailty status in older patients [1, 5].

Prevalence of Anemia in the Elderly

The prevalence of anemia increases with advancing age, especially after age ≥60–65 years, and rises sharply after the age of ≥80 years [5, 11]. In this population, anemia currently represents a public health problem in developed countries. In the USA, results from the third *National Health and Nutrition Examination Survey* (*NHANES III*) indicate that the prevalence of anemia among elderly individuals, living in towns, aged 75 or more and 85 or more, were 15.7% in men and 10.3% in women and 26.1% for men and 20.1% in women, respectively [11]. Survey findings indicate further that most anemias among the elderly are mild. In fact, only 2.8% of women and 1.6% of men had an Hb <11 g/dL [12]. Results from the *NHANES III* also indicate that nutrient-deficiency anemia represents at least one third of all causes of anemia [11]. In the USA, results from the Framingham cohort indicate a lower prevalence of anemia among 1016 subjects within 67–96 years of age. In this group, the prevalence of anemia in men and women were 6.1% and 10.5%, respectively [13]. In this study, in addition to anemia of inflammation and of renal failure, nutritional anemia was also a major cause of anemia. In a French nationwide study of 1351 patients hospitalized in several departments of internal medicine, anemia was present in 874 (65%) patients according to the *WHO* definition, and 573 (42%) patients had an Hb levels of <11 g/dL (<11 g/L) [14].

Causes of Anemia in the Elderly

In elderly patients, causes of anemia are separated into three main broad groups: (1) "nutrient-deficiency or nutritional anemia," mainly in relation with iron-deficiency anemia; (2) "anemia of chronic disease," including anemia related to chronic renal failure, chronic inflammation, and chronic heart failure; and (3) "unexplained anemia" [2, 9]. However in this later situation, an inadequate diagnostic work-up for the patient could be or may be suspected, for example, the use of invasive exams (e.g., bone marrow biopsy) [4]. Moreover, a subtle underlying inflammation had been at least associated with or responsible for anemia or "lazy" hematopoiesis in elderly patient [1]. This process of "inflammaging" is characterized by an age-associated chronic upregulation of the inflammatory immune response with increased levels of proinflammatory cytokines like interleukin-1 (IL-1), IL-6, and tumor necrosis factor (TNF) [2, 7, 9]. In the aforementioned *NHANES III* study, 34% of all anemia in adults and elderly patients were caused by iron, vitamin B9 (folate), and vitamin B12 (cobalamin) deficiency, alone or in combination (nutrient-deficiency anemia) [11]. In this study, 12% of all anemias were related, perhaps at least associated, with renal insufficiency, 20% with chronic diseases, and in 34% of the cases, the cause of anemia remained unexplained. Up to half of all elderly anemic patients have

Table 11.1 Cause of anemia in patients older than 65 years ($n = 300$), hospitalized in an internal medicine department (tertiary reference center)

Cause	Prevalence (%)
Chronic inflammation (chronic disease)	23.0
Iron deficiency	18
Renal failure	9
Liver disease and endocrine disease (chronic disease)	7
Posthemorrhagic	7
Folate deficiency	6
Myelodysplasia	5
Vitamin B12 deficiency	4
Unexplained causes	21

multifactorial anemia, characterized by a combination of underlying problems such as iron deficiency, chronic inflammation, chronic renal failure, folate deficiency, and/or vitamin B12 deficiency. In practice, because elderly patients often have several associated comorbid conditions and are commonly taking a variety of medications, some of which may contribute to anemia, the precise etiology of anemia is frequently difficult to determine, even after extensive investigations, including bone marrow biopsy [1, 3, 14]. Thus according to the literatures and in our own experience, etiology of anemia can be identified in only approximately 80% of the cases, in spite of the use of new tools such as video capsule [3, 15]. In Table 11.1, we report our personal experience of the cause of anemia in elderly patients (at least ≥65 years old) hospitalized in the University Hospital of Strasbourg (Strasbourg, France) [3]. Importantly, a significant proportion of these elderly anemic patients, around 30–50%, are presumed to have multiple causes for their anemia as we have previously demonstrated [14].

Nutritional Anemias in the Elderly

In recent studies, around 60% of nutritional anemias are associated with or related to iron deficiency, and most of those cases are the result of chronic blood loss from gastrointestinal lesions in developed countries [1, 4]. The remaining cases of nutrient-deficiency anemia are usually associated with or related to vitamin B9 deficiency, around 10% in view of the concerned geriatric population, and/or vitamin B12 deficiency, 4–5% according to the population studied [4]. Importantly, all these nutritional anemias are easily treated. Rare unknown causes of nutrient-deficiency anemias include several other vitamin deficiencies (e.g., vitamins A, B2, B3, C, and E), selenium, zinc, or copper [8]. These later etiologies are nevertheless not well-studied in the literature, and to date, few not-well documented data are available, except for the theoretical and pathological aspects of anemia [4].

Iron-Deficiency Anemia in the Elderly

Iron-deficiency anemia (IDA) is the most common cause of anemia in the elderly [1, 17]. In this population, IDA results usually from chronic gastrointestinal (GI) blood loss mainly caused by esophagitis; gastritis; ulcer, related or not related to nonsteroidal anti-inflammatory drug intake and/or chronic *Helicobacter pylori* infections; varices (portal hypertension); premalignant polyps; colorectal cancer; or angiodysplasia (idiopathic angiodysplasia, Heyde's syndrome [association between aortic stenosis, an acquired von Willebrand's disease type IIA disease, IDA anemia due to bleeding from intestinal angiodysplasia, and mechanic anemia due to aortic stenosis], rarely Rendu-Osler's disease [hereditary hemorrhagic telangiectasia]) [1, 4, 18]. In this setting, GI blood loss is often occult and is not ruled out by negative fecal blood tests. In elderly, GI tract abnormalities can be identified with appropriate investigations (mainly invasive and requires general anesthesia) in the majority of patients with IDA [5, 16]. In 40–60% of patients, the source is in the upper GI tract and the identified cause of GI blood loss is benign [18–20]. In 15–30% of patients, the source of GI blood loss is in the colon, here also with mainly benign lesions. Table 11.2 presents our experience of the evaluation of the GI tract in 90 elderly patients (all patients' ≥65 years old) with chronic blood loss during their follow-up in an internal medicine department (in a referral center) [3, 4]. Chronic blood loss from the genitourinary tract and chronic hemoptysis can be exceptionally responsible for IDA [4, 17]. In elderly patients, bleeding disorders and particularly anticoagulant and antiplatelet medications may promote the development of IDA in the elderly (around 20% in our experience) [3, 4]. The source of bleeding is not found in the remaining 10–40% of patients, particularly with GI blood loss. Fortunately, these patients do well with iron replacement, and thus, to our opinion, repeat investigation may be only proposed in "to good health" elderly patients [1, 7]. In these patients, repeat GI investigation with upper and/or lower

Table 11.2 Results of the evaluation of the gastrointestinal tract in elderly patients (≥65 years) with chronic blood loss (*n* = 90), hospitalized in an internal medicine department

Etiology	Prevalence (%)
Esophagitis and Mallory-Weiss syndrome	4.4
Gastritis, atrophic gastritis, and ulcer related or not related to NSAID use and/or *Helicobacter pylori* infection	30
Varices related to portal hypertension	9
Angiodysplasia	2.25
Colon diverticula	4.5
Colorectal benign and premalignant polyps	5.5
Colorectal cancer	5.5
Inflammatory bowel disease	2.25
Unexplained causes	36.6

NSAID nonsteroidal anti-inflammatory drug

endoscopy and video capsule may be of interest, with the detection of the etiology of bleeding in an additional 20% of cases [18, 20, 21]. It is important because one third of the IDA is related to GI malignancies. In our experience, repeat investigation is not recommended in frailty elderly patients [22]. In this setting, ruling out of several disorders is required, as *Helicobacter pylori* infection, chronic gastritis (especially atrophic gastritis), and celiac disease. In fact, these disorders are often diagnosed of "unexplained GI iron deficiency anemia" [23, 24]. More rarely, a large amount of tea (at least 2 liters per day), vegetarian, and theoretically long-term antiacid medication intake are also associated with this condition [4]. In practice, any elderly subject whose dietary intake is poor (especially institutionalized elderly patients, particularly in psychiatry, or elderly patients with limited financial resources) and has recent unexplained weight loss is a candidate for increased medical surveillance [25].

Vitamin B9 (Folate)-Deficiency Anemia in the Elderly

Vitamin B deficiencies are common among elderly, e.g., occurring in at least 10% of the patients for the vitamin B9, also known as folic acid [4, 12]. The Framingham study demonstrated an incidence of 12% among elderly people living in the community [26]. Vitamin B9 deficiency usually develops as a result of inadequate dietary intake and malnutrition [4]. This latter may be frequent in frailty elderly patients; institutionalized elderly patients, especially in psychiatric institutions; or socially isolated elderly patients or without a lot of financial resources. In fact, a regular diet contains 500–700 µg of vitamin B9, and the body contains very little vitamin B9, with stocks expected to last 4–6 months [4]. The affected patients usually have a history of weight loss, poor weight gain, and weakness. This is particularly the case in Alzheimer's patient, in patients with advanced dementia or in patients with repetitive swallowing disorders ("false roads"). True malabsorption, as in the case of celiac disease, for example, is much less common in elderly patients [5, 12]. In addition to malnutrition, several drugs (methotrexate, cotrimoxazole, sulfasalazine, anticonvulsants) and alcohol – even in elderly – usually may cause deficiency of folic acid or may be at least associated with this deficiency [4].

Vitamin B12-Deficiency Anemia in the Elderly

Vitamin B12 deficiencies are even common among elderly, occurring in at least 5% of the patients [15, 17]. In elderly patients, the etiologies of vitamin B12 deficiency are mainly represented by food-cobalamin malabsorption (FCM) and Biermer's disease [4, 27]. The FCM is not a real malabsorption in view of physiopathology but a maldigestion of cobalamin (linked to food) [28]. More rarely, the etiologies of

Fig. 11.1 Etiologies of cobalamin deficiency in 172 elderly patients hospitalized in University Hospital of Strasbourg, France

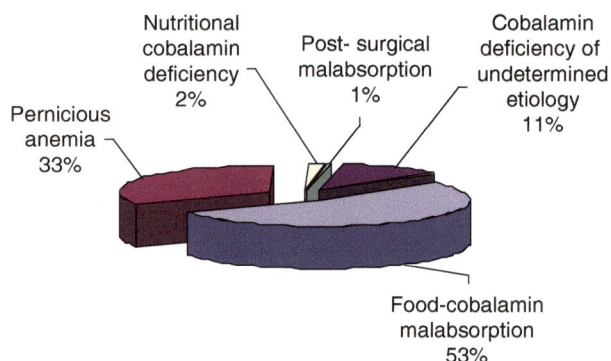

vitamin B12 deficiency include intake deficiency (reserve in the body from 5 to 10 years) and true malabsorption, related, for example, to digestive tract surgery (in particular, because resection surgery in the stomach has become infrequent since the availability of proton pump inhibitors) [28]. In a study by our group ($n = 200$), FCM accounted for about 60–70% of the etiologies of vitamin B12 deficiency and about 15–25% in Biermer's disease [28, 29]. Figure 11.1 presents the principal causes of vitamin B12 deficiency in 172 elderly patients (median age: 70 years) hospitalized in the University Hospital of Strasbourg, France [30]. FCM is characterized by the inability to release cobalamin from food and/or intestinal transport proteins, particularly in case of hypochlorhydria, where the absorption of "unbound" cobalamin is normal ("maldigestion" of the food-cobalamin) [31]. As we have recently indicated, this syndrome is defined by cobalamin deficiency despite sufficient cobalamin intake from food and a normal Schilling test, where the later rules out malabsorption or pernicious anemia [28]. FCM is caused primarily by atrophic gastritis [28, 31]. Other factors that commonly contribute to FCM in elderly people include chronic carriage and infection of *H. pylori*, intestinal microbial proliferation, long-term ingestion of antacids (e.g., proton pump inhibitors) and biguanides (metformin), chronic alcoholism, surgery or gastric reconstruction (e.g., bypass surgery for obesity), and partial and pancreatic exocrine failure [31]. It should be emphasized that Carmel first believed that FCM was associated with moderate cobalamin deficiency, leading to only "subtle" clinical symptoms ("subtle cobalamin deficiency") [31]. However in our experience, the clinical manifestations of FCM are not very different from those of cobalamin deficiencies associated with other causes, e.g., Biermer's disease [29]. Biermer's disease (Addison's disease or pernicious anemia) is caused by impaired absorption of vitamin B12 due to the neutralization of intrinsic factor action in the setting of immune atrophic gastritis (loss of intrinsic factor in genetic form) [15, 32]. In practice, diagnosis of Biermer's disease is based on the presence of (i) intrinsic factor antibodies in serum (specificity, >98%; sensibility, around 50%) and/or (ii) autoimmune atrophic gastritis (the presence of *H. pylori* infection in gastric biopsies is an exclusion factor) [3, 32]. It is to note that Biermer's disease is associated with other immunological diseases, even in the elderly, such as Sjögren's syndrome, Hashimoto's disease, type 1 diabetes mellitus, or celiac disease.

Clinical Presentation of Anemia in Elderly Patient

Anemia is a particularly common finding in elderly patients. It is associated with fatigue, impaired functional capacity, an increased risk for mortality, a longer hospitalization for elective procedures, and a decreased quality of life [1, 3, 7]. In older people, the onset of anemic symptoms (fatigue, asthenia) and signs (pallor, palpitations) is usually insidious because the majority of these patients adjust their physical activities, stay at home, and take several drugs which mask the anemic symptomatology [33]. Thus, these symptoms may be overlooked and undiagnosed [6, 12]. In elderly, anemia may be revealed by the exacerbation of chronic-associated conditions or disorders, as dyspnea or edema of the legs related to worsening of cardiac failure. Anemia has also been reported to worsen angina, cognitive dysfunction related to cerebrovascular insufficiency [33].

In the setting of nutritional anemias, iron, vitamin B9 (folate), and vitamin B12 deficiencies may be associated with specific symptoms and clinical manifestations [34, 35]. Table 11.3 presents features related to vitamin B12 deficiency in elderly patients [28]. The features of vitamin B9 deficiency are nearly indistinguishable from those of vitamin B12 deficiency, although the symptomatology is generally less severe. Iron deficiency is responsible for changes in hair (hair loss), nails (koilonychias), glossitis, dermatitis herpetiformis, photodermatitis, restless legs syndrome, and/or Plummer's syndrome [34].

Table 11.3 Manifestations related to vitamin B12 deficiency (in addition to hematological manifestations)

Neuropsychiatric manifestations	Digestive manifestations	Other manifestations
Frequent: polyneurites (especially sensitive ones), ataxia, Babinski's phenomenon	Classic: Hunter's glossitis, jaundice, LDH, and bilirubin elevation ("intramedullary destruction")	Under study: atrophy of the vaginal mucosa and chronic vaginal and urinary infections (especially mycosis), venous thromboembolic disease, angina (hyperhomocysteinemia)
Classic: combined sclerosis of the spinal cord		
Rare: cerebellar syndromes affecting the cranial nerves including optic neuritis, optic atrophy, urinary, and/or fecal incontinence	Debatable: abdominal pain, dyspepsia, nausea, vomiting, diarrhea, disturbances in intestinal functioning	
Under study: changes in the higher functions, even dementia, stroke and atherosclerosis (hyperhomocysteinemia), parkinsonian syndromes, depression, multiple sclerosis	Rare: resistant and recurring mucocutaneous ulcers cobalamin deficiency	

Biological Abnormalities Related to Nutritional Anemia

In elderly, the anemia is frequently "mild" with an Hb levels between 10 and 12 g/dL and "normocytic," with a mean erythrocyte cell volume (MECV) between 80 and 100 fL [3, 15]. Patients with established nutritional anemia often have mild to moderate anemia, with Hb levels around 10 g/dL [2, 4]. This anemia is generally hyporegenerative, with a low reticulocyte count (<50 × 10⁹/L). This represents the consequence of the reduced activity of the hematopoietic system to replace the peripheral blood loss or deficiency [15]. This normocytic nature of the anemia is related to the multifactorial etiologies of anemia [16]. In exclusive iron deficiency, the erythrocytes are usually "microcytic," with a MECV <80 fL (main differential diagnoses: chronic inflammation, thalassemia) [15]. In exclusive vitamin B9 and/or vitamin B12 deficiency, the erythrocytes are usually "macrocytic," with a MECV >120 fL (main differential diagnoses: alcohol, hypothyroidism, and myelodysplastic syndromes) [4, 15]. Other hematological abnormalities and manifestations may also be associated with cobalamin deficiency as listed in Table 11.4 [35].

Iron deficiency is documented by a low serum iron level, an increased total iron-binding capacity, and a low serum ferritin level (<15 ng/mL) [15, 36]. In cases associated with chronic inflammation, the transferrin receptor–ferritin index appears to be the most appropriate parameter to discriminate between the two disorders [18]. Vitamin B12 deficiency is usually documented by a low serum vitamin B12 level

Table 11.4 Hematological manifestations in patients with documented cobalamin deficiency ($n = 201$), hospitalized in an internal medicine department (tertiary reference center)

Parameters	Values
Hemoglobin level (g/dL)	10.3 ± 0.4 (4.9–15.1)
Mean erythrocyte cell volume (fL)	98.9 ± 25.6 (76–142)
Reticulocyte count (%)	15.2 (1–32)
White cell count (/mm³)	6200 ± 4100 (500–20.000)
Platelet count (10³/mm³)	146 ± 42 (27–580)
Anemia with Hb level <12 g/dL	37%
Anemia with Hb level <6 g/dL	2.5%
Anemia and macrocytosis (MECV >100 fL)	33.8%
Isolated macrocytosis (MECV >100 fL)	17%
Microcytosis (MECV <80 fL)	5%
White cell count <4000/mm³	14%
Neutrophile count <1000/mm³	3%
Thrombopenia (<150 × 10³/mm³)	10%
Neutrophile hypersegmentation	32%
Megaloblastosis	60%
Life-threatening manifestations	9%

MECV mean erythrocyte cell volume

(<200 pg/mL). An increase of the serum methylmalonic acid or homocysteine levels should be established to exclude a false-negative result for vitamin B12 [27, 31]. In elderly patients, Clarke et al. have reported good results with serum holotranscobalamin (HoloTC) [37]. In this study, HoloTC has a modestly superior diagnostic accuracy compared with conventional vitamin B12 for the detection of vitamin B12 deficiency. In vitamin B9 deficiency, the red cell vitamin B9 concentration is the recommended investigation [2, 15].

Treatment of Nutritional Anemia in the Elderly

The management of anemia requires the authentication of the cause of this anemia, even in the elderly [2, 3, 15]. In this context, a reflection must be made regarding the benefit and the risk taken for the exploration and documentation of the cause [3]. This is true regardless of the type of anemia. In the setting of nutritional anemia, there is usually no need to institute emergency treatment, anemia being usually mild and of very gradual installation (adaptation of the body to a gradual decline in Hb) [2, 17]. Attempts to identify suggested Hb levels for blood transfusion therapy have been confounded for elderly patients with their comorbidities. Since no specific recommended Hb threshold has stood the test of time, prudent transfusion practices to maintain Hb thresholds of 9–10 g/dL in the elderly are indicated, unless or until evidence emerges to indicate otherwise [4]. In IDA, iron supplementation should be initiated in association with the treatment of the underlying cause of bleeding [33]. Treatment of nutritional anemia requires particular attention to establish the correct cause in all patients, particularly in elderly patients in very good general condition of the body or mind [15]. Standard therapy for iron deficiency is oral administration of 200–300 mg of ferrous sulfate (60 mg of elemental iron) [15, 33]. Oral iron supplementation is usually the first choice for the treatment of iron-deficiency anemia because of its effectiveness and low cost. Vitamin C enhances iron absorption. Intravenous iron replacement may be reserved for patients with iron deficiency that fails to respond to oral replacement or in patients with documented malabsorption, inflammatory bowel diseases, malignancies, renal failure, and also perhaps in anemic patients with chronic heart failure. Parenteral iron supplementation may also be used when there is intolerance or non-compliance with oral preparations. Intravenous iron sucrose is reasonably well tolerated, even when administered in boluses [38]. In elderly patients, vitamin B12-deficiency anemia may be treated by vitamin B12 supplementation, parenterally (commonly intramuscular) or orally [39–40]. Our team (*CAREnce en vitamin B12* [Care B12]) in the University Hospital of Strasbourg (France) has developed an effective oral treatment for cobalamin deficiency, therapeutic modality extremely useful in patients on anticoagulants or antiplatelet agents and who avoids pain related to intramuscular injections [40]. The main results of our protocol of oral cobalamin therapy studies are summarized in Table 11.5. A systematic review conducted under the auspices of the *Cochrane Metabolic and*

Table 11.5 Study by our team on oral cobalamin therapy: results on hematological manifestations

Study characteristics (number of patients)	Therapeutic modalities	Results
Open prospective study of well-documented vitamin B12 deficiency related to food-cobalamin malabsorption ($n = 10$)	Oral crystalline cyanocobalamin: 650 µg per day, during the condition and continue at least 3 months	Normalization of serum vitamin B12 levels in 80% of the patients Significant increase of Hb levels (mean of 1.9 g/dL) and decrease of MECV (mean of 7.8 fL)
Open prospective study of low vitamin B12 levels not related to pernicious anemia ($n = 20$)	Oral crystalline cyanocobalamin: 1000 µg per day during the condition and continue at least 1 week	Normalization of serum vitamin B12 levels in 85% of the patients
Open prospective study of well-documented vitamin B12 deficiency related to food-cobalamin malabsorption ($n = 30$)	Oral crystalline cyanocobalamin: between 1000 and 250 µg per day, during the condition and continue at least 1 month	Normalization of serum vitamin B12 levels in 87% of the patients Significant increase of Hb levels (mean of 0.6 g/dL) and decrease of MECV (mean of 3 fL); normalization of Hb levels and MECV in 54% and 100% of the patients, respectively Dose effect – effectiveness dose of vitamin B12 ≥500 µg per day
Open prospective study of low vitamin B12 levels not related to pernicious anemia ($n = 30$)	Oral crystalline cyanocobalamin: between 1000 and 125 µg per day during the condition and continue at least 1 week	Normalization of serum vitamin B12 levels in all patients with at least a dose of vitamin ≥250 µg per day Dose effect – effectiveness dose of vitamin B12 ≥500 µg per day
Open prospective study of low vitamin B12 levels related to pernicious anemia ($n = 10$)	Oral crystalline cyanocobalamin: 1000 µg per day, during the condition and continue at least 3 months	Significant increase of serum vitamin B12 levels in 90% of the patients (mean of 117.4 pg/mL Significant increase of Hb levels (mean of 2.45 g/dL) and decrease of MECV (mean of 10.4 fL)

Hb hemoglobin, *MECV* mean erythrocyte cell volume

Endocrine Disorders Review Group also supports the efficacy of oral cobalamin therapy [41, 42]. The recommended treatment regimen is based on (1) a daily dose of 2000 and 1000 µg for 1 month of crystalline cyanocobalamin for FCM and Biermer's disease and (2) thereafter a weekly dose between 2000 and 1000 µg of vitamin B12 for FCM and a daily dose of 1000 µg (for all the life) in case of Biermer's disease [39, 41]. In vitamin B9 deficiency, therapeutic doses of vitamin B9 vary between 1 to 5 mg per day [43]. Usually, supplementation is continued for at least 3–6 months, provided that the underlying causes of the deficiencies have been corrected. Food sources of nutrients are best for prevention of nutritional anemia, but often supplementation is necessary, especially for the elderly [44]. The *US National Academy of Sciences* recommends that vitamin B9 and vitamin B12 standardized supplementation should be done (fortified cereal) in elderly.

Conclusions

Anemia is a particularly common finding in geriatric population. In elderly patients, nutritional anemia represents 30–40% of all anemias. About two thirds of these nutritional anemias are related to iron deficiency. IDA is mainly the result of chronic blood loss from gastrointestinal lesions (with benign lesions in two third of the cases). The remaining cases of nutritional anemia are usually associated with vitamin B12 and/or vitamin B9 deficiency. In elderly patients, vitamin B12 deficiency is most frequently related to food-cobalamin malabsorption and Biermer's disease. Vitamin B9 is related to inadequate dietary intake or malnutrition, several drugs (as methotrexate, cotrimoxazole) and chronic alcohol intake. Treatment of nutritional anemia is simple and involves replacement of the deficient nutrient but requires particular attention to discerning the cause.

Conflict of Interest *None related to the content of the present chapter.*

References

1. Eisenstaedt R, Penninx BW, Woodman RC. Anemia in the elderly: current understanding and emerging concepts. Blood Rev. 2006;20:213–26.
2. Goodnough LT, Schrier SL. Evaluation and management of anemia in the elderly. Am J Hematol. 2014;89:88–96.
3. Andrès E, Serraj K, Federici L, Vogel T, Kaltenbach G. Anemia in elderly patients: new insight into an old disorder. Geriatr Gerontol Int. 2013;13:519–27.
4. Andrès E, Federici L, Serraj K, Kaltenbach G. Update of nutrient-deficiency anemia in elderly patients. Eur J Intern Med. 2008;19:488–93.
5. Woodman R, Ferrucci L, Guralnik J. Anemia in older adults. Curr Opin Hematol. 2005;12:123–8.
6. Izaks GJ, Westendorp RG, Knook DL. The definition of anemia in older persons. JAMA. 1999;281:1714–7.
7. Balducci L, Ershler WB, Krantz S. Anemia in the elderly. Clinical findings and impact on health. Crit Rev Oncol Hematol. 2006;58:156–65.
8. Fishman SM, Christian P, Keith PW. The role of vitamins in the prevention and control of anaemia. Public Health Nutr. 2000;3.125–50.
9. Röhrig G. Anemia in the frail, elderly patient. Clin Interv Aging. 2016;11:319–26.
10. Zulfiqar AA, Sui Seng X, Gillibert A, Kadri N, Doucet J, Andrès E. Anémie chez le sujet âgé: étude des liens avec les critères gériatriques. Hématologie. 2017;23:379–90.
11. National Health and Nutrition Examination Survey. Anthropometric Reference Data, United States. 1988–1994. http://www.cdc.gov/nchs/about/major/nhanes/Anthropometric%20 Measures. January 7, 2018.
12. Guralnik JM, Eisenstaedt RS, Ferrucci L, Klein HG, Woodman RC. Prevalence of anemia in persons 65 years and older in the United States: evidence for a high rate of unexplained anemia. Blood. 2004;104:2263–8.
13. Fleming DJ, Jacques PF, Tucker KL, Massaro JM, D'Agostino RB, Wilson PW, et al. Iron status of the free-living, elderly Framingham heart study cohort: an iron-replete population with a high prevalence of elevated iron stores. Am J Clin Nutr. 2001;73:638–46.
14. Terrier B, Resche-Rigon M, Andrès E, Bonnet F, Hachulla E, Marie I, et al.; On behalf of the Groupe de Recherche sur les Anémies en Médecine Interne (GRAMI) Prevalence,

characteristics and prognostic significance of anemia in daily practice: results from a French nationwide cross-sectional and prospective longitudinal study. QJM. 2012;105:345–54.
15. Carmel R. Anemia and aging: an overview of clinical, diagnostic and biological issues. Blood Rev. 2001;15:9–18.
16. Petrosyan I, Blaison G, Andrès E, Federici L. Anemia in the elderly: etiologic profile in a prospective cohort of 95 hospitalized patients. Eur J Intern Med. 2012;23:524–8.
17. Joosten E, Pelemans W, Hiele M, Noyen J, Verhaeghe R, Boogaerts MA. Prevalence and causes of anaemia in a geriatric hospitalization population. Gerontology. 1992;38:111–7.
18. Rimon E, Levy S, Sapir A, Gelzer G, Peled R, Ergas D, et al. Diagnosis of iron deficiency anemia in the elderly by transferrin receptor-ferritin index. Arch Intern Med. 2002;162:445–9.
19. Rockey DC. Occult and obscure gastrointestinal bleeding: causes and clinical management. Nat Rev Gastroenterol Hepatol. 2010;7:265–79.
20. Liu K, Kaffes AJ. Iron deficiency anaemia: a review of diagnosis, investigation and management. Eur J Gastroenterol Hepatol. 2012;24:109–16.
21. Muhammad A, Vidyarthi G, Brady P. Role of small bowel capsule endoscopy in the diagnosis and management of iron deficiency anemia in elderly: a comprehensive review of the current literature. World J Gastroenterol. 2014;20:8416–23.
22. Camaschella C. Iron-deficiency anemia. N Engl J Med. 2015;372:1832–43.
23. Nahon S, Lahmek P, Massard J, Lesgourgues B, Mariaud de Serre N, Traissac L, et al. Helicobacter pylori-associated chronic gastritis and unexplained iron deficiency anemia: a reliable association? Helicobacter. 2003;8:573–7.
24. Suzuki H, Marshall BJ, Hibi T. Overview: helicobacter pylori and extragastric disease. Int J Hematol. 2006;84:291–300.
25. Milman N, Pedersen AN, Ovesen L, Schroll M. Iron status in 358 apparently healthy 80- year-old Danish men and women: relation to food composition and dietary and supplemental iron intake. Ann Hematol. 2004;83:423–9.
26. Lindenbaum J, Rosenberg IH, Wilson PW, Tabler SP, Allen RH. Prevalence of cobalamin deficiency in the Framingham elderly population. Am J Clin Nutr. 1994;60:2–11.
27. Andrès E, Loukili NH, Noel E, Kaltenbach G, Ben Abdelgheni M, Perrin AE, et al. Vitamin B12 (cobalamin) deficiency in elderly patients. CAMJ. 2004;171:251–60.
28. Andrès E, Affenberger S, Vinzio S, Kurtz JE, Noel E, Kaltenbach G, et al. Food-cobalamin malabsorption in elderly patients: clinical manifestations and treatment. Am J Med. 2005;118:1154–9.
29. Andrès E, Perrin AE, Demangeat C, Kurtz JE, Vinzio S, Grunenberger F, et al. The syndrome of food-cobalamin malabsorption revisited in a Department of Internal Medicine. A monocentric cohort study of 80 patients. Eur J Intern Med. 2003;14:221–6.
30. Andrès E, Serraj K, Mecili M, Kaltenbach G, Vogel T. The syndrome of food-cobalamin malabsorption: a personal view in a perspective of clinical practice. J Blood Disord Transfus. 2011;2:108. https://doi.org/10.4172/2155-9864.1,000108.
31. Carmel R. Diagnosis and management of clinical and subclinical cobalamin deficiencies: why controversies persist in the age of sensitive metabolic testing. Biochimie. 2013;95:1047–55.
32. Zulfiqar AA, Serraj K, Pennaforte JL, Andrès E. Maladie de Biermer: de la physiopathologie à la clinique. Médecine Thérapeutique. 2012;18:21–9.
33. Gabrilove J. Anemia and the elderly: clinical considerations. Best Pract Res Clin Haematol. 2005;18:417–22.
34. Sato S. Iron deficiency: structural and microchemical changes in hair, nails, and skin. Semin Dermatol. 1991;10:313–9.
35. Federici L, Loukili NH, Zimmer J, Affenberger S, Maloisel F, Andrès E. Manifestations hématologiques de la carence en vitamine B12: données personnelles et revue de la littérature. Rev Med Interne. 2007;28:225–31.
36. Umbreit J. Iron deficiency: a concise review. Am J Hematol. 2005;78:225–31.
37. Clarke R, Sherliker P, Hin H, Nexo E, Hvas AM, Schneede J, et al. Detection of vitamin B12 deficiency in older people by measuring vitamin B12 or the active fraction of vitamin B12, holotranscobalamin. Clin Chem. 2007;53:963–70.

38. Avni T, Bieber A, Grossman A, Green H, Leibovici L, Gafter-Gvili A. The safety of intravenous iron preparations: systematic review and meta-analysis. Mayo Clin Proc. 2015;90:12–23.
39. Andrès E. Oral cobalamin (vitamin B12) therapy: from empiricism and personal experience to evidence based medicine and perspective of recommendations and guideline. J Blood Disord Transfus. 2012;3:e102. https://doi.org/10.4172/2155-9864.1,000e102.
40. Andrès E, Fothergill H, Mecili M. Efficacy of oral cobalamin (vitamin B12) therapy. Expert Opin Pharmacother. 2010;11:249–56.
41. Andrès E, Mourot-Cottet R, Keller O, Vogel T, Kaltenbach G. Review of oral vitamin B12 (cobalamin) therapy. Intern Med Rev. 2016;11:1–13.
42. Vidal-Araball J, Butler CC, Cannings-John R, Goringe A, Hood K, McCaddon A, et al. Oral vitamin B12 versus intramuscular vitamin B12 for vitamin B12 deficiency. Cochrane Database Syst Rev. 2005;(20):CD004655.
43. Wickramasinghe SN. Diagnosis of megaloblastic anaemias. Blood Rev. 2006;20:299–318.
44. Yen PK. Nutritional anemia. Geriatr Nurs. 2000;21:111–2.

Chapter 12
Clonal Hematopoiesis and Cytopenias in the Elderly

Daniel Guy, Amber Afzal, and Meagan A. Jacoby

Introduction

Somatic mutations in hematopoietic stem and progenitor cells (HSPCs) occur randomly throughout an individual's lifetime, resulting in a heterogeneous HSPC pool composed of cells with mutations unique to that individual. Most somatic age-related mutations are random "passenger" mutations that are benign [1]. However, the advent of massively parallel, digital sequencing studies has shown that somatic mutations that are associated with myeloid malignancies are detectable in the peripheral blood of apparently healthy individuals, with a prevalence that is age-dependent. This observation suggests that these mutations confer a competitive advantage that enables clonal expansion of that HSPC, resulting in its contribution to a significant fraction of blood production. Such a process is termed clonal hematopoiesis. It has been proposed that the term clonal hematopoiesis of indeterminate potential (CHIP) be applied to individuals with somatic mutations that are associated with myeloid malignancies but do not meet the diagnostic criteria for a hematologic malignancy [2]. Because the development of clonal hematopoiesis increases with age, the term age-related clonal hematopoiesis (ARCH) has also been proposed to describe this process [3]. In this chapter, we will discuss the observations that led to the identification of clonal hematopoiesis in apparently healthy individuals, how the use of massively parallel sequencing to describe genes recurrently mutated in myeloid malignancies led to a molecular understanding of clonal hematopoiesis, and the various clinical implications of clonal hematopoiesis.

D. Guy · A. Afzal · M. A. Jacoby (✉)
Division of Oncology, Department of Internal Medicine, Washington University School of Medicine, St. Louis, MO, USA
e-mail: mjacoby@wustl.edu

© Springer Nature Switzerland AG 2019
R. T. Means Jr. (ed.), *Anemia in the Young and Old*,
https://doi.org/10.1007/978-3-319-96487-4_12

Early Evidence of Clonal Hematopoiesis

Studies showing a skewed pattern of X-chromosome inactivation of polymorphic X-linked genes in chronic myelocytic leukemia [4] and polycythemia vera [5] provided early evidence of the clonal origin of myeloid neoplasms. However, several studies of X-inactivation patterns in the peripheral blood demonstrated that somatic clonal expansion can occur with aging in healthy women (Fig. 12.1).

For example, a study investigating clonality in the peripheral blood showed that 21 of 105 normal woman showed extreme X-inactivation skewing (XIS), consistent with a clonal expansion of hematopoietic cells [6]. This finding was more predominant in older individuals, present in up to 40% of women aged 75–96 years [6]. Similarly, in a study investigating clonal expansion across different age groups (neonates, 28–32 years, and ≥60 years), extreme skewing increased with age, found in 38% of elderly women versus 8.6% of neonates [7].

Later studies made use of advances in genomics to detect clonal hematopoiesis defined by acquired structural variants (Fig. 12.1). Chromosomal copy number

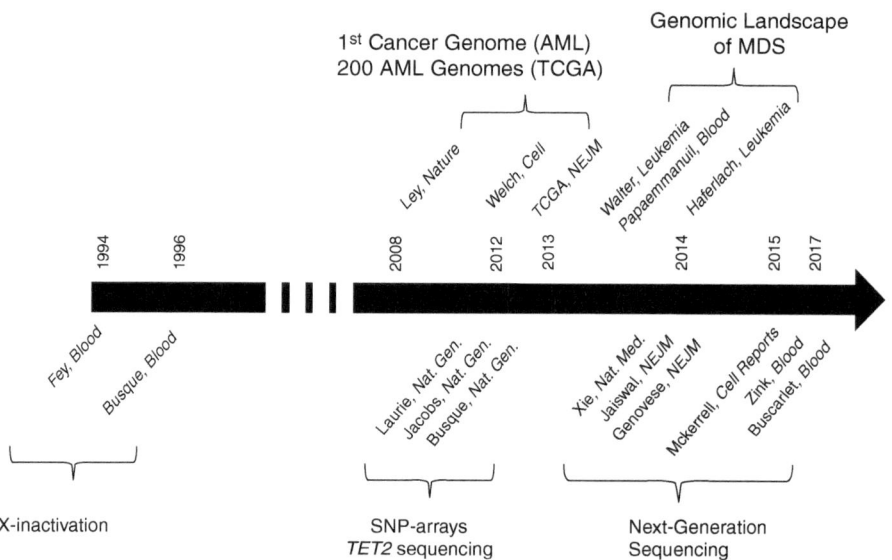

Fig. 12.1 Representative studies of clonal hematopoiesis in the pre- and post-genomic sequencing era. Early studies used X-chromosome inactivation skewing in women to demonstrate clonal hematopoiesis. Description of the genomic landscape and appreciation of the prevalence of clonal hematopoiesis occurred nearly two decades later with advances in genomic techniques. SNP arrays identified clonal hematopoiesis characterized by structural variants, including copy number alterations and copy-neutral loss of heterozygosity. Massively parallel digital sequencing led to the discovery of recurrently mutated genes in myeloid malignancies, which was translated into the identification of clonal hematopoiesis harboring myeloid malignancy-associated genes that demonstrated an age-dependent increase in prevalence in individuals with normal blood counts. AML acute myeloid leukemia, TCGA The Cancer Genome Atlas, MDS the myelodysplastic syndromes, SNP single nucleotide polymorphism

alterations (duplications, deletions) and copy number neutral loss of heterozygosity were studied using single nucleotide polymorphism (SNP) array analysis in two studies of subjects enrolled in genome-wide association studies (GWAS) [8, 9]. Because of the relative lack of sensitivity of SNP array analysis (the abnormality must be present in 5–10% of cells), the detection of a structural variant implies the presence of clonal hematopoiesis. Both studies detected somatic subclonal populations in the peripheral blood. The frequency of clonal hematopoiesis increased with age and was present in ≈2–3% of the elderly subjects [8, 9]. Of note, structural variants associated with hematologic malignancies were commonly detected, including deletions on chromosome 4q (containing the gene *TET2*) and 2p (containing the gene *DNMT3A*) [8]. The presence of clonal hematopoiesis increased the risk of subsequently developing a hematologic malignancy in patients without a prior diagnosis about tenfold [hazard ratio 10.1, (95% CI = 5.8–17.7), $p > 0.001$], although the incidence rates were relatively low (about 14% over 10 years) [8]. These observations raised the possibility that these genetic changes represented early events predisposing to disease development.

Discovery of the Genomic Landscape of Myeloid Malignancies

While the above studies focused on detection of large chromosomal changes, data at the gene level was lacking. Advances in massively parallel, high-resolution digital sequencing (commonly referred to as next-generation sequencing) resulted in the ability to survey an entire genome at the single base-pair level through whole-genome or whole-exome sequencing and the ability to rapidly sequence, with relatively high-coverage, large (100–200 gene) gene panels [10] (Fig. 12.1). In addition, digital read data provide the ability to determine (sub)clonal heterogeneity and estimate the level of tumor burden by determining the variant allele fraction (VAF), which is estimated by dividing the number of variant reads by the total (variant + reference) reads, where the variant is the acquired somatic alteration [10]. In 2008, the world of cancer genomics was revolutionized with the first report of the whole-genome sequencing of a human cancer, acute myeloid leukemia (AML) [11]. The Cancer Genome Atlas (TCGA) Research Network effort subsequently described the genomic landscapes of many cancers, including AML [12]. Studies of the genomic determinants of other clonal myeloid disorders, including the myelodysplastic syndrome(s) (MDS), the myeloproliferative neoplasms, and chronic myelomonocytic leukemia, demonstrated that there are a set of genes that are recurrently mutated in myeloid malignancies, implying that these genes have an important role in pathogenesis [13–17]. MDS is the most common myeloid malignancy in the elderly, with a median age of diagnosis of MDS of 70–75 years [18–20] and an estimated 75–162 cases per 100,000, although this may be underreported [21]. MDS is a clonal stem cell disorder associated with ineffective hematopoiesis, peripheral cytopenias, and a propensity to evolve to secondary AML. The prevalence of anemia in MDS patients is 54% [22]. There

Pathway	Genes
Splicing factors	*SF3B1, SRSF2, U2AF1, ZRSR2*
DNA methylation	*TET2, DNMT3A, IDH1/2*
Histone modification	*ASXL1, EZH2, BCOR, EP300*
Cohesins	*STAG2, RAD21, SMC1A, SMC3*
Transcription factors	*RUNX1, ETV6, CUX1, GATA2*
Signal transduction	*CBL, JAK2, KRAS, MPL1, NF1, PTPN11, KIT, FLT3*
P53 pathway	*TP53, PPM1D*

Table 12.1 Selected recurrently mutated genes in MDS by pathway

are approximately 40–50 recurrently mutated genes in MDS, which tend to be involved in cellular pathways such as epigenetic regulation (*DNMT3A, TET2, ASXL1*), RNA splicing, transcriptional regulation, signal transduction, or *TP53* [13–15, 23], reviewed in [24] (Table 12.1). There is substantial overlap in the genes and pathways affected in AML, MDS, CMML, and the myeloproliferative neoplasms (MPNs) [16, 17] (Table 12.2). Like MDS, myelofibrosis (MF) commonly presents as anemia in the elderly, present in 38% of the MF patients at diagnosis and 50% of the patients at the time of referral to a tertiary care center [25, 26] (Table 12.2). The identification of recurrently mutated genes in myeloid malignancies provided the framework to understand the significance of the variants identified in genome-/exome-wide sequencing studies of age-dependent clonal hematopoiesis and informed the design of candidate gene panels used in targeted studies.

Identifying Clonal Hematopoiesis in the Era of Next-Generation Sequencing and Genomic Discovery

Extending on earlier XIS studies, exome sequencing performed on three elderly women with extreme XIS identified somatic mutations in five genes, including *DNMT3A* and *TET2* [27]. Candidate gene resequencing in a larger cohort found *TET2* mutations in 5.6% of healthy women with XIS aged >65 years and noted that one of seven *TET2* mutation-positive subjects developed a myeloid malignancy within 5 years of follow-up [27]. This early observation linked genes associated with myeloid malignancies to age-dependent clonal hematopoiesis and suggested these individuals may have a predisposition to myeloid malignancies, with *TET2* acting as an initiating lesion [27].

Subsequently, multiple sequencing studies of large cohorts have demonstrated consistently that clonal expansions harboring mutations associated with myeloid malignancies are present in subjects without a clinically apparent myeloid neoplasm and that the prevalence of clonal hematopoiesis increases with age [28–33] (Figs. 12.1, 12.2, and 12.3).

Table 12.2 Selected recurrently mutated genes in myeloproliferative neoplasms

Gene function and symbol	Location	Frequency
Signaling MPN driver		
JAK2V617F	9p224	95%PV, 50–60% PMF, and ET
JAK2exon 12		3%PV
MPL	1p34	2–3% ET, 3–5% PMF
CALR	19p13	20–25%ET, 25–30% PMF
Other signaling		
LNK	12q24	1% ET, 2% PMF
CBL	11q23;3	4% PMF
NRAS	1p13.2	Rare PMF
NF1	17q11	Rare PMF
FLT3	13q12	MPN <3%
DNA methylation		
TET2	4q24	10–20% of all MPNs
DNMT3A	2p23	5–10% of all MPNS
IDH1	2q33.3	1–3% PMF
IDH2	15q26.1	1–3% PMF
Histone modifications		
EZH2	7q35–36	5–10% PMF
ASXL1	20q11	25% PMF
Transcription factors		
TP53	17p13.1	<5% of all MPNs
CUX1	7q22	<3%
IKZF1	7p12.2	<3%
ETV6	12p13	<3%
RUNX1	21q22.3	<3%
RNA splicing		
SRSF2	17q25.1	<2% ET, 10–15% PMF
SF3B1	2q33.1	<3% ET
U2AF1	21q22.3	10–15% PMF

Adapted from Vainchenker and Kralovics [17]

Abbreviations: *MPN* myeloproliferative neoplasm, *ET* essential thrombocythemia, *PMF* primary myelofibrosis, *PV* polycythemia vera

Whole exome and targeted amplicon sequencing interrogating 160 genetic variants known to be associated with hematologic cancers was performed on blood samples of over 17,000 patients from case/case-control cohorts in type 2 diabetes and heart studies [29]. While mutations were rare in persons under 40 years of age, their prevalence increased with each decade of life, such that they were detected in 18.4% (95% CI, 12.1–27.0) of patients >90 years of age (Fig. 12.2). The most common mutations were in *DNMT3A*, *TET2*, and *ASXL1* [29] (Fig. 12.3). Longitudinal follow-up was available for 3342 patients with a median follow-up time of 95 months. Patients with clonal hematopoiesis had an 11.1-fold (95%CI, 3.9–32.6)

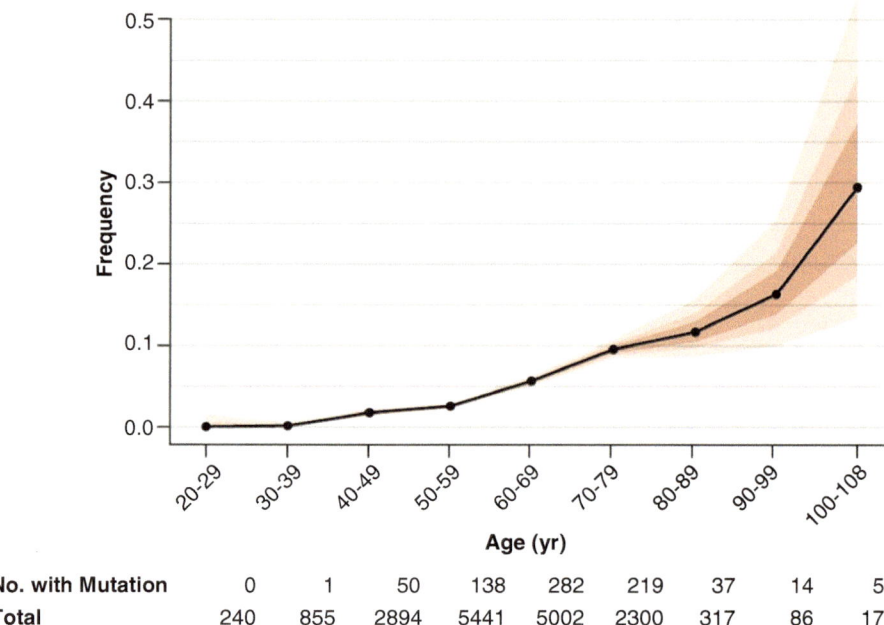

No. with Mutation	0	1	50	138	282	219	37	14	5
Total		240	855	2894	5441	5002	2300	317	86	17

Fig. 12.2 The prevalence of somatic mutations associated with clonal hematopoiesis according to age. Representative figure showing that the detection of clonal hematopoiesis increases with age, a finding that has been replicated across multiple studies [28–34]. Colored bands, in increasingly lighter shades, represent the 50th, 75th, and 95th percentiles. (From Jaiswal et al. [29]. Copyright © (2014) Massachusetts Medical Society. Reprinted with permission from Massachusetts Medical Society)

increase in the risk of developing hematologic malignancies, which translated to an absolute risk of about 0.5% per year [29]. The risk was even higher for patients with variant allele fractions of more than 10% [29]. Similarly, analysis of blood samples from a Swedish registry of 12,380 patients with no evidence of malignancy revealed a strong age-dependent increase in the frequency of mutations known to contribute to hematologic malignancies [30]. Only 0.9% of the patients <50 years of age, but 10.5% of the patients >65 years of age, had evidence of clonal hematopoiesis. In agreement with the previously described studies, the most commonly identified mutations were in *DNMT3A*, *ASXL1*, and *TET2* [30] as well as the gene *PPM1D* (Fig. 12.3). Follow-up data revealed that beginning 6 months after the sampling, patients with evidence of clonal hematopoiesis had a 12.9-fold increase (95%CI, 5.8–28.7) in the risk of developing hematologic malignancies, which translated to an absolute risk of about 1% per year. Samples available from two patients who developed leukemia demonstrated expansions and clonal evolution of the cells harboring clonal hematopoiesis, thus directly linking the clonal hematopoiesis clone to the leukemia clone [30].

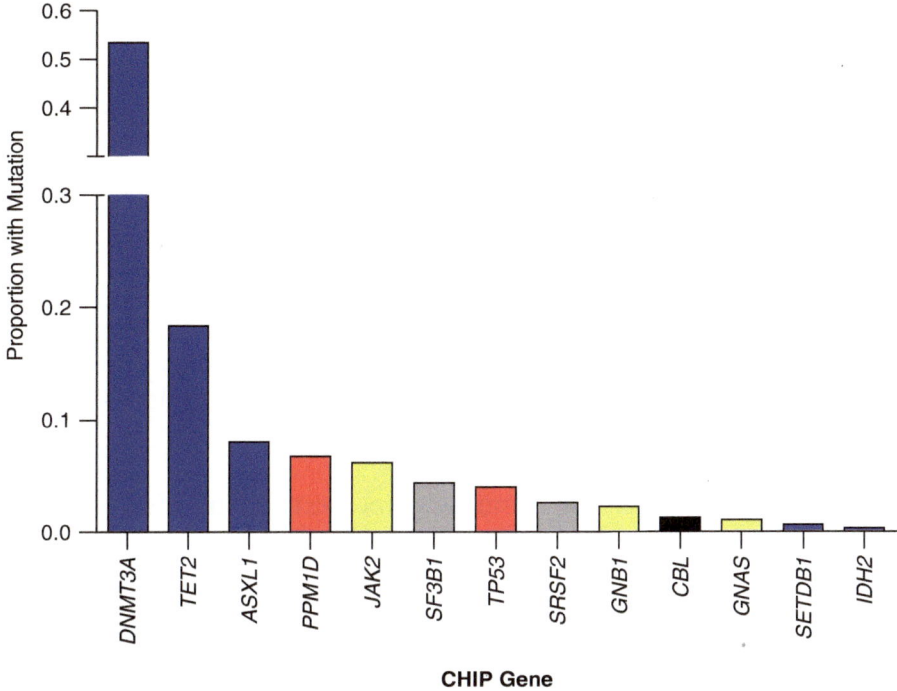

Fig. 12.3 Genes commonly mutated in individuals with clonal hematopoiesis of indeterminate potential. The proportion of individuals with clonal hematopoiesis that harbor a somatic mutation in each gene is shown, based on data from six large population studies of individuals without a known hematologic malignancy [28–33]. Blue, epigenetic regulators; red, *TP53* pathway; yellow, cell signaling; gray, spliceosome genes; black, others. CHIP clonal hematopoiesis of indeterminate potential

The McDonnell Genome Institute at Washington University analyzed 2728 samples from the TCGA cohort who had previously untreated, non-hematologic malignancies [28]. In agreement with the other large-scale sequencing studies, *DNMT3A*, *TET2*, and *ASXL1* were among the most commonly mutated genes, and mutation frequency increased with age from about 1.2% of the patients in the fifth decade of life to 6.8% of the patients in their ninth decade [28]. Interestingly, in this cohort, no mutations were found in genes such as *IDH1*, *NRAS*, *RUNX1*, *NPM1*, and *FLT3*, which are commonly mutated in AML [12]. Based on these data, it was proposed that clonal hematopoiesis with mutations in genes such as *DNMT3A*, *TET2*, *ASXL1*, and *PPM1D* may represent premalignant events leading to clonal hematopoietic expansion and that the development of overt myeloid malignancies requires cooperating mutations in genes such as *FLT3*, *NPM*, *IDH1*, *NRAS*, *RUNX1*, and others [12, 28, 30]. A later study using ultra-deep sequencing of a large population showed *NPM1* is not detectable in age-dependent clonal hematopoiesis, consistent with its acquisition leading to frank malignancy [34]. Two additional large population-based studies observed an age-dependent increase in clonal hematopoiesis, again with mutations in *DNMT3A*, *TET2*, and *ASXL1* among the most common, accounting for the vast majority of mutations [32, 33]. Association with the C > T mutational signature characteristic of aging [32] and an increased risk for hematologic malignancy were also observed, in agreement with previous studies [33]. In summary, multiple large population-based series of individuals without known blood disorders have shown an age-dependent increase in clonal hematopoiesis with genes that are known to be recurrent in myeloid malignancies such as MDS and AML. Figure 12.3 shows the 13 most frequently mutated genes reported in these seminal studies. The most frequently affected cellular pathways include epigenetic regulators, the *TP53* pathway, cell signaling, and spliceosome genes (Fig. 12.3). Of note, the minimum required variant allele fraction (VAF) used in these studies to define clonal hematopoiesis ranged from 0.8% to 10% [28–33].

Mutations in Epigenetic Modifiers Account for the Majority of Age-Dependent Clonal Hematopoiesis

Together, *DNMT3A*, *TET2*, and *ASXL1* are found in >90% of age-related clonal hematopoiesis (Fig. 12.3). *DNMT3A* catalyzes the addition of methyl groups to cytosine residues of DNA molecules at CpG dinucleotides and is critical for de novo methylation. Mutations in *DNMT3A* occur in 18–22% of all acute myeloid leukemia [35, 36] and about 10% of patients with MDS [24, 37]. *TET2* is a DNA oxidase that catalyzes the conversion of 5-methylcytosine to 5-hydroxymethylcytosine, which is thought to be involved in DNA demethylation (reviewed in [36]). *TET2* mutations are found in 9–23% of acute myeloid leukemia [36, 38] and ≈20% of patients with MDS (reviewed in [24]). Mutations in genes encoding *DNMT3A* and *TET2* result in altered regulation of gene expression [39]. *ASXL1* is a protein thought to be involved in epigenetic regulation, although its precise mechanism of action is not fully understood (reviewed in [40]). *ASXL1* mutations occur in 5–11% of all acute myeloid leukemia [36] and about 15% of MDS (reviewed in [24]). The mechanism by which epigenetic dysregulation confers a competitive advantage in HSPC harboring these genes is incompletely understood, although work in mice has shown that loss-of-function mutations in *Dnmt3a* and *Tet2* can increase hematopoietic stem cell self-renewal [41, 42] .

Increased Prevalence of Clonal Hematopoiesis-Associated Mutations Detected by Ultra-deep Sequencing

Based on sensitivities of mutation detection in the large studies with associated outcomes data, expert opinion has suggested that a mutation must be present at a minimum VAF of 2% (0.02) in the peripheral blood to meet the definition of clonal hematopoiesis [2]. Two recent studies using ultra-deep targeted sequencing suggest that clonal hematopoiesis-associated genes may be detectable at lower thresholds, and at higher prevalence, than previously appreciated. Using an assay with a sensitivity of 0.001 VAF, it was shown that clonal hematopoiesis was detectable in 3% of individuals aged 20–29 and in up to 20% of patients aged 60–69 years; however, myeloid malignancy outcomes were not reported, so it is unclear what VAF threshold confers an increased risk for subsequent development of myeloid cancers [34]. In agreement with a previous study showing the spliceosome mutations *SF3B1* and *SRSF2* were found only in those over 70 years [31], the authors reported differential mutation patterns in individuals with clonal hematopoiesis based on age [34]. For example, *DNMT3A* and *JAK2* mutations were found across all ages, while *GNB1* and *IDH2*, as well as the spliceosome mutations *U2AF1* and *SF3B1*, were exclusively found in subjects over the age of 60 years [34].

In addition, a study examining the peripheral blood of healthy 50–60-year-olds using ultra-deep, error-corrected sequencing to detect rare variants at VAF thresholds below the error rate of next-generation sequencing ($\approx$0.0003 VAF) showed that clonal hematopoiesis, predominantly with mutations in *DNMT3A* and *TET2,* could be detected in in 95% of the participants [43]. The median detected VAF was 0.0024 [43]. Temporal stability of the clonal hematopoiesis was demonstrated using paired blood samples obtained approximately 10 years apart. The authors suggest that clinically silent, low-level clonal hematopoiesis may be present in many individuals by middle age and that progression to overt hematologic malignancy is a rare occurrence that requires further mutations leading to clonal expansion [43].

Clonal Hematopoiesis in the Setting of Cytopenias

Clonal hematopoiesis can be present in healthy individuals with normal blood counts but confers an increased risk of developing hematologic cancers and an increased all-cause mortality (discussed below). As such, it is recognized that while the detection of a myeloid malignancy-associated mutation is not pathognomonic of malignancy, clonal hematopoiesis may not be completely benign. The term "clonal hematopoiesis of indeterminate potential" (CHIP) was proposed to describe the acquisition of a somatic mutation with a VAF $\geq$2% (0.02) in a gene that is recurrently mutated in myeloid malignancies, in a patient without cytopenias and/or a clear diagnosis of a hematologic malignancy [2]. "Age-related clonal hematopoiesis" (ARCH) has also been proposed to describe this process [3]. The list of CHIP/ARCH defining genetic lesions and the minimal variant allele fractions (reflective of the clonal burden) required to meet the definition of clonal hematopoiesis continues to evolve [2, 3].

Distinguishing secondary cytopenias from a clonal bone marrow process often proves difficult. For example, the definitive diagnosis of MDS can be challenging as it relies on the subjective finding of morphologic dysplasia in the marrow [44], and diagnostic discrepancies can occur in up to 12% of patients at the time of initial presentation [45]. Anemia is a significant health problem in the elderly with a preva-lence estimated to be 10–12% [46, 47]. Approximately one-third of the cases remain unexplained [46], although a significant proportion of the unexplained anemia in population studies has been attributed to clonal disorders. As discussed above, MDS and MF often present with significant anemia. For example, in an Italian study, almost one-third of the unexplained anemia was thought to be secondary to MDS with MDS being defined by macrocytic anemia, leukopenia, and thrombocytopenia, although definitive diagnosis was precluded by lack of a bone marrow biopsy [47]. The traditional definition of "idiopathic cytopenias of unknown significance" (ICUS) has been used to describe cytopenias in patients who do not meet diagnostic criteria for a myeloid malignancy and/or have comorbidities characterized by the propensity for cytopenias, such as liver disease, etc. Clonal cytopenias of undeter-mined significance (CCUS) has been suggested to specify that group of patients with evidence of clonal hematopoiesis and decreased blood counts, in the absence of an overt hematologic malignancy, thus dividing the traditional category of ICUS into clonal and non-clonal processes [2]. With the advent of next-generation sequencing panels to identify genes associated with myeloid malignancies and their increasingly routine use in clinical practice, the diagnosis of CHIP/CCUS will likely become more commonplace.

Several studies have investigated the prevalence and clinical significance of clonal hematopoiesis in patients with unexplained cytopenia(s) (i.e., CCUS). The presence of somatic mutations in a cohort of patients with unexplained cytopenias was investigated by interrogating a panel of genes known to be recurrently mutated in myeloid malignancies in a subset of patients with ICUS and some evidence of dysplasia and a subset with ICUS and no dysplasia [48]. Overall, approximately one-third of patients with ICUS had clonal hematopoiesis, including up to 27% of patients with no dysplasia. Thus, CCUS was fairly common among patients with unexplained cytopenias; furthermore, the majority of patients had VAFs greater than 10% [48]. Additional studies examined the risk of developing a hematologic malig-nancy in patients determined to have CCUS, again using sequencing to identify mutations in genes known to be recurrently mutated in myeloid malignancies. Duncavage and colleagues determined the presence of CCUS in a small cohort of patients with equivocal or no dysplasia in the setting of cytopenia(s) and showed that ~75% subsequently developed or were treated for MDS [49]. A larger study of patients who carried the provisional diagnosis of ICUS showed that 36% had evi-dence of clonal hematopoiesis, thus meeting the definition of CCUS [50]. Compared to those without evidence of clonal hematopoiesis, patients with CCUS had a higher risk of developing a myeloid malignancy with a hazard ratio of 13.9 (95% CI, 5.4–35.91) and a 10-year cumulative probability of progression 9% versus 95% ($p < 0.001$) [50]. Furthermore, patients who had mutations in spliceosome genes or in *TET2*, *ASXL1*, and *DNMT3A* with co-mutations had positive predictive values for developing a myeloid neoplasm, ranging from 0.86 to 1.0 [50]. Thus, clonal hema-topoiesis, especially in the setting of cytopenia(s), is likely to be an important clini-cal entity. Currently, there is no clinical consensus as to the approach to patients with CHIP or CCUS, although most clinicians agree that patients with CCUS require periodic follow-up with complete blood counts [3]. Longitudinal natural history studies of CHIP and CCUS and studies to determine how to incorporate evidence-based interventions to prevent the evolution of CCUS into a myeloid malignancy are likely to be an intensive area of future investigation. Studies to determine the association of clonal hematopoiesis with the approximately one-third of elderly anemia cases that remain unexplained are also needed.

The Role of Age in Promoting Clonal Hematopoiesis

Some authors suggest that clonal expansions harboring somatic mutations are a universal aspect of human aging [34, 43]. Indeed, in a 115-year-old woman with no blood dyscrasias, whole-genome sequencing detected 450 somatic variants in the peripheral blood, and it was estimated that the entirety of her blood pool was derived from two HSPC clones [51]. Why might somatic mutations increase with age? Welch and colleagues used whole-exome sequencing to demonstrate that HSPCs normally acquire mutations over the lifespan of the individual [1]. Approximately 5–10 acquired single nucleotide variants (SNVs) were detectable by the fifth to eighth decade of life in the HSPCs of healthy volunteers, suggesting that normal, self-renewing HSPCs accumulate random background mutations as a function of time, at a rate of ≈0.13 +/−0.02 exonic mutations per year [1]. This has been extrapolated to equal about five mutations/year in the whole genome, consistent with the somatic variant burden reported for the 115-year-old woman [51]. The mutational spectrum in normal subjects' exomes was identical to that of AML, with the majority C > T transitions [1]. The C > T variant has been noted to be the most common base-pair change in several clonal hematopoiesis studies as well [29, 43].

Aged HSPCs have reduced self-renewal and skewed differentiation potential, alterations in their interactions with the stem cell niche, and altered epigenetic signatures (reviewed in [52]). In addition, there may also be extrinsic HSPC stressors, such as autoimmunity, chemotherapy/radiation, and infection/inflammation that may stress the aging bone marrow (reviewed in [53]). The acquisition of a CHIP mutation may increase fitness and self-renewal in the setting of a dwindling functional HSPC pool in order to maintain hematopoiesis, thus leading to clonal expansion. While most extrinsic marrow stressors are poorly understood, there has been progress in understanding the effect of cytotoxic chemotherapy and radiation, which may serve as a proof-of-principle model of the role of clonal hematopoiesis in the stress response of the aging bone marrow.

Several studies have examined clonal hematopoiesis that results from the "stressor" of cytotoxic chemotherapy and its role in therapy-related myeloid neoplasms (t-MN) [54–61]. Wong and colleagues showed that clonal hematopoiesis harboring TP53 mutations found at the diagnosis of t-MN predated disease development by 3–6 years and could be detected, in some cases, prior to any chemotherapy exposure, implying pre-existing TP53 mutations (i.e., not resulting from mutagenic therapy) in HSPCs confer resistance to chemotherapy and result in preferential expansion after treatment [54]. Supporting the hypothesis that age-related *TP53* clonal hematopoiesis exists, functional *TP53* mutations could be detected in the peripheral blood of healthy elderly individuals [54]. Clonal expansions harboring other genes recurrently mutated in myeloid malignancies after chemotherapy have also been reported. A study of 15 patients with genetic clearance of AML post-induction therapy demonstrated clonal hematopoiesis with a rising clone harboring myeloid malignancy-associated genes such as *TP53*, *TET2*, *DNMT3A*, and *ASXL1* [55]. The rising clone was detectable at low levels prior to cytotoxic therapy, implying these CHIP genes provided a fitness advantage [55]. In addition, retrospective case-control cohort studies demonstrated that patients with t-MN were more likely to have CHIP prior to the t-MN diagnosis than those that did not develop t-MN, which in some cases was detectable prior to chemo/radiation therapy [58, 59], in keeping with previous observations [54]. Clonal hematopoiesis at the time of autologous stem cell transplantation (ASCT) of lymphoma patients has been shown to increase the rate of t-MN (10-year cumulative incidence, 14.1% vs 4.3% for CHIP vs no CHIP, respectively, $p = 0.002$) and confer inferior overall survival [61]. Finally, a large series using paired tumor and blood samples examined therapy-related clonal hematopoiesis in patients with solid tumors and found that clonal hematopoiesis in non-hematologic cancer patients was common, increased with age, tobacco use, and prior RT exposure, and increased the risk of hematologic cancers [57]. The most commonly observed mutated genes were *DNMT3A*, *TET2*, *PPM1D*, *ASXL1*, *ATM*, and *TP53*, and clonal expansions harboring mutations in *TP53* and *PPM1D* mutations were associated with prior chemotherapy [57]. The finding that cytotoxic chemotherapy results in *TP53* and *PPM1D* clonal expansions has been observed in an additional study [56].

A Model of Clonal Hematopoiesis of Indeterminate Potential: From Age-Related Mutations to Myeloid Malignancies

The data suggest that HSPCs acquire random mutations distributed throughout the genome that accumulate over the lifetime of the individual. An age-related, acquired mutation in a gene that is recurrently mutated in myeloid malignancies can lead to CHIP. However, some patients with clonal hematopoiesis harboring CHIP mutations may never have overt expansion or progression, with low-level clonal hematopoiesis that remains stable over time [43], underscoring that additional genetic changes or selection pressures must be present for clonal expansion to occur. Clonal expansion may be an initiating event, resulting in a premalignant clone that predisposes the individual to the development of a myeloid malignancy. Although the exact mechanism is not completely understood, development of a myeloid malignancy presumably requires clonal evolution through acquisition of cooperating gene mutations or structural variants, and/or strong selection pressure such as

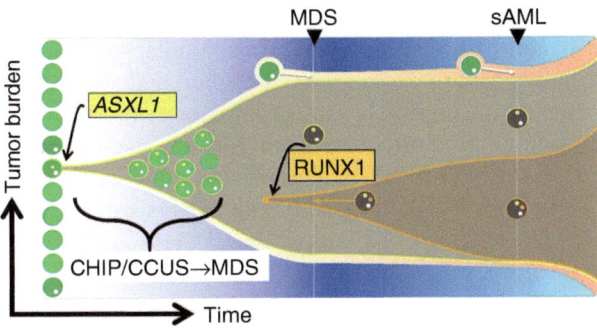

Fig. 12.4 A model of clonal hematopoiesis from age-related mutations to secondary AML. Normal hematopoietic stem and progenitor cells (HSPCs) are represented by green cells. The self-renewing HSPCs acquire random, benign mutations during normal aging (white dot). A mutation occurs in a gene (yellow dot, *ASXL1*) which confers a competitive advantage to the HSPC, perhaps secondary to increased self-renewal which results in clonal expansion and overrepresentation of the mutant cell in the HSPC pool. This process is termed CHIP, or clonal hematopoiesis of indeterminate potential. The common CHIP genes are also recurrently mutated in myeloid malignancies. Clonal evolution occurs in the expanded CHIP clone through the acquisition of cooperating mutations, epigenetic changes, and/or strong selection pressure (such as chemotherapy), giving rise to MDS (gray cells) carrying forward both the CHIP gene (yellow dot) and its unique set of age-related mutations, which are "passengers" (white dot). Clonal hematopoiesis in the setting of a cytopenia (CCUS, or clonal cytopenias of undetermined significance) is associated with a high risk of progression. The MDS clone transforms to secondary AML (sAML), after acquiring a mutation in the transcriptional regulator *RUNX1* (orange dot)

cytotoxic chemotherapy. Indeed, the risk of progression to malignancy increases with the number of mutations in an individual with clonal hematopoiesis [29], and patients with AML and MDS typically harbor multiple cooperating mutations [12–15].

Overall, clonal evolution is likely a multifactorial process, dependent on processes intrinsic to the aging stem cell, the nature and number of initiating lesions (e.g., epigenetic regulators versus *TP53*), cooperating mutations (such as *NRAS* and *FLT3*), and pressures exerted by age-related bone marrow stressors. A model of clonal evolution is shown in Fig. 12.4.

Additional Adverse Health Outcomes Associated with Clonal Hematopoiesis

The presence of clonal hematopoiesis has been linked with increases in overall mortality [29, 30, 62]. Follow-up data from the Swedish registry study and the case cohort study published by Jaiswal and colleagues demonstrated an increase in all-cause mortality in patients with CHIP (hazard ratio 1.4, 95% CI, 1.0–1.8 and hazard ratio 1.4, 95% CI, 1.1–1.8, respectively) [29, 30]. Unexpectedly, the increased mortality was attributed to an increase in cardiovascular disease, manifested as an increase in events related to coronary heart disease and strokes [29]. This correlation between clonal hematopoiesis and cardiovascular morbidity was further demonstrated in a follow-up study. Data from two prospective case-control cohorts showed that carriers of CHIP had an increased risk of coronary heart disease (hazard ratio 1.9, 95% CI 1.4–2.7) [62]. Similarly, analysis of two retrospective case-control cohorts showed that individuals with CHIP had an increased risk of early-onset myocardial infarction (hazard ratio 4.0, 95% CI 2.4–6.7) [62]. It was also shown that patients with CHIP had higher coronary calcification scores on cardiac CT, which was more pronounced in patients with higher allele frequency [62]. Mutations in *DNMT3A*, *TET2*, *ASXL1*, and *JAK2* were associated with heart disease in this study [62].

Recent studies have investigated whether certain CHIP genes could have a causal role in development of cardiovascular disease using atherosclerotic-prone LDL-receptor knockout mice that underwent irradiation and bone marrow transplantation with HSPCs with a loss-of-function *Tet2* gene [62]. This was not associated with changes in blood counts or lipid profiles but resulted in increased size and number of atherosclerotic plaques. It was also shown that these mice had an increase in inflammatory cytokines [62, 63]. Similarly, human subjects with *TET2*-associated clonal hematopoiesis had an increase in the pro-inflammatory cytokine interleukin-8 [62]. The role of other mutations associated with clonal hematopoiesis and their link to cardiovascular morbidity is unclear.

Summary

Multiple large sequencing studies of asymptomatic populations without known blood disorders have consistently demonstrated an age-dependent increase in the prevalence of clonally restricted hematopoiesis, in which genes known to be recurrently mutated in myeloid malignancies, including MDS and AML, can be detected in the peripheral blood. The presence of clonal hematopoiesis is associated with an increased risk of developing a hematologic malignancy, an increased risk of cardiovascular disease, and a higher all-cause mortality rate and is thus termed "clonal hematopoiesis of indeterminate potential" (CHIP). Individuals with clonal hematopoiesis and the presence of a cytopenia are at a particularly increased risk of developing a subsequent hematologic malignancy. However, clonal hematopoiesis and blood counts can remain stable over many years, suggesting that although CHIP may be an early, initiating step in myeloid malignancies, clonal evolution through the acquisition of cooperating mutations and/or selection pressure is required for disease. The mechanism by which CHIP genes promote clonal expansion is unclear but may be related to conferring increased fitness to the aging HSPC in a cell pool that is shrinking from the cumulative age-related effects on the bone marrow. The CHIP-defining genes and minimal required variant allele fractions required to meet the definition continue to evolve. Future studies will help define the full clinical consequences of CHIP, including if, when, and how to intervene preemptively to prevent clonal evolution of CHIP/ CCUS into a myeloid malignancy.

References

1. Welch JS, Ley TJ, Link DC, Miller CA, Larson DE, Koboldt DC, et al. The origin and evolution of mutations in acute myeloid leukemia. Cell. 2012;150(2):264–78.
2. Steensma DP, Bejar R, Jaiswal S, Lindsley RC, Sekeres MA, Hasserjian RP, et al. Clonal hematopoiesis of indeterminate potential and its distinction from myelodysplastic syndromes. Blood. 2015;126(1):9–16.
3. Shlush LI. Age-related clonal hematopoiesis. Blood. 2018;131(5):496–504.
4. Barr RD, Fialkow PJ. Clonal origin of chronic myelocytic leukemia. N Engl J Med. 1973;289(6):307–9.
5. Adamson JW, Fialkow PJ, Murphy S, Prchal JF, Steinmann L. Polycythemia vera: stem-cell and probable clonal origin of the disease. N Engl J Med. 1976;295(17):913–6.
6. Fey MF, Liechti-Gallati S, von Rohr A, Borisch B, Theilkas L, Schneider V, et al. Clonality and X-inactivation patterns in hematopoietic cell populations detected by the highly informative M27 beta DNA probe. Blood. 1994;83(4):931–8.
7. Busque L, Mio R, Mattioli J, Brais E, Blais N, Lalonde Y, et al. Nonrandom X-inactivation patterns in normal females: lyonization ratios vary with age. Blood. 1996;88(1):59–65.
8. Laurie CC, Laurie CA, Rice K, Doheny KF, Zelnick LR, McHugh CP, et al. Detectable clonal mosaicism from birth to old age and its relationship to cancer. Nat Genet. 2012;44(6):642–50.
9. Jacobs KB, Yeager M, Zhou W, Wacholder S, Wang Z, Rodriguez-Santiago B, et al. Detectable clonal mosaicism and its relationship to aging and cancer. Nat Genet. 2012;44(6):651–8.
10. Jacoby MA, Duncavage EJ, Walter MJ. Implications of tumor clonal heterogeneity in the era of next-generation sequencing. Trends Cancer. 2015;1(4):231–41.
11. Ley TJ, Mardis ER, Ding L, Fulton B, McLellan MD, Chen K, et al. DNA sequencing of a cytogenetically normal acute myeloid leukaemia genome. Nature. 2008;456(7218):66–72.
12. Cancer Genome Atlas Research N, Ley TJ, Miller C, Ding L, Raphael BJ, Mungall AJ, et al. Genomic and epigenomic landscapes of adult de novo acute myeloid leukemia. N Engl J Med. 2013;368(22):2059 74.
13. Walter MJ, Shen D, Shao J, Ding L, White BS, Kandoth C, et al. Clonal diversity of recurrently mutated genes in myelodysplastic syndromes. Leukemia. 2013;27(6):1275–82.
14. Papaemmanuil E, Gerstung M, Malcovati L, Tauro S, Gundem G, Van Loo P, et al. Clinical and biological implications of driver mutations in myelodysplastic syndromes. Blood. 2013;122(22):3616–27. quiz 99
15. Haferlach T, Nagata Y, Grossmann V, Okuno Y, Bacher U, Nagae G, et al. Landscape of genetic lesions in 944 patients with myelodysplastic syndromes. Leukemia. 2014;28(2):241–7.
16. Patel BJ, Przychodzen B, Thota S, Radivoyevitch T, Visconte V, Kuzmanovic T, et al. Genomic determinants of chronic myelomonocytic leukemia. Leukemia. 2017;31(12):2815–23.
17. Vainchenker W, Kralovics R. Genetic basis and molecular pathophysiology of classical myeloproliferative neoplasms. Blood. 2017;129(6):667–79.
18. Foran JM, Shammo JM. Clinical presentation, diagnosis, and prognosis of myelodysplastic syndromes. Am J Med. 2012;125(7 Suppl):S6–13.
19. Ma X, Does M, Raza A, Mayne ST. Myelodysplastic syndromes. Cancer. 2007;109(8): 1536–42.

20. Rollison DE, Howlader N, Smith MT, Strom SS, Merritt WD, Ries LA, et al. Epidemiology of myelodysplastic syndromes and chronic myeloproliferative disorders in the United States, 2001-2004, using data from the NAACCR and SEER programs. Blood. 2008;112(1):45–52.
21. Cogle CR. Incidence and burden of the myelodysplastic syndromes. Curr Hematol Malig Rep. 2015;10(3):272–81.
22. Greenberg P, Cox C, LeBeau MM, Fenaux P, Morel P, Sanz G, et al. International scoring system for evaluating prognosis in myelodysplastic syndromes. Blood. 1997;89(6):2079–88.
23. Makishima H, Yoshizato T, Yoshida K, Sekeres MA, Radivoyevitch T, Suzuki H, et al. Dynamics of clonal evolution in myelodysplastic syndromes. Nat Genet. 2017;49(2):204–12.
24. Bejar R, Steensma DP. Recent developments in myelodysplastic syndromes. Blood. 2014;124(18):2793–803.
25. Tefferi A, Lasho TL, Jimma T, Finke CM, Gangat N, Vaidya R, et al. One thousand patients with primary myelofibrosis: the mayo clinic experience. Mayo Clin Proc. 2012;87(1):25–33.
26. Barraco D, Elala YC, Lasho TL, Begna KH, Gangat N, Finke C, et al. Molecular correlates of anemia in primary myelofibrosis: a significant and independent association with U2AF1 mutations. Blood Cancer J. 2016;6:e415.
27. Busque L, Patel JP, Figueroa ME, Vasanthakumar A, Provost S, Hamilou Z, et al. Recurrent somatic TET2 mutations in normal elderly individuals with clonal hematopoiesis. Nat Genet. 2012;44(11):1179–81.
28. Xie M, Lu C, Wang J, McLellan MD, Johnson KJ, Wendl MC, et al. Age-related mutations associated with clonal hematopoietic expansion and malignancies. Nat Med. 2014;20(12):1472–8.
29. Jaiswal S, Fontanillas P, Flannick J, Manning A, Grauman PV, Mar BG, et al. Age-related clonal hematopoiesis associated with adverse outcomes. N Engl J Med. 2014;371(26):2488–98.
30. Genovese G, Kahler AK, Handsaker RE, Lindberg J, Rose SA, Bakhoum SF, et al. Clonal hematopoiesis and blood-cancer risk inferred from blood DNA sequence. N Engl J Med. 2014;371(26):2477–87.
31. McKerrell T, Park N, Moreno T, Grove CS, Ponstingl H, Stephens J, et al. Leukemia-associated somatic mutations drive distinct patterns of age-related clonal hemopoiesis. Cell Rep. 2015;10(8):1239–45.
32. Buscarlet M, Provost S, Zada YF, Barhdadi A, Bourgoin V, Lepine G, et al. DNMT3A and TET2 dominate clonal hematopoiesis and demonstrate benign phenotypes and different genetic predispositions. Blood. 2017;130(6):753–62.
33. Zink F, Stacey SN, Norddahl GL, Frigge ML, Magnusson OT, Jonsdottir I, et al. Clonal hematopoiesis, with and without candidate driver mutations, is common in the elderly. Blood. 2017;130(6):742–52.
34. Acuna-Hidalgo R, Sengul H, Steehouwer M, van de Vorst M, Vermeulen SH, Kiemeney L, et al. Ultra-sensitive sequencing identifies high prevalence of clonal hematopoiesis-associated mutations throughout adult life. Am J Hum Genet. 2017;101(1):50–64.
35. Ley TJ, Ding L, Walter MJ, McLellan MD, Lamprecht T, Larson DE, et al. DNMT3A mutations in acute myeloid leukemia. N Engl J Med. 2010;363(25):2424–33.
36. Medinger M, Passweg JR. Acute myeloid leukaemia genomics. Br J Haematol. 2017;179(4):530–42.
37. Walter MJ, Ding L, Shen D, Shao J, Grillot M, McLellan M, et al. Recurrent DNMT3A mutations in patients with myelodysplastic syndromes. Leukemia. 2011;25(7):1153–8.
38. Kunimoto H, Nakajima H. Epigenetic dysregulation of hematopoietic stem cells and preleukemic state. Int J Hematol. 2017;106(1):34–44.
39. Im AP, Sehgal AR, Carroll MP, Smith BD, Tefferi A, Johnson DE, et al. DNMT3A and IDH mutations in acute myeloid leukemia and other myeloid malignancies: associations with prognosis and potential treatment strategies. Leukemia. 2014;28(9):1774–83.
40. Micol JB, Abdel-Wahab O. The role of additional sex combs-like proteins in cancer. Cold Spring Harb Perspect Med. 2016;6(10).
41. Challen GA, Sun D, Jeong M, Luo M, Jelinek J, Berg JS, et al. Dnmt3a is essential for hematopoietic stem cell differentiation. Nat Genet. 2011;44(1):23–31.

42. Moran-Crusio K, Reavie L, Shih A, Abdel-Wahab O, Ndiaye-Lobry D, Lobry C, et al. Tet2 loss leads to increased hematopoietic stem cell self-renewal and myeloid transformation. Cancer Cell. 2011;20(1):11–24.
43. Young AL, Challen GA, Birmann BM, Druley TE. Clonal haematopoiesis harbouring AML-associated mutations is ubiquitous in healthy adults. Nat Commun. 2016;7:12484.
44. Arber DA, Orazi A, Hasserjian R, Thiele J, Borowitz MJ, Le Beau MM, et al. The 2016 revision to the World Health Organization classification of myeloid neoplasms and acute leukemia. Blood. 2016;127(20):2391–405.
45. Naqvi K, Jabbour E, Bueso-Ramos C, Pierce S, Borthakur G, Estrov Z, et al. Implications of discrepancy in morphologic diagnosis of myelodysplastic syndrome between referral and tertiary care centers. Blood. 2011;118(17):4690–3.
46. Guralnik JM, Eisenstaedt RS, Ferrucci L, Klein HG, Woodman RC. Prevalence of anemia in persons 65 years and older in the United States: evidence for a high rate of unexplained anemia. Blood. 2004;104(8):2263–8.
47. Tettamanti M, Lucca U, Gandini F, Recchia A, Mosconi P, Apolone G, et al. Prevalence, incidence and types of mild anemia in the elderly: the "Health and Anemia" population-based study. Haematologica. 2010;95(11):1849–56.
48. Kwok B, Hall JM, Witte JS, Xu Y, Reddy P, Lin K, et al. MDS-associated somatic mutations and clonal hematopoiesis are common in idiopathic cytopenias of undetermined significance. Blood. 2015;126(21):2355–61.
49. Duncavage EJ, O'Brien J, Vij K, Miller CA, Chang GS, Shao J, et al. Targeted sequencing informs the evaluation of normal karyotype cytopenic patients for low-grade myelodysplastic syndrome. Leukemia. 2016;30(12):2422–6.
50. Malcovati L, Galli A, Travaglino E, Ambaglio I, Rizzo E, Molteni E, et al. Clinical significance of somatic mutation in unexplained blood cytopenia. Blood. 2017;129(25):3371–8.
51. Holstege H, Pfeiffer W, Sie D, Hulsman M, Nicholas TJ, Lee CC, et al. Somatic mutations found in the healthy blood compartment of a 115-yr-old woman demonstrate oligoclonal hematopoiesis. Genome Res. 2014;24(5):733–42.
52. Geiger H, de Haan G, Florian MC. The ageing haematopoietic stem cell compartment. Nat Rev Immunol. 2013;13(5):376–89.
53. Link DC, Walter MJ. 'CHIP'ping away at clonal hematopoiesis. Leukemia. 2016;30(8):1633–5.
54. Wong TN, Ramsingh G, Young AL, Miller CA, Touma W, Welch JS, et al. Role of TP53 mutations in the origin and evolution of therapy-related acute myeloid leukaemia. Nature. 2015;518(7540):552–5.
55. Wong TN, Miller CA, Klco JM, Petti A, Demeter R, Helton NM, et al. Rapid expansion of pre-existing non-leukemic hematopoietic clones frequently follows induction therapy for de novo AML. Blood. 2015.
56. Wong TN, Miller CA, Jotte MRM, Bagegni N, Baty JD, Schmidt AP, et al. Cellular stressors contribute to the expansion of hematopoietic clones of varying leukemic potential. Nat Commun. 2018;9(1):455.
57. Coombs CC, Zehir A, Devlin SM, Kishtagari A, Syed A, Jonsson P, et al. Therapy-related clonal hematopoiesis in patients with non-hematologic cancers is common and associated with adverse clinical outcomes. Cell Stem Cell. 2017;21(3):374–82. e4
58. Gillis NK, Ball M, Zhang Q, Ma Z, Zhao Y, Yoder SJ, et al. Clonal haemopoiesis and therapy-related myeloid malignancies in elderly patients: a proof-of-concept, case-control study. Lancet Oncol. 2017;18(1):112–21.
59. Takahashi K, Wang F, Kantarjian H, Doss D, Khanna K, Thompson E, et al. Preleukaemic clonal haemopoiesis and risk of therapy-related myeloid neoplasms: a case-control study. Lancet Oncol. 2017;18(1):100–11.
60. Takahashi K, Wang F, Kantarjian H, Song X, Patel K, Neelapu S, et al. Copy number alterations detected as clonal hematopoiesis of indeterminate potential. Blood Adv. 2017;1(15):1031–6.

61. Gibson CJ, Lindsley RC, Tchekmedyian V, Mar BG, Shi J, Jaiswal S, et al. Clonal hematopoiesis associated with adverse outcomes after autologous stem-cell transplantation for lymphoma. J Clin Oncol. 2017;35(14):1598–605.
62. Jaiswal S, Natarajan P, Silver AJ, Gibson CJ, Bick AG, Shvartz E, et al. Clonal hematopoiesis and risk of atherosclerotic cardiovascular disease. N Engl J Med. 2017;377(2):111–21.
63. Fuster JJ, MacLauchlan S, Zuriaga MA, Polackal MN, Ostriker AC, Chakraborty R, et al. Clonal hematopoiesis associated with TET2 deficiency accelerates atherosclerosis development in mice. Science. 2017;355(6327):842–7.

Index

© Springer Nature Switzerland AG 2019
R. T. Means Jr. (ed.), *Anemia in the Young and Old*,
https://doi.org/10.1007/978-3-319-96487-4